GENETICS, SYNDROMES, AND COMMUNICATION DISORDERS

GENETICS, SYNDROMES, AND COMMUNICATION DISORDERS

Robert J. Shprintzen, Ph.D.

Professor and Director
Communication Disorder Unit
Center for the Diagnosis, Study, and Treatment of Velo-Cardio-Facial Syndrome
Center for Genetic Communicative Disorders
Department of Otolaryngology and Communication Science
State University of New York Health Science Center
Syracuse, New York, USA

SINGULAR PUBLISHING GROUP, INC.
SAN DIEGO · LONDON

Singular Publishing Group, Inc.
401 West "A" Street, Suite 325
San Diego, California 92101-7904

Singular Publishing Ltd.
19 Compton Terrace
London, N1 2UN, UK

e-mail: singpub@mail.cerfnet.com
Website: http://www.singpub.com

© 1997 by Singular Publishing Group, Inc.

Typeset in 10/12 Palatino by So Cal Graphics
Printed in the United States of America by McNaughton and Gunn

Library of Congress Cataloging-in-Publication Data

Shprintzen, Robert J.
    Genetics, syndromes, and communication disorders / Robert J.
Shprintzen.
       p. cm.
    Includes bibliographical references and index.
    ISBN 1–56593–620–5
    1. Genetic disorders. 2. Communicative Disorders—Genetic
aspects. I. Title.
    [DNLM: 1. Genetics, Medical. 2. Communicative Disorders—
genetics. 3. Syndrome. QZ 50 S559g 1997]
RB155.5.S57 1997
616.85'5042—dc21
DNLM/DLC
for Library of Congress
                                                                 97–20621
                                                                 CIP

CONTENTS

PREFACE

How many times have you heard the expression, "the acorn doesn't fall far from the tree"? I have heard this quaint adage applied in two ways. It is often used when a child strongly resembles a parent physically. Those of us who are parents can often see ourselves in our children's faces, and even beyond two generations, we sometimes see a strong resemblance between our children and other "blood relatives" such as grandparents, aunts, uncles, or first cousins. These are all individuals who share our gene pool so we do not tend to be surprised at these physical connections between close relatives. I have also heard the "acorn-tree" colloquialism used when a child's behavior pattern resembles that of a parent. For example, if a boy is a "troublemaker" and it is known that his father was the same as a boy, no one is necessarily surprised, even though the father is no longer troublesome as an adult. People have probably always accepted that an offspring's temperament and overall behavior will be similar to a parent's, much like their physical appearance. It is common for a parent to report that their child's behavior is just like theirs was when they were young without registering astonishment or entertaining the suggestion that it was somehow taught to the child.

Are all human behaviors subject to this type of hereditary influence? Is nature a stronger force than nurture in the way our children will develop and grow up? In the early days of the communication sciences, it was generally believed and taught that the greatest influences on the development of speech and language were those from the "nurture" (i.e., parental and sibling models, learning opportunities, amount of stimulation, reinforcement, etc.) side rather than the influence of "nature." If two brothers both had an interdental lisp, it was often assumed that the younger brother was learning the pattern from his elder sibling. This type of conclusion should not be surprising for a behavioral science whose founding members typically came from the fields of education and psychology rather than from the biological sciences.

When human genetics was a fledgling field, the connection between our genes and our behavior would not necessarily be made. All sorts of abnormal human behaviors have been attributed to external influences. To Freud, mental illness was a product of upbringing and interrelationships between child and parent at both the conscious and subconscious level. Today, many psychiatrists accept that at least some, if not most, mental illness is of genetic and biologic origin, including schizophrenia, bipolar disorder, and even more ordinary problems like anxiety and violent behavior. Perhaps the acceptance of genetics as a powerful force influencing human behavior has grown along with the incredible expansion of the science of genetics. Unfortunately, those of us working in the field of communicative science have been left behind. As others involved in health care science have integrated both clinical and molecular genetics into their fields of endeavor, speech-language pathologists and audiologists have been slow to do so. Genetics is rarely a part of undergraduate or graduate curricula, and if it is, it is included as a small subsection of another course, perhaps a single lecture. Without the proper educational background, the amalgamation of the communicative sciences and genetics becomes essentially impossible.

Conversely, scientists who work in the genetic sciences probably know as little about speech, language, and hearing as communication scientists know about genetics. Clinicians assessing patients tend to focus on physical anomalies because their medical backgrounds make this familiar territory. Molecular geneticists who spend their time in the laboratory and who often observe the effects of mutated genomes on animals ranging from fruit flies to mice do not have the opportunity to interact with disorders of communication or people who study them. Thus, while cancer researchers are finding genes that cause breast and colon cancer, neuroscientists are studying the effects of the genes that cause Huntington and Alzheimer's diseases. With the exception of a relatively few genes which have been found to cause deafness, few scientists in the area of communication disorders have been deeply involved in the most active and growing field in the health sciences today: human genetics.

The purpose of this book is to introduce the reader to the basics of both clinical and molecular genetics. This text is meant to be introductory and perhaps will provide an impetus for speech-language pathologists and audiologists to learn more and establish relationships with genetic counselors, clinical geneticists, dysmorphologists, cytogeneticists, and molecular geneticists in their region. Stated simply, almost all human disorders, with the possible exception of trauma and infection, have some type of genetic component. This includes speech, language, and hearing disorders. Hopefully, this text will provide a starting point for additional interaction between the communicative sciences and the genetic sciences. This interaction is long overdue and should be encouraged. Towards that end, this text describes the basics of heredity, how genes work and are expressed in people, how to gather information that might reveal a genetic basis for a communicative impairment, and the importance of understanding that basis. An extensive, but not all-inclusive, appendix of disorders is included. Because there are scant data on communicative impairments in multiple anomaly syndromes, we cannot yet know the true extent of these associations. Perhaps within the next few years, we will.

ACKNOWLEDGMENTS

I have had the great good fortune to be exposed to some of the greatest minds of our era who introduced me to the study of communication disorders, craniofacial anomalies, and genetics. During my studies at Syracuse University and Upstate Medical Center (now the SUNY Health Science Center at Syracuse), Gerald N. McCall, Ph.D., and M. Leon Skolnick, M.D., exposed me to the speech and physiological aspects of children with cleft palate and taught me concepts that have remained valuable to this day. With the assistance of Betty Jane McWilliams, Ph.D., another true intellectual giant, I was able to secure a position directing a large craniofacial center in New York City. There, under the tutelage of some remarkable clinicians and scientists, too numerous to mention, I learned about the morphologic errors of the head and neck which, in those days, we called birth defects. At that time, my Chairman was Michael L. Lewin, M.D., a plastic surgeon of rare quality. Michael was a humble and kind man who knew how to ignite intellectual curiosity. With his insistence that I learn something new, I was able to turn my attention to the growing field of what we referred to in those days as syndromology (today, dysmorphology).

My first contact in 1974 was with David W. Smith, M.D. David was one of a few early distinguished and eminent clinicians who recognized how patterns of anomalies in children actually made sense relative to their origin. I was fortunate to have known him for those years prior to his untimely death because he introduced me to the study of unusual children, teaching me how to recognize the common thread and relevant patterns of anomalies. It was through David that I met a colleague of his at the University of Washington in Seattle, M. Michael Cohen, Jr. Mike, who has become a good friend and mentor, took David's knack for pattern recognition to new heights for me. A man of encyclopedic knowledge and enormous good humor, Mike taught me that diagnosis is both science and art and that we must always question our previous certainties because genetics is a continuously fluid science with new discoveries every day. I was then introduced to the new and perplexing field of molecular genetics by the remarkable Raju Kucherlapati, Ph.D. Raju, a blend of scholar, statesman, and gentleman, showed enormous patience with me while I tried to fumble around the new terminology, concepts, and tenets of molecular genetics.

To allow the study of these new discoveries within the framework of the communicative sciences, my current Chairman, Robert Kellman, M.D., deserves enormous credit for providing me the opportunity to expand investigations and services at a time when most academic medical centers are contracting. It is with enormous gratitude that I thank these remarkable individuals for allowing me to stand on their shoulders so I might climb to peek over the wall that obscures our ability to see what might be ahead which is valuable to know.

Through it all, I have had the steadfast encouragement of my family, even though my own pursuits often took time away from them. Fortunately, my wife Debby, daughter Jodi, and son Adam all have their own admirable intellectual curiosities, although each is in a different direction. However, in spite of our divergent intellectual pursuits, our cohesiveness makes anyone's achievement a shared one.

Finally, I must mention that the early groundwork for my curiosity came from my parents who were able to push me without shoving. I dedicate this book to my father who understands the value of unlimited energy, and the blessed memory of my mother who was never without a book in her hands. They provided the model for me to emulate while my friends, colleagues, wife, and children provided me with the opportunity to write this book.

CHAPTER

1

INTRODUCTION

No single scientific discipline has had more impact on the understanding of diseases and disorders in humans than genetics. In fact, it is fair to say that the progress made in all phases of human genetics over the past 5 years has been astonishing. One might describe each new stage of advance in genetics as an exponential increase over the previous discovery. Nearly all professionals involved in the delivery of health care have embraced genetics and incorporated it into their study of human abnormality. This seems a natural extension of disciplines that study congenital malformations and structural anomalies and their effects on human growth and development. However, even professionals who study human behavior, such as psychiatrists, psychologists, and neuropsychologists, have begun to expand outward from their previous theories, which touted experience and child rearing as determiners of behavioral abnormalities, to the study of genetic factors as the basis for mental illness, mood disturbances, aggression, depression, cognitive dysfunction, and learning disorders. Unfortunately, professionals involved in the study of communication disorders have been left far behind in the study and incorporation of genetics into their clinical practices and scientific investigations. Although the genetic bases for some forms of hearing loss have been defined and specific genes found, the same is not true for the overwhelming majority of communicative disorders such as language, speech, and voice abnormalities. It is also fair to say that the progress made in the study of deafness has come from medical professionals and molecular geneticists rather than from audiologists and other communicative specialists.

The time has come to recognize that nearly every condition of human disability and disease (with the possible exception of trauma) has a genetic component, either direct or indirect. The purpose of this book is to acquaint specialists in the communicative disorders with the basics of human genetics;

to describe the mechanisms by which genetics can cause speech, language, hearing, cognitive, and behavioral disorders; and to show how an understanding of genetics will lead to the more efficient implementation of treatment.

WHAT IS GENETICS?

The word gene is derived from the same root that gives us *genesis* and *generation*. It means to be derived from, or to begin with. The concept of genetics began with the observation that traits ran in families and children looked like their parents. The word was actually coined in the work of Darwin who used it in relation to his hypotheses regarding some presumed biological material that was passed from parent to child which carried heritable traits. More germane to this text is the notion that behavior runs in families (hence the old colloquialism, *the acorn doesn't fall far from the tree*). Of course, the notion that things that people do (i.e., human behavior) and even the way that people think may be partially or largely genetically based brings up the old and emotionally charged conundrum pitting **nature versus nurture**. The notion that human behavior has a basis in genetic make-up is regarded by some as anathema to the philosophical implications of individuals' responsibility for their actions and human freedom of will. Actually, these two supposedly opposing schools of thought are not necessarily mutually exclusive. It has been demonstrated that human behavioral and psychological factors such as intellect, temperament, and personality are strongly influenced by genetics. However, regardless of one's behavioral predisposition, free will is still enjoyed by most people in the free world and has a clear influence on human behavior. This brief comment will suffice as commentary on the more controversial philosophical aspects of genetics and human behavior, although some of the scientific components which provoke con-

troversy will be discussed later in this chapter and elsewhere in the text.

All science is prone to controversy, but genetics more so than most because of two factors: the association of heredity with reproduction and the guilt which can be associated with a parent passing on a genetic disease to his or her child. Reproductive choices have been a center of controversy worldwide for several decades. As genetics continues to provide an additional range of choices with regard to prenatal diagnosis and eventual fetal treatments, it can be anticipated that controversy will continue to swell. The issue of parental guilt for passing on genetic traits is often difficult to resolve because of the responsibility a parent will feel which can often lead to denial.

IS GENETICS REALLY RESPONSIBLE FOR NEARLY ALL HUMAN DISORDERS AND DISEASE?

It may seem like an overstatement to regard nearly all human disorders as being genetically based, but as the human genetic code continues to be deciphered, it is becoming clearer that many diseases which previously did not have explanations are turning out to be genetically caused. Many forms of cancer, obesity, manic-depressive illness, and other conditions not previously linked to genetic causes are now known to be based in abnormalities within the human genome. Genetic abnormalities can cause human disease in two ways: directly or indirectly.

Direct Genetic Effects

A direct effect of genetics is exemplified by a gene causing a disorder, or anomaly, by direct action on the development of the embryo or its biochemical make-up and the consequences that action has on human function. For example, the gene that causes Hurler syndrome, a recessive genetic condition which is categorized as a lysosomal storage disorder, causes a failure of the body to metabolize certain types of cellular waste products (mucopolysaccharides). As a result, these toxic waste products are retained in the body's tissues, such as the brain, and cause the effected organs to dysfunction or fail. Thus, children with Hurler syndrome have severe and progressive cognitive dysfunction as these cellular wastes continue to collect in the central nervous system. Death eventually results from generalized organ failure and chronic congestion from these waste products collecting in the lungs, bronchi, or trachea.

Indirect Genetic Influences

An indirect genetic effect is one in which a problem or abnormality results secondarily from a predisposition or anomaly directly caused by a genetic error. In other words, a gene causes an organ system to be malformed or dysfunction and that malformed or disfunctioning organ secondarily causes another anomaly which can cause an illness or disorder. This cascading effect is actually a common manner in which genetic errors can cause problems in humans. Sets of disorders known as sequences, which will be described in Chapter 3, are actually complexes of human diseases that are the result of indirect genetic influences. An example of an indirect genetic effect is the upper airway obstruction that accompanies babies born with a very small lower jaw (also often accompanied by cleft palate in a condition known as **Robin sequence** or **Pierre Robin sequence**). The effect of a gene causes the mandible (lower jaw) to be extremely small (Figure 1–1). Newborns are obligate nose breathers. This is a reflexive respiratory mechanism because babies utilize the oral cavity primarily for feeding and the nasal cavity for respiration. If the mandible is extremely small, the baby can not position the tongue anteriorly which enlarges the breathing space posteriorly. With the mouth closed, the tongue may fall back into the oropharynx and obstruct the upper airway (Figure 1–1), a condition usually called **glossoptosis**. Glossoptosis and airway obstruction is not a directly inherited genetic trait. Rather, it is secondary to the inherited genetic trait of **micrognathia**, a very small mandible.

Given this inclusive view of the possible contribution of genetics to human disorders, it can be seen why it can be stated with certainty that essentially all disorders of communication are caused directly by genetic factors or have at least some type of genetic contribution. Actually, under these parameters, even trauma (such as noise-induced hearing loss) could have a genetic predisposition. Although the high decibel noise is the direct cause of the hearing loss at 4,000 Hz, not all individuals exposed to the same level and duration of noise will develop the same hearing loss. Furthermore, even more indirectly, human aptitudes will predict the types of jobs they take (and hence the type of occupational noise to which they are exposed), the type of music they might prefer to hear, and their basic personality might determine how likely they might be to expose themselves to certain risks. There is very strong evidence to suggest that such aptitudes and personality traits are strongly influenced by genetics.

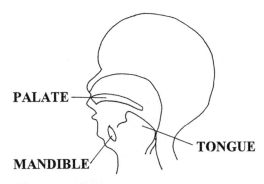

Figure 1–1. Drawing of a midsagittal section of a newborn's head showing that a small mandible causes the tongue to be retropositioned in the upper airway resulting in respiratory obstruction.

WHAT IS THE ADVANTAGE IN RECOGNIZING GENETIC CAUSES OF HUMAN DISORDERS?

There are a number of benefits as well as possible problems associated with establishing a diagnosis based on a genetic abnormality. The benefits of a correct diagnosis accrue to both the patient and the health care professional managing a patient, whereas the potential negative aspects apply only to the professionals and result from the patient's inability to deal with news they consider to be "bad" or, at the very least, unpleasant and unexpected.

THE BENEFITS OF CORRECT GENETIC DIAGNOSIS

Advantages to the Professional

The professional involved directly in patient care has the complex task of proper diagnosis, applying treatments, and counseling the patient about expected outcomes. Applying the correct diagnosis if a genetic disorder is involved, especially if the disorder is a previously described and studied multiple anomaly disorder, or syndrome, provides the clinician with three components critical to proper patient care: the **phenotypic spectrum**, **natural history**, and **prognosis**.

Phenotypic Spectrum

Phenotype refers to the physical and behavioral characteristics of an individual. For example, an individual with Down syndrome is likely to have a phenotype that includes short stature, mental retardation, a large geographic tongue, close set eyes, small ears, language delay, poor fine and gross motor coordination, and congenital heart anomalies. The **phenotypic spectrum** refers to not only anomalies that might be found in a single individual if one were to

carefully examine him or her, but also all suspected anomalies that might be found because they are known to occur in association with the syndrome. Down syndrome, as an easily recognized and well studied disorder, has a complete and thoroughly described phenotypic spectrum. When presented with a child with Down syndrome, the astute clinician is immediately armed with the knowledge provided by scientists who studied the disorder previously and published their findings in the scientific literature. Therefore, the clinician who sees a new patient can note the obvious anomalies shown by the patient, but also perform specialized examinations for anomalies that would not be obvious on routine physical examination. For example, patients with Down syndrome are known to have a higher frequency of thyroid disorders than the general population. The effects of hypothyroidism or hyperthyroidism (both of which occur in Down syndrome) may not be initially apparent, but can be detectable if specific tests to measure thyroid function are performed. If a clinician did not know that thyroid disease was a part of the phenotypic spectrum of Down syndrome, the tests would not be ordered until the individual was symptomatic.

Natural History

Natural history refers to the course of a disorder over time. Disorders may be progressive and get worse with time, remain relatively stable, and in some cases, anomalies may even improve or disappear with time. It is obviously important to understand the natural history of a disorder so that clinicians can anticipate problems that are known to occur at a specific stage of development. This not only allows for effective counseling, but also allows the clinician to anticipate the development of problems and intervene in a timely manner. Using Down syndrome as an example one more time, a high percentage of individuals with Down syndrome develop Alzheimer's disease or changes in the brain consistent with Alzheimer's. As a result, slowly progressing dementia of relatively early onset is common in Down syndrome, and premature mortality is prevalent with an average age of death of approximately 35 years (Tolksdorf & Wiedemann, 1981).

Prognosis

Prognosis refers to the predicted outcome of a disorder relative to both the quantity and quality of life. When a clinician is presented with a baby with Down syndrome, the prognosis for normal mental development is very poor, with the majority of affected children having at least mild mental retardation, although a large percentage have moderate or severe retardation. A prognosis is actually less a prediction and more a way of providing parents with a practical framework for dealing with a disorder in a realistic way. An accurate prognosis has very practical application to case management. In today's health care climate, clinicians must be accountable for the expenditure of time and money. In cases where the prognosis is poor, a decision may be made to withold treatments that have no likelihood of success while concentrating efforts in cases with better prognoses.

FOCUSING DIAGNOSTIC EFFORT

Another major advantage of correct diagnosis to the professional is the focusing of diagnostic efforts directly on treatment planning. When the clinician is unable to establish a firm diagnosis for a child with multiple anomalies, diagnostic efforts are largely hit or miss because of the uncertainty about the primary diagnosis. If the clinician has several possible diagnoses in mind, the phenotypic spectrum of each may need to be explored, which will markedly increase the number of diagnostic tests which need to be applied. If there is no specific diagnosis in mind, a less concentrated diagnostic search

will prolong the diagnostic effort (and expense) even further.

If proper diagnosis is applied to the patient, diagnostic efforts can be restricted to those features of the phenotypic spectrum that have a direct impact on plans for treatment. The clinician's efforts become focused on treating the patient, not trying to find out what the problem is. For example, a patient presents with hypernasal speech of unknown origin. Oral examination fails to show evidence of cleft palate or submucous cleft palate. The child also has learning disabilities, heart anomalies, inguinal hernias, and hypocalcemia. The clinician recognizes this pattern as consistent with the diagnosis of velo-cardio-facial syndrome and refers the patient for the genetic laboratory test to confirm the diagnosis (see Chapters 6 and 7). The test comes back positive for the deletion of genetic material on the long arm of chromosome 22, which is known to cause velo-cardio-facial syndrome. As a result, the clinician becomes immediately aware that there is a strong likelihood that the patient has an occult submucous cleft palate, hypoplasia (underdevelopment) of the adenoid, and hypotonia of the pharynx, all factors that contribute to velopharyngeal insufficiency and resultant hypernasality. Therefore, the correct diagnostic tests, such as nasopharyngoscopy and videofluoroscopy, can be scheduled to assess these problems. However, the clinician also knows that part of the phenotypic spectrum of velo-cardio-facial syndrome is an anomalous course of the internal carotid arteries which brings them close to the pharyngeal midline where they could interfere with pharyngeal flap surgery (a treatment for velopharyngeal insufficiency). Therefore, the clincian requests a magnetic resonance angiography to plot the course of the pharyngeal vessels so that proper surgical treatment can be applied. These actions by the clinician are completely dependent on establishing a genetic diagnosis and are specific to the disease suspected. Once the syndrome is defined, all efforts can be focused on treating the problems associated with the syndrome, both known and anticipated.

THE INFLUENCE OF GENES

The genetic make-up of human beings, sometimes called the gene pool, is more properly called the human **genome**. An individual's specific genetic make-up is known as his or her **genotype**. The human genome consists of approximately 100,000 genes distributed along the normal compliment of 46 chromosomes in the nucleus of the body's cells. Each gene of the 100,000 making up an individual's genome can exist in different forms. For example, a gene for eye color may exist in a form that encodes for blue eyes, or a form that encodes for green eyes, or a form that encodes for brown eyes, and so on. These differing forms of each gene are known as alleles. In other words, the eye color gene has multiple alleles, all resulting in what would be considered normal traits. Because of the variability of the many possible alleles, or gene alternatives, and the 100,000 genes it takes to produce a human being, the number of variations that can exist within the genome is for all practical purposes infinite. Therefore, an individual's genotype is essentially unique. The only exception is monozygotic (identical) twinning. Monozygotic twins are both the product of a single fertilized ovum and therefore have the same exact genotype.

What is the relationship between genotype and phenotype? Does genotype exactly predict phenotype? Is the same phenotype always the result of an identical genotype? The answer to both questions is no. Scientists have not completely figured out how identical genotypes can cause different phenotypes, but it is known that monozygotic twins can be discordant for certain traits and even abnormal genes can be expressed differently in each twin. This process will eventually be understood, but for now, the hypothesis is that environmental factors may play a role and, as will be discussed later in this text, the timing of

the action of genes is so precise that delays of even seconds in a gene's action can produce completely different effects. It is also understood that two seemingly identical (or at least very similar) phenotypes can be caused by completely different genes, or even by environmental factors. Identical phenotypes with different causes are known as **phenocopies**.

However, it is also well known that genetic influences are very strong and are the single most predictive factor in the production of traits, whether normal or abnormal. Therefore, although genotype is not perfectly predictive of phenotype, nothing has more influence on the phenotype than the genotype.

WHAT IS THE ROLE FOR THE SPECIALIST IN COMMUNICATION DISORDERS?

The implications of correct diagnosis carry enormous emotional impact for the parents of a child with a genetic disorder. Once a diagnosis with possible effects on inheritance is made, the impact is spread to all first degree relatives and even more distant kin. Although all of the advantages outlined above accrue to the patient (the provision of the phenotypic spectrum, natural history, and prognosis), there is potential for causing significant worry and other psychological trauma and stress to the parents and other relatives of the affected individual because of possible guilt, denial, or worry over the chance that another family member may be affected or pass the disease on to someone else. Because of the potential for creating enormous psychological stress, the clinician must be wary of the medico-legal implications of applying a diagnosis.

Although genetics is a relatively young science, many professionals have entered into the study of either the clinical or laboratory aspects of it. In 1989, the American

Board of Human Genetics was established to certify Medical Geneticists, Genetic Counselors, Cytogeneticists, and Molecular Geneticists. Although board certification does not prevent other specialists from applying diagnoses, it does connote a level of expertise which would signify the certified professional as a proper referral source. Inexperienced and untrained professionals must be careful about applying diagnoses without a firm base of knowledge and must also be careful not to blurt out even the possibility of a diagnosis because the recipient is likely to attach more weight to the statement than the clinician intended.

Possible Legal Implications

It is the job, or perhaps more appropriately, the responsibility of clinicians to diagnose problems. Is it sufficient for the specialist in communication disorders to diagnose the type of speech problem or the exact nature of a hearing loss? According to litigation that has already been successfully prosecuted by plaintiffs with undetected genetic conditions, the answer is a blunt no. When a genetic condition has, as a part of a broader symptom complex, a speech, language, voice, resonance, perceptual, cognitive, or hearing disorder, it is incumbent on the clinician at the very least to recognize that there may be a syndrome involved which has implications for the patient's quantity or quality of life. Even if the clinician is not qualified to render a genetic diagnosis, he or she must recognize that such a diagnosis may exist and therefore refer the patient for additional evaluation. Failure to do so could potentially result in two types of litigation: a personal injury suit for failure to diagnose a problem, or a wrongful life suit. The following hypothetical scenario illustrates a possible type of suit:

Case Study

A patient with hypernasal speech secondary to a cleft palate is referred for a speech evaluation. A speech pathologist participating in a multidisciplinary cleft palate team is asked to determine if the patient requires speech therapy, pharyngeal flap surgery, or prosthetic management. The speech pathologist performs a complete speech assessment and requests nasopharyngoscopic and videofluoroscopic studies to evaluate the velopharyngeal mechanism. In collaboration with the other team members, the speech pathologist determines that speech therapy will have no beneficial effect on the velopharyngeal insufficiency and recommends to the patient that a pharyngeal flap should be done. The patient is never seen by a geneticist or dysmorphologist. As a result, a number of anomalies are missed by the examining professionals including a small ear tag, mild asymmetry of the ears, a small dermoid cyst in the left eye, and mild mandibular asymmetry. Furthermore, an audiogram is not done prior to surgery. Had the audiogram been obtained, it would have been found that the patient had a 35 dB conductive hearing loss in the right ear, but no evidence of middle ear fluid. Additional assessment would have revealed a malformation of the ossicles and an abnormal middle ear space. In reality, the patient had oculo-auriculo-vertebral dysplasia (also known as hemifacial microsomia). Cleft palate is a common finding in oculo-auriculo-vertebral dysplasia (OAV), as is hypernasal speech which is related in large part to pharyngeal asymmetry (Shprintzen, Croft, Berkman, & Rakoff, 1980). Unfortunately, another clinical finding in OAV is cervical spine malformation. Vertebral fusion, hemivertebrae, and hypoplastic (underdeveloped) vertebrae are found in OAV, occurring in 20–35% of cases (Gorlin, Cohen, & Levin., 1990). An occipitalized atlas is found in 30% of cases (Gorlin, et al.,

(continued)

> ## *Case Study* (continued)
>
> *1990). The patient is sent to surgery and the neck is hyperextended to position the mouth appropriately for the pharyngeal flap. This patient had an occipitalized atlas and fusion of C1 and C2. Because of the fusion, the neck did not hyperextend easily, so the surgeon was more vigorous than usual in manipulating the head. This caused the atlas to torque backwards and damage the spinal cord resulting in a severe quadraplegic paralysis.*

WHAT SHOULD YOU KNOW?

Even though the study of communicative disorders has traditionally been based in behavioral science, there is no question that, with each passing year, speech-language pathologists and audiologists have become more and more involved in the management of physically based disorders and illnesses rooted in abnormal structure or biological function. To apply the sciences of genetics and dysmorphology to the communicative sciences, speech-language pathologists and audiologists must have a strong understanding of human biology (i.e., antomy and physiology), a basic understanding of cell biology, a knowledge of patterns of inheritance, and a basic understanding of DNA biochemistry and gene function. All of these factors will be discussed in this text, and it is the author's hope that the reader will seek out additional information in an effort to join the modern world of genetic study.

REFERENCES

Gorlin, R. J., Cohen, M. M. Jr., & Levin, L. S. (1990). *Syndromes of the head and neck* (3rd ed.). New York: Oxford University Press.

Shprintzen, R. J., Croft, C. B., Berkman, M. D., & Rakoff, S. J. (1980). Velopharyngeal insufficiency in the facio-auriculo-vertebral malformation complex. *Cleft Palate Journal, 17,* 132–137.

Tolksdorf, M., & Wiedemann, H.-R. (1981). Clinical aspects of Down's syndrome from infancy to adult life. In G. R. Burgio (Ed.), *Trisomy 21: An international symposium* (pp. 1–31). Heidelberg: Springer-Verlag.

CHAPTER

2

A PRIMER IN HUMAN GENETICS

The heritability of human traits certainly could not have been lost on our ancestors. In fact, the notion that somehow some physical and behavioral component of the father was passed on to his son is a central theme of many cultures where continuing a family line was a priority. However, to our predecessors, two components of the equation were missing: the understanding of the patterns of inheritance and the discovery of the genetic mechanism and material which transmitted that pattern. It was not until 1866 and the first reports of the experiments of Gregor Mendel, a 19th century Austrian monk, that patterns of inheritance which would predict the mathematical probability of the passing on of traits in flowering plants (garden peas) were discovered so that heritability could be reduced to some type of biologically governed system. Mendel was able to observe several patterns of inherited traits, including dominant traits, recessive traits, and mixed traits. In other words he was able to observe that by mating, for example, a red flower with a white flower, if the resulting offspring were red 50% of the time, dominant inheritance was occurring. If a red and white flower mating yielded pink flowers, then mixed inheritance was hypothesized. In some cases, the mating of two red flowers might yield red flowers 75% of the time, but 25% of the time, a white flower would be produced (recessive inheritance). Mendel's work was truly an advance considering that, at the time of Mendel, the exact nature of the biological components of inheritance (DNA, chromosomes, and genes) was unknown. However, Mendel's experiments with flowers to study how the traits of color and other structural aspects of the plants were passed along to progeny was a breakthrough that was largely ignored for over three decades until scientists were able to determine the mechanism for these patterns of inheritance.

Preceding Mendel's discoveries by several years was the revolutionary work of Charles Darwin who utilized the concept of genetics to explain the process of heredity. Darwin (1859) contended that heritable traits varied within species and that this variation was the foundation for evolution. Darwin believed that traits which offered an organism an advantage over other members of the same species would persist within the species, whereas those that were disadvantageous would eventually be extinguished. Darwin's view of a genetic basis to explain evolution was very sophisticated considering that he had no knowledge of Mendel's work or its implications.

In 1903, William Sutton, at the time a student working in the laboratory of famed American cytologist Edmund Wilson, connected the pattern of inheritance observed by Mendel 36 years earlier in 1866 to the microscopic observations of chromosomes in germ cells. These basic discoveries in the early years of the birth of a new scientific discipline changed the study of traits passed from one generation to the other from the science of heredity to the science of genetics. Scientists would now understand that the predictions of how traits would segregate in the offspring of animals and plants was based on the transmission of some type of genetic material located within the cell nuclei of all living beings. The concept of the gene as a biological unit of heredity was conceived in 1909 by William Johannsen.

A number of other scientists working in the first half of the 20th century began to define the biochemical nature of inheritance, including Herrmann J. Muller, George W. Beadle, Edward L. Tatum, Arthur Kornberg, and Joshua Lederberg, all of whom won Nobel prizes for their work in discovering the biochemical nature of how DNA and genes function to pass heritable traits from one generation to the next. Perhaps the most easily recognizable names in the process of unravelling the genetic code are those of J. D. Watson and F. H. C. Crick. Their hypothesis of the molecular structure of DNA as the "double helix" has captured and continues to capture the imaginations and scientific curiosity of people more than 40 years after its introduction in 1953.

Once the nature of DNA and its action became better understood, molecular biologists began to work on the more difficult problem of exactly how genes produce specific structures and functions in the body. The next logical step was the discovery of specific genes and the subsequent description of the entire complement of genes contained on the chromosomes. This process is continuing as part of a major international project known as

The Human Genome Project. It is expected that the entire human genome will be completely defined by the year 2005.

At the same time that molecular biologists were discovering the nature of genes and DNA, clinicians were becoming interested in discovering and classifying genetic diseases in humans. It was not until the late 1960s and early 1970s that clinicians began to systematically categorize children with multiple congenital anomalies and describe patterns of *syndromes*, giving birth to the clinical science of *syndromology* (now more commonly referred to as *clinical genetics, medical genetics,* or *dysmorphology*). Prior to the birth of clinical genetics as a specialty, there had been descriptions of multiple anomaly disorders (i.e., syndromes), but these early delineations of new disorders were not always accurate and were rudimentary in understanding the implications of the diagnosis. The early descriptions of syndromes tended to come from specialists who were interested in one particular aspect of a disorder that related to their own area of specialization, such as the Treacher Collins syndrome. Treacher Collins, who specialized in diseases of the eye, reported the syndrome that bears his name because of the notch that occurs in the lower eye lid, even though there is a broader and more impressive pattern of craniofacial anomalies affecting the facial skeleton, mandible, and ear (Figure 2–1). In fact, the most consistent finding in Treacher Collins syndrome is probably conductive hearing loss secondary to ossicular malformation.

As clinical genetics became a separate discipline, a wide variety of specialists became interested in delineating new syndromes. Although many, such as David Smith and Victor McKusick, came from pediatrics and medicine, others came from different areas of specialization. For example, Robert J. Gorlin, one of the driving forces behind the special interest in craniofacial genetics, was a dentist, specializing in oral pathology. This area of specialization also provided the impetus for Dr. Gorlin's student, M. Michael

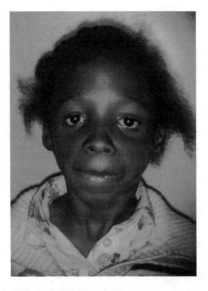

Figure 2–1. The facial appearance in Treacher Collins syndrome. Note the notch in the lower eyelid.

Cohen, Jr., who has contributed immeasurably not only to the catalogue of new syndromes, but also to the establishment of models for classification and ways of thinking of syndromes that provide a logical framework for clinicians who encounter children with multiple anomalies. Other **syndromologists** (i.e., clinical geneticists and dysmorphologists) came from many diverse fields including neurology, ophthalmology, orthodontics, orthopedics, and otolaryngology, among others.

Another approach to syndromes was provided by embryologists and developmental biologists who studied models of disease in developing embryos of animal models. This particular discipline, often called **teratology** (derived from the Greek **teratos**, meaning **monster**) was given a major emphasis by the early input of Josef Warkany. Today's generation of embryologists and developmental biologists have a far broader foundation of human disease models provided to them by the clinicians so that they can relate anomalies created in animal models to the thousands of genetic diseases which have been delineated in humans over the past three

decades. One of the most important contributions of the developmental biology approach to syndromes is the ability to know the time frame within which an insult to the developing embryo occurs.

It was not until the latter part of the 1980s that molecular genetics, clinical genetics, and developmental biology/embryology began to merge to create a more unified approach to the study of human genetic disease. As the human genetic code began to be unravelled, it became necessary to relate clinical findings to specific sequences of DNA and then to observe how these DNA sequences acted developmentally to cause anomalies. Thus, molecular genetics provided the building blocks, which then needed to be matched to a picture of the finished building (the syndrome), and the developmental biologists provided the blueprints for the building plan.

In order for the specialist in communicative disorders to become familiar with all three fields relating to genetics (i.e., molecular genetics, clinical genetics, and developmental biology), a sound foothold in the basic knowledge and nosology of each field is necessary. A good text for readers interested in learning more about the broad range of topics in genetics is *Thompson and Thompson Genetics in Medicine* (Thompson, Roderick, & Willard, 1991).

WHAT DO GENES DO?

Genes basically perform two functions. First, genes contain the basic set of instructions for putting together an organism following fertilization of the egg (ovum) by the sperm. The resulting fertilized egg, or ovum, responds to the set of instructions carried on the genes which regulates the formations of specific cell types, cell functions, and where those cells are distributed in the growing embryo. In the case of human beings, it takes approximately 100,000 genes strung along the 46 chromosomes to fulfill this task known as **morphogenesis**. The genes are actually spaced along the chromosomes in a rather irregular pattern with large segments of DNA in between which does not contain any known genes. Researchers estimate that 95% of the DNA contained on the chromosomes does not participate in the genetic code. The function of these random DNA sequences, which make up a far larger part of the total human DNA than the genes, is unknown.

Any error in the genetic instruction contained within the genes could result in a congenital anomaly, multiple anomalies, or even a nonviable organism. Approximately one of every six established pregnancies results in a spontaneous abortion primarily because the developing embryo is not viable. Therefore, it is probable that there are many genes that code for errors in morphogenesis which have not yet been discovered because the embryos never reach term.

The second purpose of genes is to regulate the function, growth, and development of the organism after birth. This regulation includes every physiologic function, such as metabolic, endocrinologic, hematologic, neurologic, and so forth. Many genetic disorders are expressed after birth when physiologic functions are disturbed by abnormal genes, such as in the group of disorders known as storage disorders, also known as lysosomal storage diseases or mucopolysaccharidoses. Hurler syndrome, Hunter syndrome, Tay-Sachs disease, and Morquio syndrome are just a few of these types of disorders. These genetic conditions, usually inherited in an autosomal recessive manner, result in the absence of basic metabolic enzymes so that certain cellular waste products cannot be broken down and end up being stored in various tissues and organs, including the skin, brain, and skeleton. At birth, children with these disorders appear normal, and their early development is also normal. However, as the waste products continue to be stored in the affected organs and tissues, physical changes occur; and if the central nervous system is involved, deterioration of behavior can also occur. In some of the lysosomal storage disorders these ef-

fects may not be obvious until the second year of life . In some other genetic metabolic disorders, such as homocystinuria, the disease may not become evident for decades. An example of a lysosomal storage disease is Sly syndrome (designated as mucopolysaccharidosis Type VII) which is inherited as an autosomal recessive genetic disorder. Affected individuals have β-Glucuronidase deficiency, resulting in a failure to degrade the cellular waste products dermatan sulfate and heparan sulfate. Development appears normal until age 2 years, at which point mental retardation begins to appear and gets progressively worse. The abnormal gene for this disorder is known to be on the long arm of chromosome 7.

It can therefore be seen that the action of genes can have both short- and long-term effects. Furthermore, abnormalities in genes may remain dormant for many years yet still cause problems very late in life. A major source of current research is the isolation of **oncogenes**, genes that can predispose someone to cancer, or directly cause cancer. Major advances have been made in isolating oncogenes for colon cancer, breast cancer, and several other forms of neoplasias that were not always considered to be genetic in nature. Genes have even been implicated in the development of Alzheimer's disease, a disorder typically associated with senility and old age (although it can begin to occur in individuals in their 40s).

THE BASIC LANGUAGE OF GENETICS

Every living cell at one time during its life contains a genetic code. Some cells, like red blood cells, contain genetic information for only part of their lives, subsequently losing it as the cell matures to perform a specific function. For the most part, however, living cells of all species of living things contain a nucleus (Figure 2–2). The nucleus contains the sum total of genetic information on the chromosomes which are structures made of DNA which can be seen with a light micro-

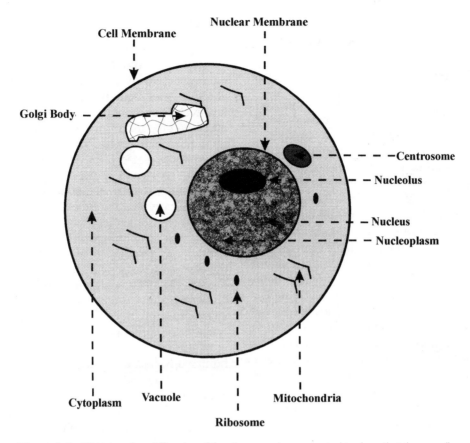

Figure 2–2. Diagram of a cell. The size of the ribosomes is exaggerated to show that they are dispersed in the cytoplasm of the cell.

scope. The chromosomes are the vehicles for carrying the genes which are a part of the chromosomes' DNA structure and contained in a specific order that is essentially the same for all normal members of the same species. Each species, from the simplest bacteria to the most complex mammals, has a set number of chromosomes in each cell, that number being the same for each normal member of that species. For example, a simple bacterium may have one chromosome, the garden pea has 14 chromosomes, the fruit fly (drosophila melanogaster) has 8 chromosomes, and each normal human cell (except for spermatozoa and ova) has 46 chromosomes.

BASIC CELL BIOLOGY

Living cells all have similar basic functions, whether they are white blood cells, neurons, or skin cells; all cells engage in metabolism and reproduction. Although cells also perform other specialized functions (e.g., neurons conduct nerve impulses and white blood cells surround and destroy disease causing agents), their basic functions of life are the same. Metabolism continues until the cell dies (in essence, without metabolism, a cell can not live). Cells do not have to reproduce in order to survive, but essentially all cells engage in some type of reproduction during a stage of its life and development. The cell's structures all play some type of role in performing these basic functions.

Cell Structure

The study of cells is known as **cytology**. Although most cells have specialized structures unique to their function or species, nearly all cells have some structures in common, including two structures critical to the genetic process: the nucleus and ribosomes (see Figure 2–2). All of the cell elements are contained within the cell membrane which is the semipermeable separation between the cell and its environment. The cell membrane allows some substances to pass through it while protecting the cell from foreign bodies or substances that cannot permeate it. The cell membrane contains the substance of the cell, the cytoplasm, and all of the structures that are contained within the cytoplasm. The nucleus, surrounded by a nuclear membrane, is filled with **chromatin,** which during cell division condenses into the chromosomes (Figure 2–3), discrete structures of varying size which contain the genes.

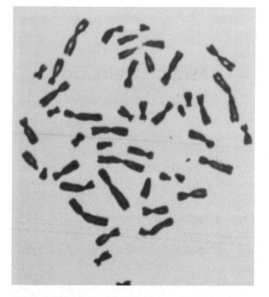

Figure 2–3. Cell nucleus during cell division.

The Chromosomes

The study of chromosomes is known as **cytogenetics,** a word derived from the combination of cytology and genetics because the chromosomes regulate genetics at the cellular level. People who study chromosomes and who prepare chromosome analyses are known as **cytogeneticists.** Chromosomes (literally translated from Greek as "colored bodies," so named because they were the only cellular structures that became purple when an early staining procedure known as the Feulgen-Rossenbeck technique was applied) consist of approximately equal parts of DNA and protein and are located within the cell's nucleus. Modern cytogenetics dates to the 1950s when procedures that allowed the chromosomes to become clearly visible by applying biological stains during cell division were first developed. It was not until 1956 that scientists confirmed that human cells had 46 chromosomes.

During their normal resting state, chromosomes are not visible as identifiable structures within the nucleus. It is only when the cell is dividing that the chromosomes become microscopically visible. The chromosomes appear as two strands joined by a structure known as the **centromere** (Figure 2–4). On either side of the centromere, the strand of chromosome is known as a **chromatid.** One chromatid is usually shorter than the other and is therefore called the **short arm,** or the **p** arm, while the longer segment is labeled the **long arm,** or **q.** At the end of each chromatid is the **telomere.**

In the early years of chromosome analysis, it was difficult to distinguish one chromosome from another because several of the chromosomes resembled each other. Early inspection of chromosomes showed that they could be grouped by relative size. Five groups were distinguished and were designated by letter in descending size order. A, B, C, D, and E group chromosomes and the sex chromosomes were the designations with the A chromosomes being the longest and the E group being the shortest (Figure 2–5).

CHROMOSOME 6

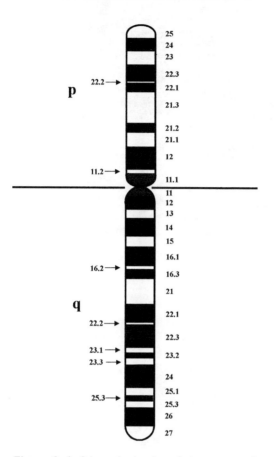

Figure 2–4. Schematic drawing of chromosome 6 showing the bands that become visible with Giemsa staining (G banding).

As chromosome analysis techniques (**kary-otypes**) improved, it became easier to distinguish one chromosome from the other and they became designated by number in descending order of size (Figure 2–6), with chromosome 1 being the longest and chromosome 22 being the shortest (actually, it is now known that chromosome 21 is slightly shorter than chromosome 22). The proper numerical designation is as written here: **chromosome 12**, not the **number 12 chromosome** or **the 12th chromosome**. The short arm of chromosome 12 is designated 12p, the long arm is designated as 12q.

It was also recognized that chromosomes had slightly different structures depending on the position of the centromere (Figure 2–7). When the centromere was near the middle of the chromosome, the chromosome was labeled **metacentric**. When the centromere was slightly off-center, the chromosome was called **submetacentric**. When the centromere is close to the end of the p arm, the chromosome is known as **acrocentric**. These are the only types of chromosomes in humans, but in other species, there is a fourth type known as **telocentric** in which the centromere is at the very end of the chromosome (which is found in mice).

In humans, the acrocentric chromosomes have an unusual structure at the top of the short arms (Figure 2–7). Chromosomes 13, 14, 15, 21, and 22 have small pods of chromatin attached to the p arm by slender stalks. These stalks contain genes that code for a type of RNA (which will be discussed later in this chapter) important in the synthesis of proteins.

Today, chromosomes can be visualized through a light microscope during certain stages of cell division. At that time, chromosomes can be stained with a variety of chemicals, the most common being giemsa which has the effect of creating alternating regions of dark and light segments known as **bands** (see Figure 2–6). Giemsa staining is referred to as G banding. Banding techniques allow tiny segments of each chromosome to be seen and counted, comparing them to the other chromosome in the pair and to the normal structure of that particular chromosome. Thus, it can be determined if more or less chromosome material is present. The number of bands present helps to distinguish one chromosome from another since several chromosomes are of similar size, such as chromosome 21 and 22. During cell division, each arm of the chromosome replicates prior to the time when each chromosome splits vertically to form two copies which then diverge into the two new cells formed during mitotic cell division.

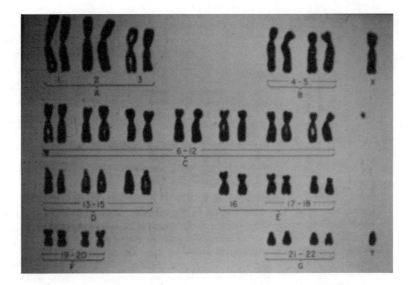

Figure 2–5. An older karyotype designating chromosomes by a letter grouping.

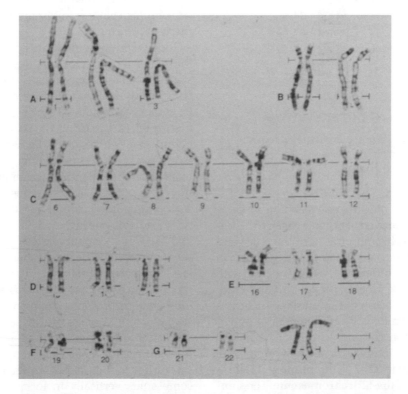

Figure 2–6. A modern high resolution karyotype with G banding designating the chromosomes by number (except for the sex chromosomes).

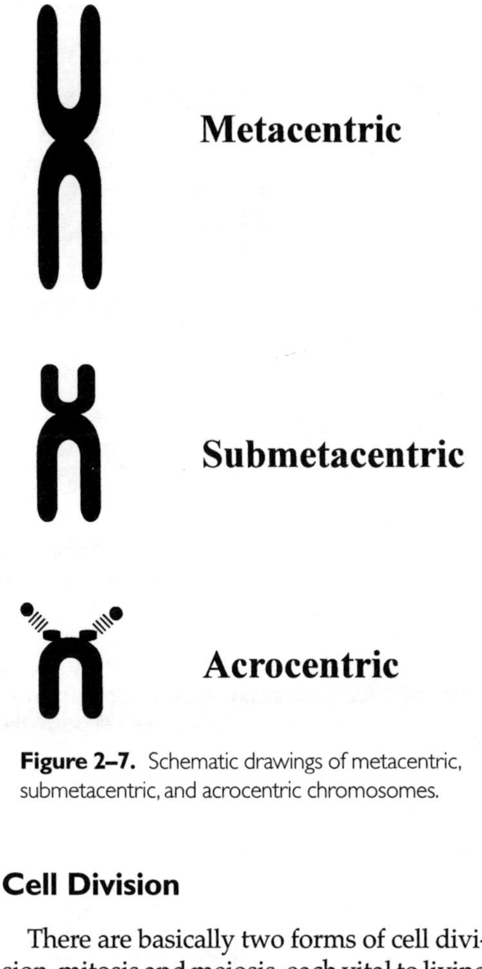

Metacentric

Submetacentric

Acrocentric

Figure 2–7. Schematic drawings of metacentric, submetacentric, and acrocentric chromosomes.

Cell Division

There are basically two forms of cell division, mitosis and meiosis, each vital to living organisms. Some scientists define *life* as the ability for an organism to respire, metabolize (i.e., eat and burn fuel for growth), and reproduce. Cell division is a key component to growth and reproduction. Growth and development are the result of mitosis. Reproduction, in the case of higher organisms (including humans), is the result of meiosis.

Mitosis

Mitosis, or mitotic cell division, allows an organism to grow in size, and also allows complex organisms like mammals to have many different types of tissues derived from a single cell. In mitosis, the cytoplasm di-

vides roughly in half so that the division of the original cell results in two smaller cells of roughly equal size. After cell division, each cell then grows larger. There are several distinct phases of cell division which can be easily observed under a microscope.

Interphase

This is the state of the cell when it is not actively dividing. The cell is actually quite active during interphase, growing, metabolizing, and performing the specific chemical actions of the cell (such as the secretion of acetylcholine in nerve cells or adrenalin from the adrenal gland cells). During interphase, the nucleus looks like a spherical mass filled with a substance resembling coffee grounds suspended in jelly (Figure 2–8). It is during interphase that the DNA in the nucleus replicates so that the chromatids of the chromosomes become intertwined double strands.

Prophase

This marks the first visible signs of cell division. In early prophase (Figure 2–9), the nucleus changes appearance from the "coffee ground" pattern to visible chromosomal strands within the nucleus. As prophase progresses, the chromosomes appear to become thicker as the duplicated chromosomal arms begin to unravel from their intertwined configuration during the DNA replication of interphase. The nucleolus, an organelle normally present within the nucleus, disappears and two structures appear, the centrioles and the spindles. The centrioles move to the poles of the cell (Figure 2–10).

Prometaphase

In prometaphase, the nuclear membrane disappears and the spindles become more prominent, looking like a grating (Figure 2–11) running across the middle of the cell. The chromosomes begin to actively move with the movement centered around the centromeres.

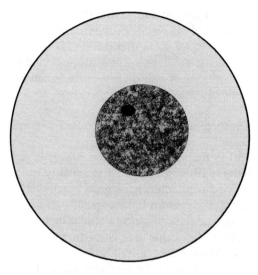

Figure 2–8. Drawing of a cell during interphase.

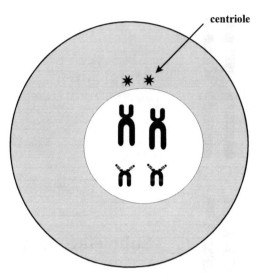

Figure 2–9. Schematic drawing of a cell during early prophase of mitosis showing only two pairs of chromosomes, one submetacentric pair and one acrocentric pair, for simplification. The chromosomes are already in the duplicated state (i.e., the chromatids have already replicated). In early mitotic prophase, the diploid number of chromosomes becomes visible as the cell begins the division process.

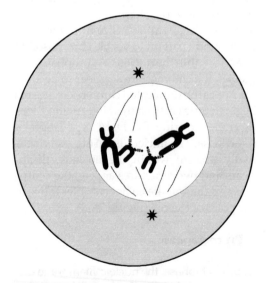

Figure 2–10. A cell during late prophase mitotis. The centrioles migrate to opposite ends of the nucleus, the spindles begin to form, and the chromosomes begin to migrate towards the center of the nucleus.

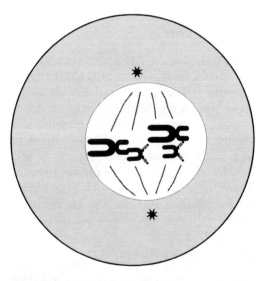

Figure 2–11. A cell during mitotic prometaphase. The spindles become more prominent, and the chromosomes begin to line up in the center of the nucleus in single file.

Metaphase

The chromosomes move in an arrangement along the center of the spindle, the centromeres appearing to be tugged to the midline where the chromosomes line up in the center of the cell (Figure 2–12). At this point, the chromosome's duplicated chromatids are still attached at the centromere so that the chromosome looks very much like an X, the center for the X being the point of attachment of the chromatids at the centromere.

Anaphase

At this point, the duplicated chromatids separate (Figure 2–13), each duplicated chromosome now with its own centromere. The chromosome, now in its normal unduplicated state, consists of single chromatids (the p and q arms) joined at the center by the centromere. Therefore, at this point where the duplicated chromosomes have separated, the cell in the process of dividing now has a double comple-

ment of chromosomes, or 92 (46 pairs) chromosomes. The separated chromosomes now begin to migrate away from each other toward the opposing poles of the spindle, being dragged by the pull on the centromeres.

Telophase

In this final stage of mitosis, events occur in the opposite order of those observed in early mitosis. After the chromosomes have migrated to the poles of the spindle, the spindle disappears and a new nuclear membrane forms around the chromosomes. The cell's protoplasm divides roughly in half creating two new cells (Figure 2–14) and the nucleus returns to the "coffee ground" appearance seen during interphase.

In mitosis, the purpose of the cell division is growth and development. Organisms and structures contained within organisms become larger by adding more cells. Tissues differentiate from early embryonic cells by dividing and changing structure, but main-

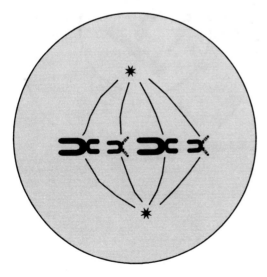

Figure 2–12. A cell during mitotic metaphase. The nuclear membrane disappears and the spindles become more prominent. The chromosomes are now lined up in the center of the cell.

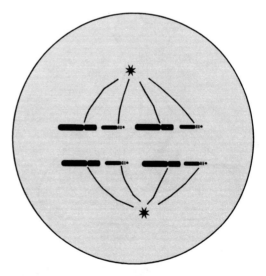

Figure 2–13. A cell during mitotic anaphase. The chromosomes split at the centromere with each pair now separating into two complete sets of nonduplicated chromatids. In humans, there would now be 92 nonduplicated chromosomes contained within the dividing cell.

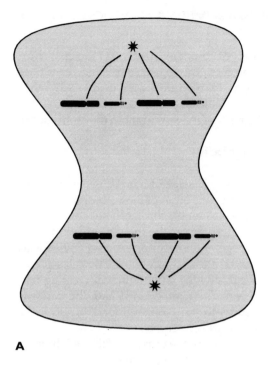

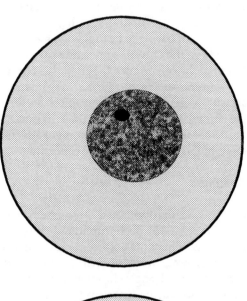

A

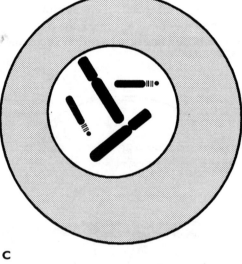

C

B

Figure 2–14. A. A cell during mitotic telophase. The spindles begin to pull each set of nonduplicated chromosomes toward the centromeres located at each pole of the cell. The cytoplasm begins to divide into two equal portions, each containing its own diploid set of chromosomes. **B.** As the cytoplasmic division continues, a new nuclear membrane appears surounding the diploid set of chromosomes, the spindles disappear, and two new cells are formed. **C.** The nucleus returns to its interphase appearance until the next division.

taining the same chromosomal complement as the rest of the organism. Mitosis is not, however, the only form of cell division. Another type is meiosis.

Meiosis

The growth and development of all organisms is the result of mitotic cell division. The process of growth and development begins with a single cell representing a fertilized egg, or **zygote** undergoing mitosis to form other cells. In higher animals, the zygote is formed when an egg, or ovum, is fertilized by a sperm. Ova and sperm are known as **gametes**. When a sperm fertilizes an ovum, the genetic material from the sperm (i.e., its chromosomes) joins with that of the ovum to create the zygote. In humans, the zygote has the normal complement of 46 chromosomes. Therefore, both the sperm and egg must have fewer than 46 chromosomes. In fact, the sperm and ovum have an equal number of chromosomes (23 in each gamete). This represents half of the total complement of human chromosomes, known as the haploid number, or haplotype. Forty-six chromosomes is the normal diploid number, or diplotype. In fact, each gamete contains one chromosome from each of the 23 pairs of chromosomes. The process by which gametes with the haploid number of chromosomes are produced from cells with the diploid number of chromosomes is known as **meiosis.**

Meiosis is the form of cell division necessary for the production of the cells that are involved in procreation (the gametes). Actually, in most animals, meiosis involves two divisions of the nucleus, but four separations of the cell so that each resulting cell has 23 chromosomes rather than 46 (Figure 2–15). The first stage of the first cell division in meiosis, or prophase I, is far longer in duration than prophase in mitosis and has several substages. At the beginning of prophase, the chromosomes are very long and thin; much thinner than ever seen in the process of mitosis (Figure 2–15a). These thin chromosome strands then line up side-by-side with the other member of the pair in a

very tight and close formation, known as **synapsis** (Figure 2–15b). During synapsis, the chromosomes of each pair are so precisely aligned that the DNA sequences from one chromosome are in direct proximity to the matching sequences from the other chromosome. Once paired, the chromosomes shorten and thicken (Figure 2–15c). Metaphase begins as the nuclear membrane disappears (Figure 2–15d and e) and the spindle forms as in mitosis. During the close proximity of the chromosome pairs, they are so tightly aligned that the strands of chromosome material actually exchange genetic material with the other member of the pair, a phenomenon known as **crossing over** (Figure 2–15f). Crossing over is a mechanism that allows the genome to alter in a way that provides greater genetic variability for the species and which may be a way to strengthen and fortify a species against the possible negative effects of inbreeding when the genetic pool (i.e., available mates) is small. The attachment of the chromosomes that allows crossing over to occur is known as a chiasma. In the first division's metaphase, or metaphase I, the chromosomes do not line up in single file in the midline as in mitosis. Each pair of chromosomes is side-by-side during the first stage of meiosis because they remain attached by the chiasmas so that each chromosome bundle is comprised of four chromatids.

The chromosomes then begin to pull apart (Figure 2–15g) and it can be seen that each chromosome has two sets of chromatids attached to a common centromere indicating duplication. The chromosomes continue to get shorter and thicker so that they are shorter and thicker than at any point during mitosis. In the first anaphase, the centromeres divide and the separated chromosomes (each with two chromatids attached to a single centromere) move towards the poles of the cell. Therefore, rather than each new cell getting a single chromatid copy of both pairs of each chromosome, each new cell will receive a duplicated chromatid copy of a single member of each chromosome pair (Figure 2–15h). In the first telophase, the new

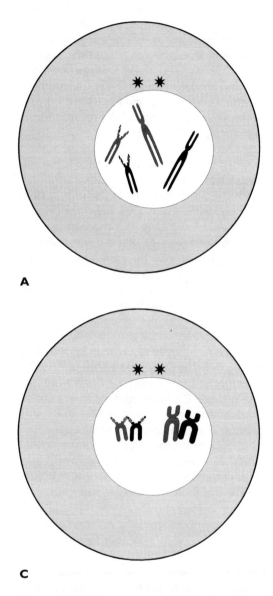

A

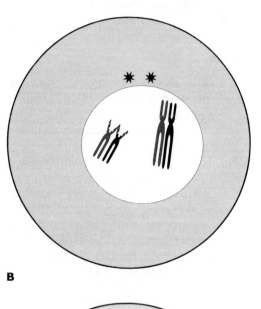

B

C

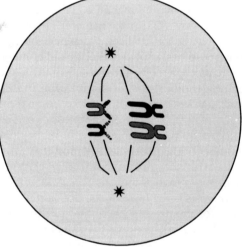

D

Figure 2–15. The stages of meiosis illustrating how primary germ cells divide to result in four cells, each with 23 chromosomes, known as the haploid number. **A**. During meiotic prophase I, the chromosomes (in their duplicated chromatid state) become visible, but unlike mitosis, the chromosomes appear longer and thinner. **B**. The chromosomes, still in their stretched appearance, pair closely with one another within the nucleus, a process known as synapsis. **C**. Once paired, the chromosomes shorten and thicken. **D** and **E**. In meiotic metaphase I, the nuclear membrane disappears, spindles form, and the chromosomes line up in the midline of the cell, but not in single file as in mitosis. In meiotic metaphase, the chromosomes line up alongside each other in their chromatid duplicated state. Because the chromosomes begin this process in the diploid state, the schematic here represents the members of each pair in different shades (one gray, one black) to indicate the genetic heterogeneity of the alleles on each chromosome (i.e., each chromosome within a pair is slightly dif-

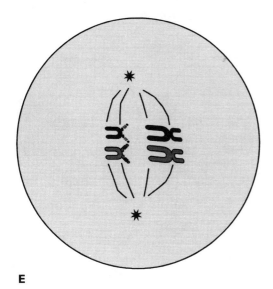

E

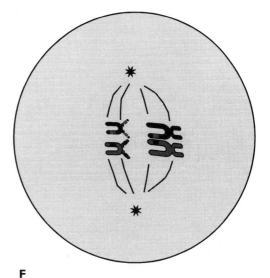

F

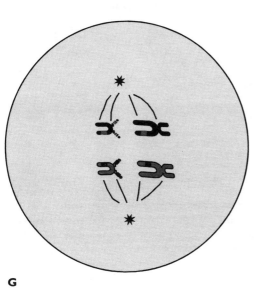

G

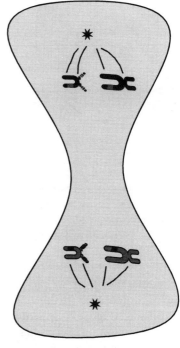

H

ferent genetically from its counterpart because one chromosome came from that individual's father and one from the mother). Therefore, multiple possible arrangements of the members of each pair are possible, demonstrated here using just two pairs showing the two different possible arrangements of the two pairs (**D** and **E**). The larger the number of chromosomes, the larger the amount of variation of the possible arrangements.

Genetic variation is also enhanced by crossing over. Using just one of the possible pairings (the one shown in e), the results of crossing over are demonstrated in **F**. **G.** In meiotic anaphase I, the still intact (i.e., chromatid duplicated) members of each pair are pulled toward opposite poles of the cell. **H.** In meiotic telophase I, the cytoplasm divides, each new cell now containing a haploid set (23 chromosomes) of chromatid duplicated

(continued)

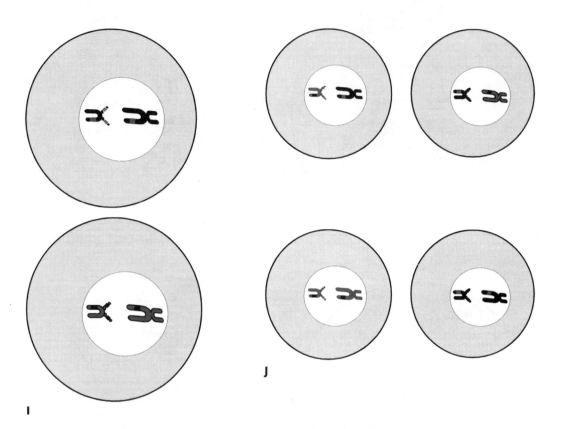

Figure 2–15. *(continued)* chromosomes (**I**). **J.** The possible distribution of chromosomes for just two chromosome pairs at the end of meiosis I. The number of variations would obviously be far greater for the 23 pairs of human chromosomes. Meiosis II is shown in **K**. In meiosis II, the haploid set of chromatid duplicated chromosomes goes through the same process as in mitotic metaphase, anaphase, and telophase in that the chromosomes split into single strand chromosomes (i.e., without duplicated chromatids). The possible segregation into resulting gametes with genetic variability is shown in the bottom row.

nuclear membranes form in each new cell with each chromosome in the nucleus already duplicated (Figure 2–15i). Interphase I (Figure 2–15j) follows anaphase and is followed, in turn, by the second cell division beginning with prophase II.

In prophase II (Figure 2–15k), the chromosomes contract and become visible as in mitosis. In metaphase II, the spindle forms and the chromosomes migrate to the midline of the cell. In anaphase II, the chromosomes separate and move towards the poles of the cell as single chromatid copies, as in mitosis (Figure 2–15k). In telophase II, as in mitosis, the cell's nucleus again becomes indistinct.

How Sperm and Ova Result from Meiosis

The process of reproductive cells being derived from meiotic divisions is known as **gametogenesis.** In males, the process is **spermatogenesis** and in females it is **oogenesis** (pronounced ō-ō-genesis).

Oogenesis

Human eggs (ova) are derived from cells called **oogonia,** which are contained in the ovary. Oogonia are the result of many mitotic divisions of cells known as **primary germ cells.** These cells are contained within the cortex of each ovary and are surrounded by a follicle which develops in the ovarian cor-

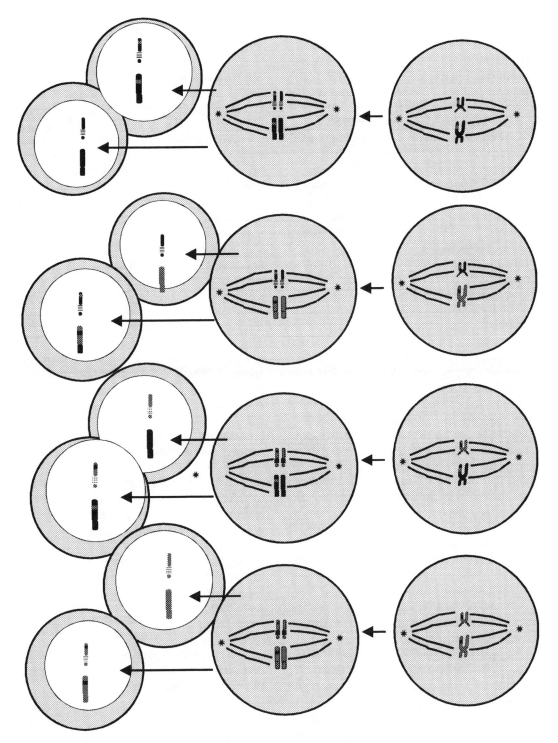

K

25

tex. This process occurs in females even before they are born with the process of oogonia formation happening in the embryonic period in the first trimester after fertilization. By the end of the first trimester, the oogonia begin to differentiate into cells known as **primary oocytes**. Meiotic cell division can begin in either the oogonia or the oocytes, but whenever meiosis begins, it becomes suspended at the first stage of meiosis (prophase I). As the fetus continues to develop, all oogonia mature into oocytes, which become suspended at prophase I embedded within a follicle in the ovarian cortex. At birth, the female child has over 2 million oocytes. The large majority of these oocytes disintegrate and their follicles become resorbed, leaving behind only about 400 oocytes which will be the female's full complement of reproductive cells with no others being produced. After puberty, the follicles begin to mature, essentially one at a time, one during the ovulatory phase of each menstrual cycle. As each follicle matures, the oocyte again becomes active, completing the first stage of meiosis. At the end of telophase I, as the primary oocyte divides in two, the two resulting cells do not have equal amounts of cytoplasm. One new cell gets the majority of the cytoplasm and cell organelles plus the haplotype of chromosomes and becomes the secondary oocyte. The other cell is called a **polar body**. It assumes a position aligned at one end of the secondary oocyte. The polar body is a smaller unit containing very little cytoplasm plus the haplotype of chromosomes.

Immediately after completion of the first stage of meiosis, meiosis II begins during ovulation and reaches metaphase II, but it will proceed no further unless fertilization occurs. If fertilization occurs, meiosis II is completed with a second polar body being formed adjacent to the first and the resulting ovum retaining the majority of the cytoplasm once again. Once meiosis has been completed, the chromosomes of the sperm and the chromosomes of the ovum merge into a single nucleus, which restores the diploid complement of chromosomes, creating the zygote (fertilized egg) which then begins mitotic cell division to create the embryo.

Spermatogenesis

Unlike oogenesis, which is essentially complete prior to the time a human female is born, spermatogenesis is an ongoing process throughout the large majority of adult male life. Spermatogenesis occurs in the testes, specifically in the seminiferous tubules. The inner lining of the seminiferous tubules are cells known as **spermatogonia**. The spermatogonia undergo mitotic cell division throughout life, but it is not until puberty and the appearance of secondary sexual characteristics in the male that these divisions give rise to a cell known as a **primary spermatocyte**. The primary spermatocyte is the cell that eventually undergoes meiotic division. The result of the first stage of meiotic division is a cell known as a secondary **spermatocyte**. The secondary spermatocyte then undergoes the second stage of meiotic division, and the resulting cells with haploid complements of chromosomes are knows as **spermatids**. Following the second stage of meiosis, spermatids are round cells that look very much like other cells in the body, but they then begin to change structurally without any additional cell divisions and become sperm cells with the characteristic appearance of a small cell head trailed by a long tail, which provides motility for the cell. The entire process of spermatogenesis from the mitotic division of the spermatogonium to the final appearance of the sperm is approximately 9 weeks. The process of spermatogenesis is continuous throughout adult life, resulting in the production of more than 10 trillion sperm in the average male. Each ejaculation in the human male contains approximately 200 million sperm.

FERTILIZATION: THE RECONSTITUTION OF THE DIPLOTYPE

Each human sperm and each human ovum has the haplotype number of chromosomes

(23). The DNA contained in these chromosomes represents half of the total genetic constitution of the mother (in the case of the ovum) or father (in the case of the sperm). Once a sperm fertilizes an ovum, the normal complement of chromosomes number, 46 (the diplotype) is restored. The fertilized ovum, now known as a zygote, contains half of the father's genetic material and half of the mother's. The zygote then begins the process of mitosis. The mitosis of the zygote is very rapid. As the cells resulting from the mitotic divisions grow in number, they also differentiate into differing tissue types, such as neurons, muscle cells, skin cells, nd so on. This process is determined and regulated by the genes on the 46 chromosomes in each cell. Although the process of meiosis and resulting mitosis of the zygote ensures that offspring will largely resemble one or both of the parents (because the offspring contains 50% of each parent's genetic make-up), the process also ensures differences between each offspring by a number of mechanisms. First, because of the process of the multiple cell divisions in meiosis, there is a different distribution of the parent's genes in each sperm or ovum. In other words, although there is a 50% contribution from each parent, there is no prediction of which 50% that will be. Second, the process of crossing-over helps to redistribute each parent's genetic material differently for each germ cell. Finally, because the genetic material is distributed in a fairly random manner from each parent, the union of a particular sperm or ovum provides an essentially unique combination of the two parents' genetic material.

HOW CHROMOSOMES AND GENES MAKE PEOPLE WHAT THEY ARE

The human genome can be compared to a computer in many ways. This analogy is not as far-fetched as one might think. Contemporary scientists have hypothesized that DNA is, in essence, a biological computer code that could be applied to most functions currently performed by even the most powerful computers. Using the computer analogy, the body is the computer, the various organs and cells are the peripherals (the printer, the CD-ROM, etc.), the chromosomes are the disk drives, the genes are the software that contains the program for performing various functions, and the DNA is the binary code, or the computer language, which allows the computer to interpret the software commands. When the computer (the body) is up and running, the software program (the genes), which is contained in a code on the disk drive (the chromosomes), issues commands in the computer language that is read by the computer (the DNA code), which sends signals to the peripherals (such as the brain, liver, arms, eyes, etc.) to develop a specific structure or perform a specific biochemical function. Failure of the process (resulting in congenital anomalies) can be caused by errors anywhere in the computer. The disk drive could be broken so that the software cannot be retrieved properly. In the case of the human computer, this is analogous to a chromosome rearrangement. If there is a corruption of the software, the program will not perform properly (a genetic mutation). If the binary computer language is not loaded properly, the software will not be interpreted properly (a transcription error). If the peripherals are broken, the proper output will not be produced (a congenital anomaly).

The human computer works by the genes transmitting information to the cells, which then create proteins, which instigate a biochemical process of growth and development. The process of genes causing cells to perform specific functions, produce specific cellular products, and grow specific organs is complex in operation, but simple in design. Using the computer analogy, instead of using a binary code of two symbols (0 and 1 in the case of a computer), genes use a code of four symbols (A, C, G, T). This code is made a bit more complicated in that each symbol of the code is paired with another symbol. This will be described in more detail in the following pages. The purpose of the code is to transmit information out of the cell's nucleus into the cytoplasm where structures known as ribosomes take the information and use it to synthesize a protein. It is the formation of the protein that leads to extracellular activities necessary for growth and development.

The DNA Connection

The reason that the nucleus and the ribosomes are important in the process of genetic determination is because of the biochemical mechanisms by which genes function. The genes on the chromosomes are portions of DNA molecules. DNA is a long complex molecule comprised of two strands of a sugar-phosphate compound, which are wound around each other in a counter-clockwise direction (the double helix). Connecting these two strands are pairs of nitrogen-containing organic bases (Figure 2–16). There are four organic bases in DNA: adenine, cytosine, guanine, and thymine (the A, C, G, and T cited above). These bases are attached (chemically bound) to a segment of the sugar-phosphate strand. The unit composed of the base, the phosphate, and the sugar is known as a **nucleotide**. Each base couples with another base like connecting rungs on a ladder, the legs of the ladder being constructed of the sugar-phosphate backbone of DNA. The four bases in DNA are divided into two types: two purines (adenine and guanine) and two pyrimidines (cytosine and thymine). Cytosine always joins with guanine; adenine always pairs with thymine. The ordering, or sequence, of these pairs of connections, called base pairs, makes up the genetic code. The diploid human genome contains approximately 7 billion base pairs strung along the 46 chromosomes. Each chromosome is actually a gigantic double macromolecule of DNA constructed together with a number of proteins, which also contribute to the structure of chromatin. Each chromosome consists of two very long strands of DNA wrapped around the structural proteins of the chromatin and around each other in a spiral. The DNA is wound

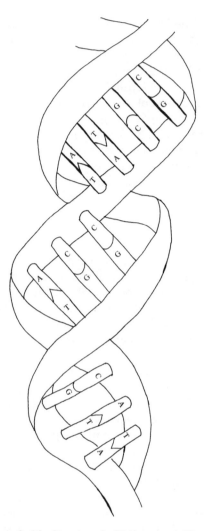

Figure 2–16. Drawing of a DNA molecule. The base pairs (adenine, thymine, guanine, and cytosine) resemble rungs on a ladder.

around the chromatin proteins (known as histones) in discrete segments, looking much like a beaded necklace so that very long segments of DNA are contained within the microscopic chromosomes. For example, if the DNA that constitutes chromosome 1 were stretched out to its maximum unwound length, it would be approximately 15 cm long (about 6 inches). In terms of base pairs, chromosome 1, the longest human chromosome, is approximately 250 million base pairs in length while the shortest, chromosome 21, is 50 million base pairs long. The winding of the DNA around the chromosomal proteins in discrete segments probably serves as a method for sequential reading of the DNA code (transcription), and is responsible for the ability to stain chromosomes in the discrete segments, which show up in banding procedures (such as G banding).

DNA sequences are of several types within the genome. The majority of DNA consists of essentially unique sequences of nucleotides that exist in a single copy, or at most, several copies within the genome (and are therefore referred to by some as single-copy DNA). Most, although not all, human genes are unique sequences. Conversely, not all of the unique sequences represent genes. In fact, most unique sequences are not genes and constitute much of the random DNA in each chromosome. Another type of DNA sequence is the "repeat." Repeat sequences of DNA, which may occur many thousands of times within the genome, often sit in between known genes. The purpose of these repetitive sequences is still not clear. Repeats often appear in groups of relatively short DNA segments arranged in mirror-image connections (i.e., a sequence of C-G-T-A-T-A-G-C will be followed by a sequence of C-G-A-T-A-T-G-C, although the sequences of DNA involved are much longer). These clusters of DNA repeat sequences are known as **tandem repeats**.

Genes

Genes are segments of DNA molecules, ranging in size from 1000 base pairs (referred to as a **kilobase**, or 1 kb) to several million base pairs (a million base pairs is a **megabase**, or mb). Not all of the DNA in the long DNA sequences on a chromosome are genes. In fact, most of the DNA sequences (over 90%) are not genes. The genes are the segments of DNA on the chromosomes that generate some type of product necessary for some type of function, such as growth and development. There are also genes located within the mitochondria, which will be discussed briefly later. However, the overwhelming

majority of the cell's DNA and genes are contained within the nuclear chromosomes.

The sequence of nucleotides in the DNA segments within the genes is known as the genetic code and must be somehow transmitted to perform a function within the cells and organs of the body. This is done by the production of proteins, which themselves respond to a code comprised of amino acids. The process by which information gets transmitted from the nuclear DNA to the cellular organelles that are responsible for protein production, the ribosomes, is known as transcription and involves a molecule similar to DNA known as RNA. The DNA sequences within the gene contain a series of instructions that are interrupted by "switches." The coding portions of the genes are known as **exons**. Exons encode for the production of amino acids, which then code for the production of a specific protein by the ribosomes. Each gene usually contains several exons interrupted by several **introns**. Introns are segments of DNA sequences that do not code for products, so that the genes are basically transcribed in segments of exons. These patterns of exons and introns within genes are largely preserved across species, thus often providing an evolutionary link down the phylogenetic scale and also allowing the observation of gene effects in species other than humans. The ability to study gene function in species other than humans is one of the methods that has allowed the rapid deciphering of the human genome.

Genes are often grouped by the products for which they code, which also allows them to be studied in other species because the development of particular substances and organs can be observed in species that reproduce and develop rapidly, such as mice. For example, there are genes that code for the production of collagen, which serves as the basis for connective tissue, and genes that code for the production of fibrillin, which plays a role in bone and connective tissue formation. These genes can be found and identified in mice or other species and their coding sequences observed. Therefore, changes in their coding sequences can also be observed in mice so that human diseases caused by fibrillin or collagen disorders resulting from gene mutations can be studied.

Specific ordering of a long series of base pairs (such as C-G,A-T,T-A, G-C,C-G,A-T, and so on) provides a template for a message to be sent from the gene to the ribosome, which in turn produces a protein that acts to perform a specific function. In order for the message to be sent, there must be a mechanism for "reading" the sequence and then sending the results of the reading to the ribosomes. This is done by a molecule similar to DNA known as **RNA**, the molecule ribonucleic acid, which exists in the nucleus of the cell, but is not part of the chromosomes. The reading of the DNA is known as **transcription**. RNA is similar in structure to DNA in that it also consists of a double strand of a sugar-phosphate molecule connected by base pairs. However, the sugar-

phosphate molecule is slightly different in structure from DNA's and the base pairs consist of adenine, cytosine, guanine, and uracil which replaces thymine. The RNA begins to transcribe the DNA sequence beginning at a specific point before each coding sequence and reads all exons and introns for the length of the gene until it is past the coding sequences. The RNA transcribes the DNA sequence by matching its own sequence of bases to the DNA bases (Figure 2–17). Because each base in the RNA can join with only one base in the DNA (RNA adenine to DNA thymine, RNA cytosine to DNA guanine, RNA guanine to DNA cytosine, and RNA uracil to DNA adenine), the resulting RNA sequence represents the complementary base pairing for the DNA sequence making up that person's genome. The RNA then goes through a process known as splicing in which the portions of RNA corresponding to the

DNA

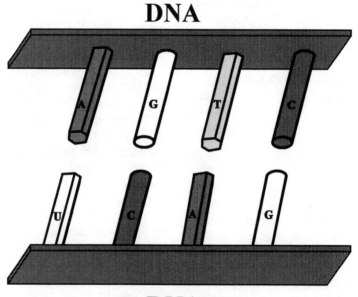

mRNA

Figure 2–17. Transcription of a DNA sequence by mRNA. Note that the bases in the mRNA (uracil, cytosine, adenine, and guanine) can pair only with their obligatory DNA partners (adenine, guanine, thymine, and cytosine, respectively), thus making a reciprocal exact copy of the DNA sequence except for the substitution of uracil for thymine in the mRNA.

introns are deleted from the RNA molecule and only the sequences corresponding to exons remain. The resulting RNA molecule is known as **messenger RNA**, or **mRNA**. The mRNA then leaves the nucleus, enters the cytoplasm, and enters a ribosome where a process known as **translation** occurs.

Translation is the process by which the mRNA code is read and rendered into a sequence of amino acids that are strung together to form a polypeptide chain. Polypeptide chains in turn are strung together to form a protein. Proteins may consist of a single large polypeptide chain or two or more polypeptides. Each amino acid formed is determined by a sequence of three organic bases called a **codon**. Twenty possible amino acids can be formed, even though there are 64 possible combinations of bases (there are four bases, adenine, cytosine, guanine, and uracil, which can be sequenced to form a combination of three, such as A-A-A, A-C-A, A-A-C, A-G-A, A-U-A, A-U-U, A-G-U, A-U-G, C-A-A, C-A-G, etc.). Therefore, some amino acids are formed from the translation of more than one sequence of bases. For example, the amino acid cysteine can be formed from the translation of the sequences U-G-U and U-G-C. Table 2–1 lists the possible sequences of mRNA and the corresponding amino acids for which they code. The translation process is mediated by another form of RNA known as **transfer RNA** or **tRNA**. Molecules of tRNA are short compared to DNA, RNA, and mRNA molecules. Each tRNA molecule is 100 or fewer base pairs in length. Amino acids from the cytoplasm are transferred to the mRNA by the tRNA. Remember, the mRNA is the carrier of the genetic code from the nucleus, so that the tRNA matches a specific amino acid determined by the instructions from the nuclear chromosomal DNA. As each short segment of tRNA delivers the amino acid from the codons determined by the nuclear genetic code, a chain of amino acids is added to an expanding polypeptide chain that is synthesized into a protein by the ribosomes.

A logical question to be asked is how the translation process is started and stopped?

In other words, as the tRNA begins the process of utilizing the genetic code to bring the components of the protein together, how is this information divided into discrete components? Genes are specific to a particular function, so it is important that the information be delivered in components that perform the function intended. The answer is that there are codons which serve to initiate and terminate the reading of the sequence by the tRNA. Table 2–1 shows the mRNA sequences of three bases, or codons, that code for a stopping point. There are three codon sequences known as **stops**: UAA, UGA, and UGC. The starting point in a sequence producing a string of amino acids is always the codon AUG, which translates to the amino acid methionine. Therefore, methionine is the first amino acid in any polypeptide chain and a stop codon is the last. Methionine is one of only 2 of the 20 amino acids that has a single codon sequence (Table 2–1), the other being tryptophan.

After the chain of amino acids is transformed into a protein within the ribosome, it is then passed into the cell's cytoplasm to perform a specific function in the development of the organism. Such functions may relate to specific cellular functions, such as changing the form of a specific type of cell to a neuron; sending a message to a particular group of cells to migrate to another point in the developing embryo; or instructing a group of cells to form a particular organ, such the liver or heart. There is an elegant orchestration of the events that form the developing baby from these sets of computerlike instructions emanating from the nuclear chromosomal DNA. The process of embryo formation depends on very precise timing of the events prompted by the 100,000 genes in the human genome. The process of growth and development begins from the moment of fertilization and continues not only throughout the prenatal period, but throughout postnatal life, as well. Genes have been identified that cause Alzheimer's disease, colon cancer, and other illnesses of late adult life. Genes also mediate the process of sexual maturation (puberty)

TABLE 2–1. The Possible Sequences of a mRNA and the Corresponding Amino Acids for Which They Code

Codon Sequence	Amino Acid	Codon Sequence	Amino Acid
UUU	PHENYLALANINE	GAG	GLUTAMIC ACID
UUC	PHENYLALANINE	UGU	CYSTEINE
UUA	LEUCINE	UGC	CYSTEINE
UUG	LEUCINE	UGG	TRYPTOPHAN
CUU	LEUCINE	CGU	ARGININE
CUC	LEUCINE	CGC	ARGININE
CUA	LEUCINE	CGA	ARGININE
CUG	LEUCINE	CGG	ARGININE
AUU	ISOLEUCINE	AGA	ARGININE
AUC	ISOLEUCINE	AGG	ARGININE
AUA	ISOLEUCINE	AGU	SERINE
AUG	METHIONINE	AGC	SERINE
GUU	VALINE	UCU	SERINE
GUC	VALINE	UCC	SERINE
GUA	VALINE	UCA	SERINE
GUG	VALINE	UCG	SERINE
UAU	TYROSINE	GGU	GLYCINE
UAC	TYROSINE	GGC	GLYCINE
UAA	STOP CODON	GGA	GLYCINE
UAG	STOP CODON	GGG	GLYCINE
UGA	STOP CODON	CCU	PROLINE
CAU	HISTIDINE	CCC	PROLINE
CAC	HISTIDINE	CCA	PROLINE
CAA	GLUTAMINE	CCG	PROLINE
CAG	GLUTAMINE	ACU	THREONINE
AAU	ASPARAGINE	ACC	THREONINE
AAC	ASPARAGINE	ACG	THREONINE
AAA	LYSINE	ACA	THREONINE
AAG	LYSINE	GCC	ALANINE
GAU	ASPARTIC ACID	GCA	ALANINE
GAC	ASPARTIC ACID	GCG	ALANINE
GAA	GLUTAMIC ACID	GCU	ALANINE

and aging. Therefore, the process of DNA, RNA, mRNA, and tRNA activity continues for as long as life does.

Gene Penetrance and Expression

In the past, prior to the advent of molecular genetics, pedigree analysis served as the primary method for tracing genetic traits and diseases. Clinicians and scientists observed that not all traits followed the Mendelian patterns of inheritance with exactitude. Even though the traits were known to be autosomal dominant, autosomal recessive, or X-linked (see Chapter 3), the trait would not always show up as predicted by mathematical probability. For example, autosomal dominant traits should not skip generations. If a child is affected and the child's paternal grandfather is affected, then the child's father must be the person who transmitted the gene to the child (see Chapter 3). However, cases have been observed where the father did not express the trait, even though he was an obligate gene carrier and the trait was dominant so that it should have been expressed. In such cases, the gene has been labeled **nonpenetrant**. **Penetrance** of a gene is calculated based on many observations of how often the gene is expressed in people who are known to be obligate carriers who should express it.

Another important concept is gene expression. **Variable expression** is a concept of extreme importance in clinical genetics. It is possible, using probability theory and the principles of Mendelian inheritance, to determine if an individual is likely to inherit a gene. This calculation is known as **recurrence risk**. However, even though an individual can be counseled for the risk or probability of inheritance, it is not possible to counsel for how severe the trait or disease will be. Although genetic traits all share basic similarities in individuals who have

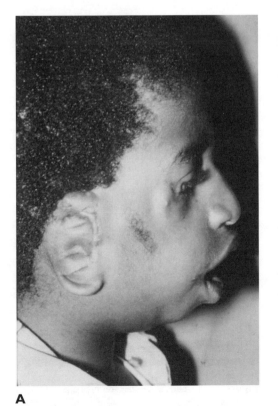

A

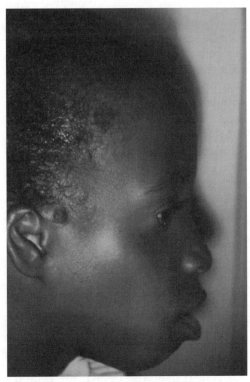

B

Figure 2–18. Two patients with Treacher Collins syndrome showing a severe expression (**A**) and a mild expression (**B**).

them, they do not render affected individuals carbon-copy identical. Figure 2–18 shows an example of variable expression in two individuals with the same genetic disease, Treacher Collins syndrome. In one case, the expression is severe (Figure 2–18a), and in the other, the expression is so mild that the individual is essentially normal in appearance, requiring a skilled clinician to note that the disorder is present (Figure 2–18b).

Actually, variable expression is not unique to genetic diseases. Essentially all diseases show some degree of variability in how they are expressed. Genetic disorders are no different even though there are basic similarities in people who have them. For example, one need look only as far as one of the most common childhood diseases, chicken pox, to see the principles of variable expression. Chicken pox is caused by a virus, varicella. I recall when I was a child that my brother got chicken pox. He was 9 years old, I was 4. He developed a very slight fever, had only several small pox, and within several days he was out and about as if he had never been ill. Ten days later, the incubation period for varicella, I came down with chicken pox, but unlike my brother, I developed a very high fever, was covered with pox from head to toe, and was sick for over a week. This was the same virus (the fact that I became ill 10 days after my brother indicates he gave me the exact same virus), and my brother and I are genetically very similar, yet the virus was expressed very differently in the two of us. This same pattern of possible variable expression is also true in genetic disorders.

The mechanisms of how genes are expressed are not yet completely understood. Some clinicians do not believe that there is actually nonpenetrance of genes which should predictably cause a disorder. It may be that the problem is not that the gene is not expressed, but rather that the expression of the gene is so mild that clinicians can not detect it. It may also be that the gene is expressed in an area of the body or a tissue that is not obvious to clinical examination

and requires special laboratory tests or examination techniques, which would not normally be ordered unless the expression were obvious. For example, the individual shown in Figure 2–18b with Treacher Collins syndrome is essentially normal in appearance, but has two traits that are consistent with Treacher Collins syndrome for which the diagnosis is dependent on specialty tests. This individual has a mild to moderate conductive hearing loss resulting from minor ossicular anomalies. He also has a typical pattern of mandibular growth characteristic of Treacher Collins syndrome, known as antegonial notching of the body of the mandible (Figure 2–19). Therefore, without an audiogram and a cephalometric radiograph, the diagnosis might not be made. In this case, suspicion was raised by the fact that there were other affected family members who had more severe expressions of the syndrome (including a complete microtia of the ears, which is a more severe manifesta-

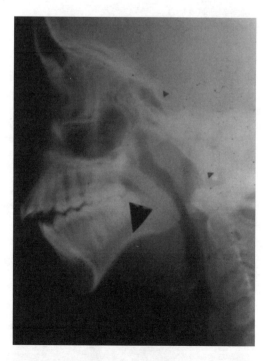

Figure 2–19. Lateral cephalograph of a patient with Treacher Collins syndrome showing antegonial notching of the body of the mandible (*arrow*).

tion of the ear anomalies in this syndrome).

In summary, the exact mechanisms of gene expression with respect to variability are not yet fully understood. Although it is possible to counsel for gene inheritance, it is not usually possible to counsel for the severity of the disorder once it is inherited (for an exception, see the portion of Chapter 3 related to imprinting). There are, however, some factors that contribute to how a gene is expressed which can be identified. They include the timing of expression and type of the gene.

Timing of Expression

The transcription and translation of genes follow a pattern of timing that is important to the developmental process. Obviously, **embryogenesis,** the process of formation of the embryo, does not happen all at once. Embryogenesis must follow a delicately choreographed scenario in order for necessary biological structures and functions to intermesh so that the organism will live and grow. The earlier in the process of embryogenesis that genes are switched on, the more widespread their effect will be because fewer tissues and structures are already formed. Early embryonic structures and tissues typically develop subsequently into multiple structures or large components of the body. For example, in very early embryogenesis, there is a layer of cells that sits atop the developing neural tube. This layer of cells is known as the neural crest. Neural crest cells migrate very early in embryogenesis to become parts of nearly every major structure and organ in the body. Neural crest cells make up parts of the face, the limbs, the gut, and the sensory organs. Therefore, in the case of genetic errors, the earlier faulty genes are expressed, the more likely their effects will be very widespread in the organism with many diverse parts of the body affected.

Types of Genes

A number of different types of genes play roles necessary to both the growth and development of the organism, as well as the regulation of the process of the expression of the genome. There are **structural genes**, **homeobox genes**, and **regulatory genes**.

Structural Genes

Structural genes are those that code for RNA, which subsequently leads to the production of a protein. Structural genes have a direct impact on growth and development because the proteins that result from their translation and the transcription of the resulting RNA are responsible for the formation of a particular body part (such as a specific part of the heart, or one of the bones in the hand), tissue, or metabolic function (such as the maintenance of the normal balance of blood electrolytes or basal metabolic rate). Therefore, abnormalities or mutations of these genes will have a direct impact on that particular structure or function but not on other unrelated structures or functions. However, some structural genes code for the production of a specific substance or type of tissue. For example, there are genes that code for the production of various types of collagen, which is a necessary component of connective tissues and skeletal structures. These genes may be expressed very early in embryonic development; and as a result, when that particular type of collagen is important to the development of multiple anatomic structures, their effect may be widespread throughout the organism.

It is possible to trace the effect of structural genes by tracing the types of tissues in which they are expressed. This type of process allows molecular geneticists to determine gene effect by knowing where in the body the protein products of the gene action are distributed. Genes may be expressed in single tissue types, single places in the body, or in multiple tissue types and multiple places. Collagen II, a type of collagen necessary to connective tissue, cartilage, fibrous tissue, and skeletal formation, may be expressed in all of those tissues and in body parts as diverse as the eyes, the spine, the palate, and the inner ear. Another gene, known as COMT (which will be discussed in more detail later in this text) is located on the long arm of chromosome 22. COMT is an acronym for catechol-o-methyl transferase. COMT is necessary for the production of a group of chemicals that metabolize dopamines, chemicals found in the brain. Therefore, COMT is expressed in the brain. If COMT is not present, the dopamines in the brain are not fully metabolized and are present in excess levels, a condition known to be present in various psychiatric illnesses and in children with attention deficit disorder.

Regulatory Genes

Regulatory genes are, as the name implies, genes that "supervise" the expression of structural genes. Rather than coding for structural proteins, regulatory genes code for RNA and its protein derivatives, which influence how other genes are expressed. Therefore, the action of regulatory genes may have a far more widespread effect than the action of structural genes. Abnormalities in the function of a regulatory gene may disrupt the normal function of many genes located throughout the genome rather than be simply isolated to a single chromosomal locus. Because some genes may be present in more than one copy in the genome, the effect of regulatory genes may cover not only a large area of the developing embryo, but also a wide time frame because not all genes act at the same time (see the section on timing below).

Homeobox Genes

Homeobox genes are a special group of a very small number of genes that play an important role in embryonic development. Homeobox genes are remarkably well preserved across most animal species from fruit flies (*Drosophila melanogaster*) to humans. The group of homeobox genes in humans are structurally much like homeobox genes in mice, hamsters, and fruit flies. All homeobox genes contain a region of DNA known as a homeobox, which encodes for a specific set of 60 amino acids that govern specific aspects of embryonic development, such as

the formation of the eye, the leg, or the brain. Because of their involvement with embryonic development, homeobox genes begin to act very early in the developmental process. Genes that contain homeoboxes include HOX genes, which are distributed on the long arm of chromosome 2, short arm of chromosome 7, the long arm of chromosome 12, and the long arm of chromosome 17.

Mitochondrial Genes

Mitochondrial genes, because they reside only in the cytoplasm of the cell, not in the nucleus, are transmitted only through the mother because the sperm provides essentially no cytoplasm and no mitochondria to the fertilized zygote. Most human cells contain several hundred mitochondria, each of which contains a small chromosome which is 16 kb long (much smaller than even the smallest nuclear chromosome) with 13 genes. Mutations can occur in mitochondrial genes, which result in a number of disease conditions, particularly a small number of rare neuromuscular diseases. Unlike Mendelian modes of inheritance (autosomal dominant, autosomal recessive, X-linked recessive, and X-linked dominant), mitochondrial diseases are always inherited from the mother because the abnormal gene that affects cell function is contained within the cell's cytoplasm, not the nucleus. All of a child's cytoplasm, and hence all of the child's mitochondria, are inherited from the mother. Therefore, affected mothers can pass the trait on to either their sons or daughters, but affected fathers cannot pass on the trait to any offspring.

Mutations

Mutations are simply defined as changes in genetic structure. In strictest terms, mutations include chromosome rearrangements, but the term is most often reserved for genetic errors that are not microscopically visible and occur in single genes or very tiny regions of DNA. Mutations are actually occurring all of the time within the human genome. DNA has a degree of intrinsic instability, which is, in part, responsible for both congenital anomalies and the process of evolution. Congenital anomalies occur far more frequently than major evolutionary changes because so many mutations in the human DNA sequence are either incompatible with life or cause errors in growth and development that are perceived to be abnormal.

Mutations in genetic structure are of essentially three types: deletions, additions, and changes in the DNA sequence without the addition or deletion of genetic material. Deletions involve the absence of one or more base pairs of DNA, which therefore alters the genetic code of that particular gene. Deletions may be quite large, involving large segments of DNA, sometimes involving segments larger than a single gene, in which case the resulting congenital anomalies represent a **contiguous gene syndrome**. Of course, deletions also can involve such large segments of DNA that a karyotype will reveal a microscopically visible deletion (see below).

Just as deletions alter the genetic code, so do additions of DNA. Additions within single genes usually involve very small segments of DNA, such as several base pairs. Even the addition of a single base pair can cause an error in the code significant enough to result in a complex of congenital anomalies. Additional chromosomal material also can be present as a result of errors in cell division known as nondisjunction, which will be described later in this chapter.

Changes in the DNA sequence are isolated to a single gene, although it is certainly possible that more than one gene within a person's genome could mutate. However, mutation of multiple genes in different locations within the genome rarely occurs. Changes in the DNA sequence could involve one or more base pairs. However, as in deletions and additions, any change in the sequence represents a change in the code sufficient to cause an abnormality in the translation and transcription of the DNA sequence. The result of the alteration will cause a different or defective polypeptide chain to form, which in turn will affect the process or structure to be determined by the gene.

Somatic mutations

Sometimes, genetic mutations occur after fertilization and the early development of the embryo. In such cases, the mutations do not reside in every cell in the body, but only in cells and tissues derived from the cell where the mutation originally occurred. Depending on when the mutation occurred in the embryonic process, the number of cells and tissues affected will vary. For example, the mutation may only be found in the cells of the liver, or the left arm, or even the skin. Somatic mutations will not be detected by studying peripheral blood, but can be isolated by studying the affected tissues by biopsy.

PROBLEMS OF GENETIC STRUCTURE

The descriptions of cell biology, cell division, DNA, chromosomes, genes, transcription, translation, and the genetic code in the preceding pages represent a very complicated process of interacting elements that depend on precise codes, careful timing, and movements of microscopic and submicroscopic structures. Opportunities for errors or malfunctions in the process are many. When errors occur in any step of the process, the possibility exists that the genetic code will not be delivered intact so that the correct proteins will not be produced for a specific process of growth and development. Errors could occur in meiotic cell division, fertilization, mitotic cell division of the zygote or embryo, or in the genetic code itself. Errors that occur during meiosis, fertilization, or zygote mitosis are usually reflected in abnormalities of chromosome number and/or structure. Errors that occur in the genetic code are referred to as **mutations** and have several different forms.

Errors of Chromosome Structure and Number

Karyotypes may show a variety of errors of chromosome number or structure in individuals who have congenital anomalies. It is also possible to have certain types of chromosome rearrangements known as balanced translocations (to be described later in this chapter) without resulting malformations, but with risk to offspring. In general, chromosome rearrangements are called **aneuploidies**. The clinical ramifications of aneuploidies are discussed in additional detail in Chapter 3. Chromosome rearrangements can occur as a result of simple chromosome breakage, an error in cell division known as **nondisjunction**, or during the process of crossing over.

Monosomy

A monosomy is the deletion of an entire chromosome from the normal chromosome complement of 46. Because each chromosome is normally present in duplicate for all cells except gametes (the diploid number, or disomy), a monosomy would result in a cell having 45 chromosomes. Monosomies usually result from nondisjunction during meiosis in either the male or female gametes. Nondisjunction refers to the failure of one or more chromosomes to separate normally during an anaphase separation of the chromosomes. One of the chromosomes may fail to separate from its partner so that, of the two resulting cells, one cell gets an additional chromosome, and the other cell is missing a chromosome. Nondisjunction is often likely to occur during one of the two anaphases during meiosis (Figure 2–20). In living individuals, nondisjunction is most often likely to result in monosomies or trisomies (see

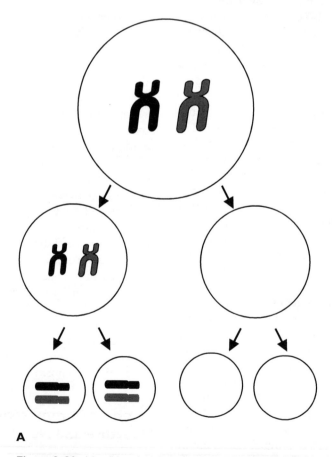

A

Figure 2–20. Nondisjunction during meiosis. In **A.**, the nondisjunction occurs during meiosis I so that the two resulting cells from the first stage of meiosis have unbalanced numbers of chromosomes. Using a

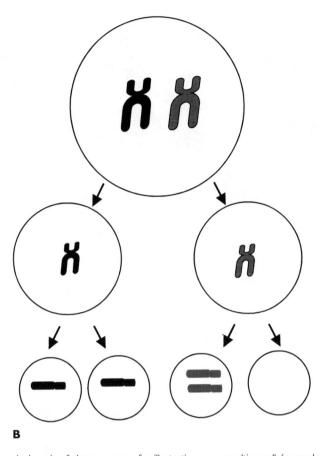

B

single pair of chromosomes for illustration, one resulting cell (second row) gets two copies of the same chromosome, the other none. After meiosis II, two cells have extra chromosomes, two cells are missing this chromosome. In **B.**, if the nondisjunction occurs during meiosis II, two resulting gametes get the normal complement of chromosomes, one gets an extra chromosome, and one is missing that chromosome *(bottom row)*.

below) in which there is either one missing or one extra chromosome. However, nondisjunction can happen to more than one chromosome and may even result in the failure for an entire set of chromosomes (i.e., a complete haploid set) to disjoin (see polypoloidy below).

An individual with a monosomy will be missing one entire set of genes contained on the missing chromosome. Therefore, the coding instructions for that chromosome will also be missing which is likely to cause many errors in growth and development. It is likely that many pregnancies involving fetuses with monosomies do not come to term and

undergo spontaneous abortion (miscarriage) as a result of nonviability of the fetus.

Trisomy

As in monosomies, trisomies are also the result of nondisjunction with the resulting fertilized zygote having 47 chromosomes rather than the normal 46 as the result of nondisjunction in one of the gametes (Figure 2–21). In this case, the developmental process is disturbed by the presence of extra DNA and coding sequences, which disrupt the normal process of morphogenesis. Down syndrome is a trisomy (trisomy 21) and is proba-

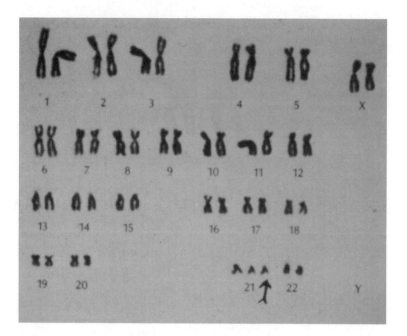

Figure 2–21. Karyotype showing trisomy 21 (written as 47XX, +21 in this female karyotype), diagnostic for Down syndrome.

bly the most common multiple anomaly syndrome in humans.

Polyploidy

A polyploidy is the presence of one or more extra complete sets of chromosomes, the most common being triploidy in which the affected individual has 69 chromosomes (the equivalent of the diploid set plus an additional haploid set of chromosomes). Again, nondisjunction of an entire set of chromosomes during an anaphase stage of division is likely to be the contributing factor to the aneuploidy.

Deletions

A deletion is the absence of a segment of a chromosome that should normally be present. There are two types of deletions: terminal deletions and interstitial deletions (Figure 2–22). Terminal deletions are those where the chromosomal material is missing from one of the ends of the chromosome (i.e., the end of the p arm or q arm). An interstitial deletion is the absence of a segment of normally present chromosomal material from somewhere between the ends of the chromosome. Deletions have three possible causes. Deletions may be the result of simple breakage of the chromosome. They may also be caused by an unequal distribution of chromosomal material during the process of crossing over, as described earlier in this chapter. The third explanation for the presence of deletions is the consequences of a mating involving someone with a balanced translocation, which will be described in additional detail below. Deletions large enough to be seen on a karyotype must involve the loss of multiple genes so that the coding process will be disturbed by the addition of a fairly large segment of DNA and its resulting code.

Translocations

Translocations are rearrangements of chromosomes in which a segment of one chromosome breaks and attaches to another chromosome. For example, a segment of the long arm of chromosome 1 may break and become

CHROMOSOME 5

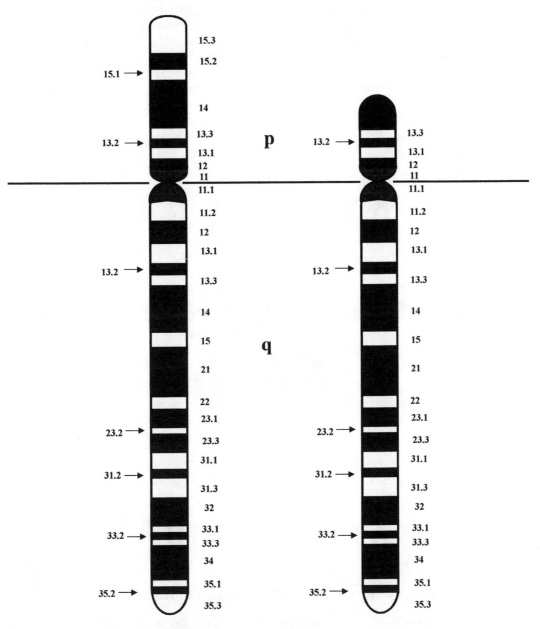

Figure 2–22. Schematic of a deletion of the short arm of chromosome 5 in a female (written as 46XX del (5)(p14)). This karyotype is consistent with the diagnosis of cri-du-chat syndrome.

attached to the short arm of chromosome 18. There are several different categories of translocations, which are descriptive of the types of rearrangements and the integrity of the genome. One of the two types of translocation categories is related to the completeness of the genome and has two types: balanced and unbalanced. In balanced translocations, chromosomal material is rearranged, but no chromosomal material or genes are lost. Individuals with balanced translocations are phenotypically normal, because all of their genome is intact and the process of transcription and translation is unimpeded. In unbalanced translocations, genetic material is lost so that the genome is missing some genes and there are resulting anomalies, as described above in the section on deletions.

Although individuals with balanced translocations are phenotypically normal, they do run the risk of having children with major anomalies because in meiotic divisions of the primary germ cells, there will be an abnormal segregation of genetic material (Figure 2–23).

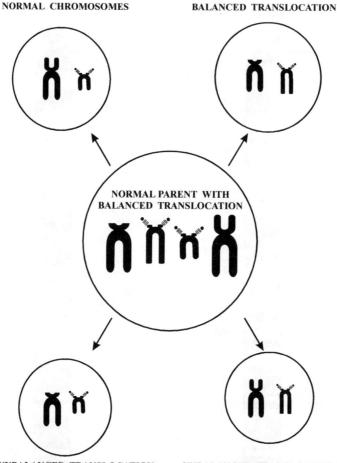

Figure 2–23. A schematic representation using only two pair of chromosomes to show the possible causes of unbalanced translocations when segregation of chromosomal material during meiosis in an individual with a balanced translocation can result in gametes with a balanced rearrangement, cells with a normal chromosome complement, and cells with unbalanced translocations resulting in congenital malformations.

As shown in Figure 2–23, a mother with a balanced translocation involving a piece of the long arm of chromosome 6 having broken off and becoming attached to the short arm of chromosome 15 is phenotypically normal. In her diploid state, all chromosomal material is present so that she has no loss of genetic material. However, as a result of meiosis, half of her resulting ova will have a chromosome 6 missing a segment of the long arm (a 6q- deletion). Of those ova, half will have the chromosome 15 with the translocated chromosome 6 so that all genomic DNA will be present. However, the other half, or 25% of all of the resulting ova, will have a 6q- without the normal chromosome 15 (Figure 2–23). The individual who results from the fertilization of the ovum with the 6q- will develop the phenotype associated with this chromosomal aneuploidy, which includes limb anomalies, mental retardation, and cleft palate, among other anomalies.

In some instances, a balanced translocation may result in congenital malformations if the breakpoint for the translocation interrupts a gene. Therefore, even if no chromosomal material is lost, the break in the gene's sequence prevents the proper signals to start and stop the gene action from being decoded in the normal sequenced manner. Thus, the gene's code cannot be correctly interpreted and errors are likely to result. These types of balanced translocations cannot be seen on a karyotype, but can be discovered using molecular genetics techniques (see Chapter 7).

Other translocation classifications include reciprocal and Robertsonian translocations. In reciprocal translocations, there is an ex-

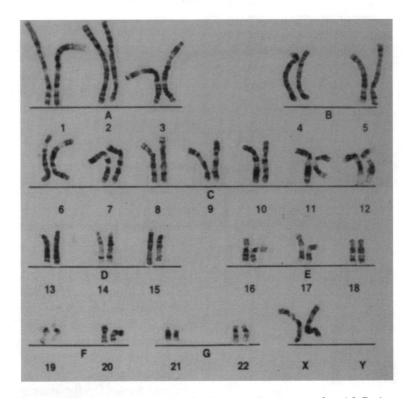

Figure 2–24. A reciprocal translocation between chromosomes 2 and 8. During meiosis, these balanced translocations may result in unbalanced segregation of chromosomal material.

change of chromosomal material between two chromosomes not of the same pair (Figure 2–24). For example, chromosome 2 and chromosome 8 could exchange material without loss of DNA or genes. Individuals who have balanced reciprocal translocations are phenotypically normal, but during the process of meiosis, there will be resulting ova that do have a loss of haplotype genetic complement thus resulting in a chromosomal deletion disorder if that ovum is fertilized (Figure 2–24).

Robertsonian translocations involve only acrocentric chromosomes (Figure 2–25). A Robertsonian translocation occurs when the short arms of two acrocentric chromosomes are lost and the remaining long arms fuse at their centromeres. Therefore, the two acrocentric chromosomes involved form one larger chromosome so that the resulting karyotype looks like it has 45 chromosomes rather than 46. Because the DNA contained in the small short arms of acrocentric chromosomes does not contain structural genes (i.e., genes that code for growth and development), but does contain genes for ribosomal DNA,

individuals with Robertsonian translocations are phenotypically normal. However, as in individuals with balanced translocations and reciprocal translocations, the normal process of chromosomal segregation during meiosis can lead to an ovum or sperm with one less chromosome than normal or one extra chromosome than normal. Because chromosome 21 is an acrocentric chromosome, it is possible for an ovum to have a normal chromosome 21 and a Robertsonian translocation with the long arm of chromosome 21 involved. When fertilized by a normal sperm with a normal chromosome 21, the resulting zygote will have a trisomy 21 (Down syndrome). In the case of a Robertsonian translocation, the trisomy is known as **translocation Down syndrome**.

Less Common Chromosome Aneuploidies

Dicentric Chromosomes

Dicentric chromosomes have two centromeres because they are made up of two broken segments of other chromosomes, each with its own centromere that fuse end-to-end (Figure 2–26).

Isochromosomes

Isochromosomes are an unusual rearrangement, which is found most often in the X chromosome, but may also occur in other chromosomes. Isochromosomes consist of both arms of the chromosome being identical (i.e., a duplication of either the long or short arm) so that one arm has been deleted. In other words, within a given pair of chromosomes, the individual with an isochromosome has three copies of one arm and only one copy of another arm, thus effectively making the person both trisomic (for one arm) and deleted (for the other arm) resulting in multiple anomalies. In the case of the X isochromosome, the long arm is usually trisomic and the short arm deleted.

ACROCENTRIC CHROMOSOMES

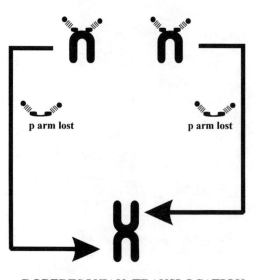

p arm lost   p arm lost

ROBERTSONIAN TRANSLOCATION

Figure 2–25. A Robertsonian translocation.

Inversions

Inversions result from an interstitial break in a chromosome where the resulting segment of chromosome is inverted 180°, so that its "north to south" orientation is reversed, rejoining with the original chromosome so that no chromosomal material is lost but the orientation of the inverted segment is opposite to its original alignment (Figure 2–27). Because there is no loss of chromosomal material or genes, individuals with inversions are phenotypically normal. There are two types of inversions depending on the position of the breaks in the chromosome. If both breaks occur on the same side of the centromere (either in the long arm or the short arm), the inversion is known as a paracentric inversion. If the breaks occur so that one break is on one side of the centromere (in the short arm) and the other is on the other side of the centromere (in the long arm), the inversion is known as pericentric (see Figure 2–27).

Inversions may occur as new rearrangements in individuals, or may be inherited.

Although inversions do not cause anomalies in individuals who have them, they may result in anomalies in offspring because the chromosomes align abnormally during the meiosis of gamete formation. As described previously in this chapter, during meiosis, the chromosomes align very closely so that corresponding genes and DNA sequences are precisely opposite each other. This precise alignment is essential to the process of crossing over and the recombination of DNA from one chromosome to the other during the first stage of meiosis. In order for the normal chromosome to align with the inverted one, it must also loop. This is possible only with larger inversions. When the inversions are small, there can be no crossing over because the normal chromosome will not be able to loop in so small a space. Therefore, offspring can inherit the inverted chromosome intact and will be phenotypically normal. However, if the inversion is large, the noninverted chromosome will loop in an attempt to match the proper DNA sequences. However, the alignment is not perfect and the recombinations between chromosomes may result in aberrant genet-

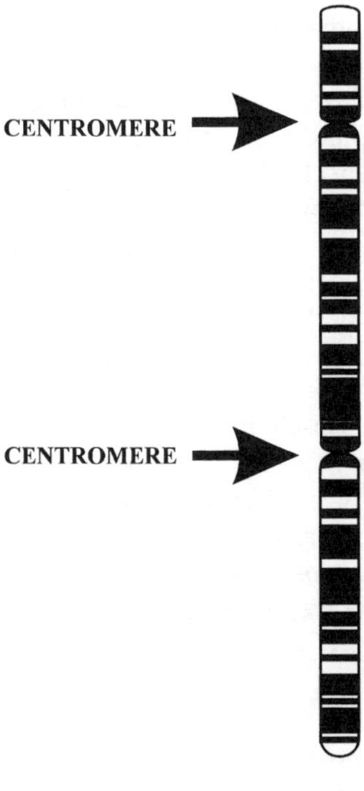

Figure 2–26. A dicentric chromosome.

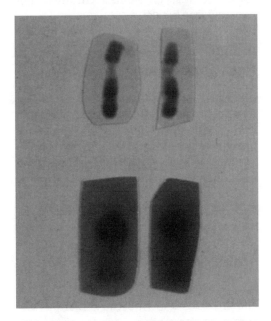

Figure 2–27. A pericentric inversion of chromosome 8.

ic patterns on the resulting chromosome pairs, thus resulting in either nonviable fetuses or major anomalies. When the inversions are pericentric, crossing over may result in unbalanced chromosome complements after meiosis, yielding duplicated or deleted segments of chromosome and subsequent anomalies. Although the risks of chromosomal aneuploidies in the offspring of people with inversions is not known precisely, it is thought to be relatively low, probably well under 10%.

Ring Chromosomes

Ring chromosomes are exactly what the name implies; chromosomes that look like rings because they are a circular chromosome formed when there are two breaks in the chromosome which then join to each other. If the breaks in the chromosome are close to the distal ends of both arms, the ring will include the centromere. Because chromosomal material containing genes important to growth and development may be lost in the breaks, ring chromosomes can be associated with anomalies. Ring chromosomes can occur with any of the human chromosomes because all human chromosomes may undergo breaks.

Frequency of Chromosome Rearrangements

Chromosome rearrangements occur with a reported frequency of 1:160 live births (Hook & Hamerton, 1977), although this number is likely to be low because the karyotypic techniques used to obtain them were not as good as the high resolution karyotypes developed over the last several years. Furthermore, there is a very high frequency of chromosome rearrangements among spontaneous abortuses. Probably more than half of all spontaneous abortions are caused by chromosome rearrangements that are either incompatible with life or severely life-threatening. This is known because many of the chromosome rearrangements found in spon-

taneous abortuses are not found in living individuals and many other chromosome rearrangements are those that cause severe malformations, such as trisomy 18. Because spontaneous abortions are common in humans (occurring in approximately one of every six established pregnancies), the total number of chromosome rearrangements in the combined sample of live births and spontaneous abortions is quite high, perhaps as frequent as just under 1% of conceptions.

Mosaicism

Most people who have chromosome rearrangements have them in every cell in their bodies. However, in some cases, aneuploidies are present in only some of the persons cells, a condition known as **mosaicism**. Mosaicism usually occurs because of an instance of nondisjunction occurring at a very early stage of cell division. As a result, some of the individual's cells will get an abnormal complement of chromosomes while others will maintain a normal karyotype. The earlier the nondisjunction occurs, the larger the number of cells that will have an abnormal chromosome complement. Individuals with mosaic conditions typically display the abnormal traits associated with the particular aneuploidy found in some of their cells, but the effect will be less severe than if all cells were involved. When the nondisjunction occurs early, prior to the point in embryogenesis where cells differentiate into a variety of different tissue types, the mosaicism will be present in most or all of the body's tissues, including peripheral blood which is usually the source for karyotypes. However, mosaics can also occur later in the mitotic divisions of the embryo so that only one or several tissues are affected. In these cases, the mosaic may not be detected by a karyotype prepared from peripheral blood.

Karyotype Symbols

As with most things in life, karyotypes tend to be reported with a series of symbols and

TABLE 2–2. Common Symbols and Terms Used to Describe Karyotypes

Symbol	Meaning	Example; Translation
46, XX	Normal female karyotype (46 chromosomes, female)	
46, XY	Normal male karyotype (46 chromosomes, male)	
47, XXY	Extra X chromosome (47 chromosomes, male)	
47, XXX	Trisomy X, an extra X chromosome (47 chromosomes, female)	
69, XXX	Triploidy (69 chromosomes, or triplets of each rather than pairs)	
45, X	Also 45, XO, or Turner syndrome, a deleted X chromosome	
p	short arm	4p; short arm of chromosome 4
q	long arm	22q; long arm of chromosome 22
−	deletion of a part or whole chromosome	46XY, (6q-); deletion of a portion of the long arm of chromosome 6
del	deletion of a part or whole chromosome (same as above)	del(11)(p13); interstitial deletion of a portion of the short arm of chromosome 11 at the p13 band
+	Duplication of a part or whole chromosome	47XX,+21; trisomy 21 1q+; duplication of a part of the long arm of chromosome 1
dup	Duplication of a part or whole chromosome (same as above)	dup(1q); duplication of a part of the long arm of chromosome 1
ter	terminal end of a chromosome	pter; terminal end of the short arm, as in dup(2q31→qter) which is duplication of the long arm of chromosome 2 from the q31 band to the terminal end of the long arm of chromosome 2
→	From one band to another	dup(17q23→17qter); duplication of 17q from band 23 to the terminal end. May also be written as (17q–17qter) or (17q17qter)
t( )	Translocation	t(10;17)(q26.6;p13.3); balanced translocation between the 26.6 band of the long arm of chromosome 10 and the short arm of chromosome 13
Mos /	Mosaicism	Mos45,X/46,XX; mosaicism with some cells having a missing X chromosome, others normal (Turner mosaic)
r	Ring chromosome	46,XX,r(19); female with ring chromosome 19
ins	Insertion of a piece of chromosome	ins(7;20)(q11.23;p11.23p12.2); insertion into chromosome 7 at the q11.23 band of a piece of chromosome 20 consisting of bands p11.23 to p12.2
inv	Inversion	inv(4)(q12.21;q22.31); inversion of the long arm of chromosome 4 from bands 12.21 to 22.31
dic	Dicentric chromosome	dic(X); a dicentric X chromosome

abbreviations which are generally accepted and recognized by both clinicians and cytogeneticists. These symbols and karyotypic abbreviations are listed in Table 2–2.

IS IT NECESSARY TO KNOW MORE?

The state-of-the-art in genetics is advancing at an astonishing pace. Both the clinical and molecular aspects of the field are advancing in a balanced tandem of interaction which allows the clinical recognition of new disorders on what seems to be a daily basis and the discovery of genes responsible for diseases at a similar pace. Therefore, the reader is urged not to regard this text as an ending point, but rather a starting block in the effort to enlist specialists in the communicative disorders to join the race to delineate the human genome and its effects on human structure and behavior. Communication scientists can play an important role in the delineation of genetic illness by studying the types of communicative impairments that occur in known genetic diseases and matching that information to gene discovery, gene biology, and gene action. By doing this, speech-language pathology and audiology will enter the new age of the study of human disease in union with other physical and behavioral sciences.

REFERENCES

Darwin, C. (1859). *The origin of the species*. New York: Mentor.

Hook, E. B., & Hamerton, J. L. (1977). The frequency of chromosome abnormalities detected in consecutive newborn studies, differences between studies, results by sex and by severity of phenotypic involvement. In E. B. Hook & I. H. Porter (Eds.), *Population cytogenetics: Studies in humans* (pp. 63–79). New York: Academic Press.

Johannsen, W. (1909). Elemente der exakten erblichkeitslehre. Translated in J. A. Peters, (Ed.), *Classic papers in genetics* (pp. 20–26). Englewood Cliffs, NJ: Prentice-Hall, 1959.

Mendel, G. (1866). Experiments in plant hybridization. Translated in J. A. Peters (Ed.), *Classic papers in genetics* (pp. 1–20). Englewood Cliffs, NJ: Prentice-Hall, 1959.

Sutton, W. S. (1903). The chromosomes in heredity. *Biological Bulletin, 4*, 231–251.

Thompson, M. W., Roderick, R. M., & Willard, H. F. (1991). *Thompson and Thompson genetics in medicine* (5th ed.). Philadelphia: W. B. Saunders.

Watson, J. D., & Crick, F. H. C. (1953). *The structure of DNA*. Cold Spring Harbor Symposia. *Quantitative Biology, 23*, 123–131.

CHAPTER

3

WHAT IS A SYNDROME AND WHY SHOULD I CARE?

The ability of specialists in communication disorders to participate in the process of syndrome delineation, diagnosis, and treatment depends in large part on their ability to communicate effectively with professionals from other disciplines who have experience in clinical genetics. This means that communicative disorder specialists must learn the "lingo" of clinical genetics and apply it to disorders of speech, language, hearing, and cognition. This is not very difficult because many of the terms applied by geneticists are commonly used in everyday language and one needs only a system for applying them. Toward that end, it becomes useful to know a system of terms agreed on by an international working group, which met in 1979 and 1980, resulting in the adoption of a basic genetics glossary, which will be described in the pages to follow. This system of nosology can be further enhanced by applying it within a framework used to classify syndromes. In my opinion, the most intuitive approach was described by Dr. M. Michael Cohen, Jr. in his excellent primer of dysmorphology and

syndromology, *The Child With Multiple Birth Defects* (1982) and recently updated and expanded (Cohen, 1997). Although there have been many major advances in the application of molecular genetics to clinical genetics over the past several years, Cohen's original system has withstood the test of time and may be applied to what is currently known about multiple anomaly congenital syndromes and is a particularly useful foundation for beginners interested in the study of individuals with multiple anomalies.

BASIC DEFINITIONS

Prior to the 1979 meeting of the international working group, abnormalities related to errors in embryogenesis that were found in children were referred to as **birth defects**. However, it is now understood that not all errors related to abnormalities in development of the human embryo are present at birth. Some abnormalities may not be present at birth because some anatomical structures are not mature enough to be properly assessed at birth, for example, the secondary dentition. In some multiple anomaly syndromes, the permanent teeth may be missing, or unusually shaped (such as peg-shaped teeth in Down syndrome). Because the first permanent tooth does not erupt until 5 or 6 years of age, it is not possible to tell if it is abnormal until that time. Even with radiographs to look at the teeth before they erupt, it would be some time after birth before abnormalities in the developing tooth buds could be detected. The term **birth defect** also does not take into account abnormalities of behavior. As discussed in Chapter 1, abnormalities of human behavior are becoming recognized as traits caused by abnormal genetic contributions, such as single gene disorders or chromosome alterations. The term **birth defect** has therefore been abandoned for the more inclusive **anomaly**.

Anomaly is defined as any deviation from normal structure, form, or function that is considered to be abnormal. There are two basic type of anomalies: malformations and deformations. **Malformations** are anomalies in which there is an intrinsic error in the development of a tissue, organ, structure, or function. In other words, from the moment embryogenesis began, that particular tissue, organ, structure, or function was destined to express a particular anomaly because of a basic intrinsic error in the code or process of growth and development. Examples include the retinitis pigmentosa associated with Usher syndrome (Figure 3–1) or the club foot associated with Stickler syndrome. Retinitis pigmentosa, which results in vision impairment and possibly blindness, is related to an abnormal organization of the cells of the retina caused by a recessive mutant gene. The club foot (turning in of the foot, also known as talipes equinovarus) occurring in Stickler syndrome, an autosomal dominant genetic condition, is caused by abnormally shaped epiphyses at the ankles (Figure 3–2) which forces the foot to be torqued inward.

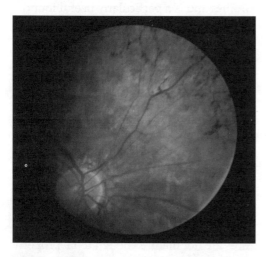

Figure 3–1. Fundoscopic examination of the retina of an individual with Usher syndrome showing areas of depigmentation characteristic of retinitis pigmentosa.

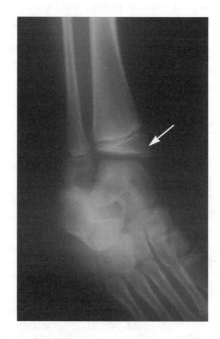

Figure 3–2. Epiphyseal dysplasia in Stickler syndrome. Note the wedge-shaped epiphysis (*arrow*).

Deformations are anomalies in which the problem is extrinsic to the tissue, organ, structure, or function. In most cases, deformations involve the bending, torquing, or warping of structures, such as limbs or the cranium. Many instances of cranial asymmetry, or plagiocephaly, are caused by intrauterine constriction, which results in torticollis (shortening of the clinomastoid muscle) and premature fusion of the cranial suture on the affected side (Figure 3–3). Of interest, club foot can also be caused by constriction of the legs of the developing fetus (Figure 3–4) when in a breech position. The constant bending force of the uterine walls on the abnormally placed fetus will cause the foot to turn in so that, symptomatically, there is little difference in the appearance of a club foot caused by the epiphyseal dysplasia of Stickler syndrome or the constricting effects of positional compression. This similarity points out the importance of careful diagnostic accuracy, which can be facilitated by a careful history as detailed in Chapter 5. The implications of the difference are even more important in relation to

genetic counseling. Deformations, because they are usually intrauterine accidents, have little or no risk of recurrence; whereas malformations caused by genetic disorders may have as high as a 50% chance of recurrence, as in Stickler syndrome.

In some cases, extrinsic forces can cause tears in the developing fetus, or prevent the fusion of the various developing processes. Such deformations are known as **disruptions**. The most recognizable type of disruption is known as **amnion rupture syndrome**. Amnion rupture syndrome occurs when the amnion, one of the membranes that surrounds the embryo and contains the amniotic fluid, the placenta, and the embryo, ruptures (either spontaneously or the result of trauma). As the amnion (which is actually a part of the embryo) begins to heal, strands of scar tissue form and may attach to the nearby embryo. They may wrap around an arm, leg, finger, or the head, or they may adhere to the forming face and prevent embryonic processes from fusing or tear weak anatomical bonds apart. These amniotic adhesions may even be swallowed and adhere

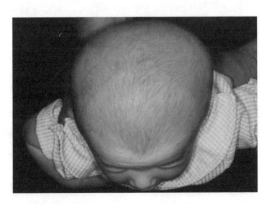

Figure 3–3. Plagiocephaly resulting from intrauterine constriction, which may also cause a torticollis.

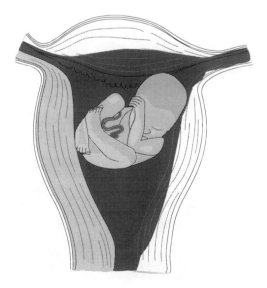

Figure 3–4. Deformational constriction of a fetus in breech position resulting in club foot.

to the palate, causing a cleft palate. The resulting baby at term may therefore present with a variety of facial clefts, ringlike constrictions of the digits or limbs, or even amputations of fingers, toes, or entire limbs (Figure 3–5).

Anomalies may also be classified according to severity. It is sometimes useful to think of anomalies as either **major** or **minor**. Minor anomalies are those that typically do not require treatment to enhance either the quantity or quality of life. Minor anomalies include missing teeth, abnormal fingernails, a small sinus tract near the ear (known as a branchial cleft), or a streak of white hair in otherwise uniformly dark colored scalp hair. Although an individual might choose electively to do something about these problems, under most circumstances they would not be considered significantly detrimental. Major anomalies are those that do require treatment. If left untreated, life or health could be threatened, or the quality of life would be significantly impaired. Major anomalies include cleft palate, congenital heart anomalies, missing digits or limbs, or metabolic abnormalities such as phenylketonuria. There are also major behavioral anomalies,

such as mental retardation, profound deafness, or hypernasal speech.

Prevalence and Incidence

It is also important to understand the value of the reporting of statistics with regard to the frequency of occurrence of specific anomalies or multiple anomaly disorders. The term incidence is used rather casually by both clinicians and the lay public. The term has several meanings in relation to how often disorders occur, but it does not really refer to how likely a person is to see a particular disorder among the general population. *Incidence* refers to the total frequency of a particular disorder either among conceptions or births. In cases where this figure is essentially the same (meaning that all or nearly all individuals with the disorder are born living), incidence refers to the total frequency of a disorder at birth. Incidence is usually expressed as a ratio, such as 1:2,000, which means that there is one affected individual for every 2,000 births. Many scientists prefer to use a fixed number, such as 1,000 or 10,000 to express this ratio, so that 1:2,000 would be expressed as 0.5:1,000, or

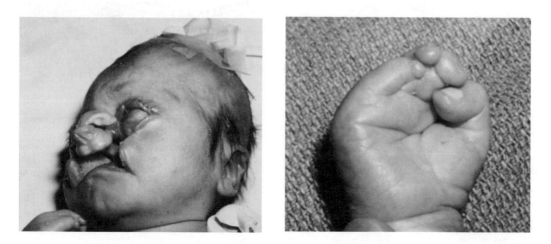

Figure 3–5. A newborn with amnion rupture sequence showing unusual facial clefts and amputations and ringlike constrictions of the fingers.

5:10,000. In cases where many conceptions do not survive to term, resulting in spontaneous abortions (often called miscarriages) or stillborn babies, the incidence of conceptions with a particular disorder will be in excess of live births with that disorder (the birth incidence). In disorders where the anomalies or syndrome result in severe health problems that may result in death, the birth incidence undoubtedly will be much higher than the frequency of individuals with that disorder found among the general population at 10 or 20 years of age. The frequency of a disorder among a specific portion of the population is known as *prevalence*. Therefore, the prevalence of, for example, trisomy 18 (a disorder almost always incompatible with life beyond the neonatal period) among the adult population of the U.S. is zero (0:1,000), but the birth incidence is approximately 1:7,000 (i.e., 0.14:1,000 or 1.4:10,000). For the purposes of clinical awareness of disorders, prevalence statistics tend to be most valuable because they provide the clinician with an estimate of how often they might see a particular disorder, especially if the symptoms fall within their area of expertise for diagnosis or treatment. Incidence statistics obviously are of major importance in order to provide accurate genetic counseling.

MULTIPLE ANOMALY DISORDERS

Anomalies may occur singly, as isolated malformations or deformations, or in combination with other anomalies. When two or more anomalies occur together, especially when the anomalies are major anomalies, the clinician must suspect that they are in some way related, or part of a multiple anomaly disorder. There are several types of multiple anomaly disorders:

▶ Syndromes
▶ Sequences, and
▶ Associations.

SYNDROMES

Syndrome is defined as the presence of multiple anomalies in the same individual with all of those anomalies having a single cause. Cohen (1982) broadly categorized syndromes into two types: known genesis and unknown genesis syndromes, the difference being the ability to isolate the cause of the syndrome. Known genesis syndromes are categorized according to the type of cause that results in the anomalies; hence there are four types: chromosomal, genetic, teratogenic, and mechanically induced.

Known Genesis Syndromes

Chromosomal Syndromes

As described in Chapter 2, chromosomes are the microscopic structures in the nuclei of cells that contain the genes responsible for the growth and development of all organisms. The genes, approximately 100,000 of them in humans, are strung along the 46 chromosomes which are normally contained in each nucleus. Syndromes are classified as chromosomal in origin if a chromosome analysis, or karyotype, reveals an abnormality in chromosome structure that can be seen under a light microscope. Multiple malformations almost always result from deviations in chromosome structure because many genes would be involved in the chromosome abnormality. There are a number of different types of chromosome rearrangements, which can occur spontaneously or can be inherited from a parent. Rearrangements of chromosome structure resulting in an abnormal amount or structure of the chromosomes is known as an *aneuploidy*. There are several types of chromosome aneuploidies, including:

▶ deletion of whole chromosomes,
▶ addition of extra whole chromosomes,
▶ deletion of parts of chromosomes,
▶ addition of parts of chromosomes,
▶ restructured chromosomes, and

▶ rearrangements of chromosomes known as unbalanced translocations.

In general, individuals with chromosome disorders have severe problems, including mental retardation, short stature, and a variety of severe malformations such as heart anomalies, brain anomalies, and limb anomalies. Essentially all individuals with chromosomal syndromes have craniofacial malformations, and the overwhelming majority have communicative impairment, most often language impairment and articulation impairment related to neurological or structural malformations of the oral cavity or jaws (including clefting).

Whole Chromosome Deletions

When whole chromosomes are missing, the problem is known as a monosomy. When the missing chromosome is a sex chromosome, the resulting individual will always have a single X chromosome, a disorder known as Turner syndrome. Monosomies are rare and it is known that many spontaneous abortions and stillbirths have chromosome abnormalities that are incompatible with life. There have been a very small number of documented cases of monosomy of chromosome 21 resulting in individuals with small stature, cleft lip and/or palate, failure-to-thrive, microcephaly, hypertonicity, short thorax, and scoliosis. Many babies with monosomy 21 die in the neonatal period and the long-term developmental prognosis is very poor.

Turner syndrome is a well recognized disorder with a varying phenotype and often presents as a mosaic (see Chapter 2), which has the effect of diluting the phenotype so that the individual has fewer of the anomalies associated with the syndrome, and those that are present tend to be less severe. In its fully expressed form, where every cell of the individual has a 45 X karyotype rather than a 46 XX or 46 XY, anomalies include agenesis of the gonads, small stature, a webbed short neck with a low posterior hair line, and occasional cardiac anomalies. There is variable cognitive functioning, with mild mental retardation in many cases. Cleft palate occurs more frequently than in the general population and may be associated with the Robin sequence. Many cases of pure 45 X chromosome complement do not reach term and result in spontaneous abortions. Therefore, many of the surviving cases of Turner syndrome represent mosaics.

Whole Chromosome Additions

When there is one extra whole chromosome so that instead of a matching pair for a particular chromosome, there are three, the disorder is known as a trisomy. Trisomies typically result in individuals with 47 rather than 46 chromosomes, except for a condition known as triploidy where the entire set of chromosomes is triplicated. Trisomy usually results from an error in meiotic cell division known as nondisjunction (see Chapter 2), an error that occurs during meiotic cell division. Trisomies of individual autosomes are rare, with the exception of the most common trisomy, and one of the most common of all disorders in humans, trisomy 21, or Down syndrome. This easily recognized disorder was probably first described by Séguin in 1846, 20 years prior to Langdon Down's theory of ethnic traits and their effect on intellect (hence the pejorative term "mongoloid idiots"). Although Down's intolerance was clearly evident in his 1866 treatise, his name has become synonymous with this very common pattern of anomalies. It was not until 1959 that LeJeune reported the cause of the syndrome to be the presence of an extra chromosome. With an entire extra chromosome, there are thousands of genes which are present in an extra copy, thus interfering with the normal code for human development. Because so many genes are involved in trisomies, typically many anomalies are present, and those that are present are very often severe in nature. Although many individuals with Down syndrome survive birth and live into adulthood, many do not reach birth, are stillborn, or die in infancy. It is likely that only about 20% of Down syndrome conceptions reach term and are born alive (Smith, 1982). Following birth, because many children with Down syndrome have severe cardiac malformations, many do not survive the neonatal period. Therefore, the frequency of trisomy 21 conceptions (i.e., the total incidence) is far higher than the birth frequency (birth incidence), which is still higher than the population prevalence (those individuals with trisomy 21 who survive beyond the neonatal period).

Other trisomies include trisomy 8, trisomy 9, trisomy 13, and trisomy 18. Individuals with trisomy 8 are usually lanky and thin and may, unlike in many chromosomal disorders, be taller than normal. Mental deficiency is variable, ranging from mild to severe. Conductive hearing loss is often found in trisomy 8, as is agenesis of the corpus callosum, language impairment, and global developmental delay. The majority of living patients with trisomy 8 represent mosaics (see Chapter 2). Many of the full trisomies do not survive infancy.

There are other trisomies of autosomes which, unlike Down syndrome and trisomy 8, are essentially always incompatible with life and present with major brain anomalies along with cardiovascular, craniofacial, and genitourinary abnormalities. Trisomy 13 and trisomy 18 are the best known and most easily recognized of these disorders. Both of these syndromes are likely to be seen in neonatal units, but life expectancy rarely exceeds infancy in either condition. Similarly, babies with trisomy 9 (again, almost always a mosaic) rarely survive infancy. When they do, they are severely retarded and rarely develop useful speech or language. The only autosomal trisomy likely to be seen by most speech-language-hearing clinicians is trisomy 21, which has many speech and language disorders and frequent serous otitis. Trisomy 8 is rare.

Trisomies of the sex chromosomes are also found in children and adults. An abnormal complement of sex chromosomes includes XXY (Klinefelter syndrome), XYY, and XXX.

Individuals with XXY and XYY are phenotypically males, whereas individuals with XXX are phenotypically females. Some clinicians classify other aneuploidies of the X chromosomes in phenotypic males as Klinefelter syndrome, so that individuals with 47XXY, 48XXXY, 48XXYY, and 49XXXXY are considered to be variants of Klinefelter syndrome.

Triploidy is the triplication of all chromosomes and may present as a 69XXX (approximately 35–40% of triploidies), 69XXY (approximately 60% of triploidies), and 69XYY (less than 5% of triploidies). Although often incompatible with life (it is estimated that 2% of all conceptions are triploidies), the incidence at birth is approximately 1:2,500. Some documented cases of triploidy have survived long term. Triploidies may result from either nondisjunction (usually in the male germ cells) or fertilization of a single ovum by two spermatozoa.

The Deletion of Parts of Chromosomes

Probably the majority of chromosomal aneuploidies resulting in living individuals are deletions of parts of chromosomes (this includes unbalanced translocations), usually referred to simply as **deletions**. Because small segments of chromosomes carry far fewer genes than whole chromosomes, the alteration of the genetic code will be less severe than in monosomies. Of course, the effect of deletions will be variable, depending on the segment of chromosome deleted and the size of the deletion. As the resolution of karyotypes continues to improve, smaller and smaller deletions are detected.

There are two types of deletion defined based on their position within the chromosome. When deletions occur at the ends of either the short (p) arm or long (q) arm, they are known as **terminal** deletions (Figure 3–6). When chromosome material is deleted from the middle of a chromosomal arm, the deletion is known as an **interstitial** deletion (Figure 3–7).

Later in this chapter, very small deletions, often too small to be seen under a micro-

Normal chromosome 18   18q-   18p-

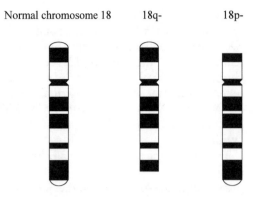

Normal chromosome 22   22q11 deletion

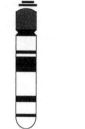

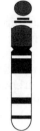

Figure 3–6. Diagram of terminal deletions of chromosome 18 compared to a normal chromosome 18. The deletion of the short arm (*top*) is known as an 18p- terminal deletion. The deletion of the long arm (*bottom*) is known as an 18q- terminal deletion.

Figure 3–7. Diagram of an interstitial deletion from the long arm of chromosome 22 at the q11 region, therefore known as a 22q11 deletion.

scope, but detectable by modern techniques of DNA analysis will be discussed. In such cases, a very small segment of chromosome, and hence genetic material, is deleted, but it still contains more than one gene (perhaps as many as 30, 40, or 50 genes). The classification of syndromes caused by this type of a deletion will be considered separately under the category of **contiguous gene syndromes.**

Syndromes caused by the deletions of parts of chromosomes are more common than monosomies (where whole chromosomes are deleted) in part because fewer genes are involved (although there are still many genes deleted) so that fewer of the resulting pregnancies are incompatible with life. In addition, chromosomes often undergo rearrangement whereas the circumstances leading to the deletion of whole chromosomes are less common.

Well recognized deletion syndromes include 4p- and 5p-, also known as **Wolf-Hirschhorn syndrome** and **cri du chat syndrome**, respectively. Newborns with a missing segment of the short arm of chromosome 4 (4p-) are severely mentally retarded, have pre- and postnatal growth deficiency, hypotonia, and seizures. Cleft lip, cleft palate, cranial asymmetry, orbital hypertelorism, stra-

bismus, scalp defects, and genital anomalies in males (hypospadias and cryptorchidism). Many die in infancy and those who survive tend to get frequent upper respiratory illnesses.

Cri du chat syndrome (meaning "cat cry" in French) is so named because affected infants have a cry that sounds very much like a cat's mew so that speech pathologists are often called to assess these early vocalizations. Caused by a deletion of the short arm of chromosome 5, these babies are small at birth and have significant postnatal growth deficiency, as well. Facial asymmetry is common, as is hypertelorism with epicanthal folds, downslanting eyes, low set ears, and strabismus. Approximately a third of infants with this deletion syndrome have congenital heart anomalies. The overwhelming majority are severely retarded with IQ rarely exceeding 30. Speech is rarely developed and language, if present, tends to be very rudimentary. Although the larynx may be developmentally small compared to other children of the same age, the size of the glottis and vocal cords is not really discordant with the rest of somatic development and is probably not related significantly to the high-pitched cry, which may be more of a central phenomenon (Manning, 1977).

Contiguous Gene Syndromes

This type of syndrome is categorized by many as "genetic," although, in reality, it is a type of chromosomal deletion syndrome. This term has come to be associated with disorders where a submicroscopic section of chromosome is known to be missing because molecular genetic analysis (see Chapter 2) shows that several or many genes are deleted, but karyotype, even of very high resolution, fails to show a visible deletion of chromosomal material (i.e., a microscopically detectable cytogenetic deletion). Key to the concept of contiguous gene syndromes is the contention that single anomalies or groups of anomalies are caused by separate genes in the deleted segment so that the size of the deletion would have a definite effect on the expression of the syndrome. It could also be assumed that, the larger the deletion, the more severe the expression. A number of syndromes have been hypothesized to be caused by the deletion of a string of genes, but to date there there are relatively few syndromes caused by submicroscopic deletions. However, many more syndromes are likely to be found to be contiguous gene syndromes in the future. In any event, the fact that a deletion cannot be seen does not make it any less a deletion. Therefore, contiguous gene syndromes might best be considered as chromosomal deletion syndromes in which the deletion is extremely small.

As an example, the velo-cardio-facial syndrome (VCFS), also known as Shprintzen syndrome, has recently been associated with the deletion of a very small segment of the long arm of chromosome 22 in a region known as 22q11.2. This deletion has been detected using high resolution karyotyping in a small percentage of cases, but in the large majority of cases, the deletion is detectable only by molecular genetics procedures (Morrow et al., 1995). It is not completely clear, however, that the syndrome is actually caused by the deletion of multiple genes strung along this specific length of chromosome. Morrow et al. (1995), studying a large sample of individuals with VCFS with sophisticated molecular genetics procedures, found no relationship between the size of the deletion and the expression of the syndrome. Individuals were found with deletions measuring over 2 megabases in length and some as small as 400 kilobases (one fifth the size of the 2 megabase deletions) with no significant difference in the severity of expression. Although some scientists believe that VCFS is a contiguous gene syndrome, the fact that its variable expression is not related to the size of the deletion is more consistent with a single gene causing the disorder. Clearly, these types of mysteries will be unraveled within a very short time frame as the Human Genome Project continues to make the astounding progress for which it has been noteworthy over the past several years.

Genetic Disorders

The largest group of multiple congenital anomalies falls into the category of genetic causation. Although it is true that chromosomally caused syndromes are really genetically based, most dysmorphologists prefer to think of chromosomally caused syndromes as those that are diagnosed by visible microscopically chromosomal rearrangements. Genetic syndromes are usually thought of as those that do not have visible cytogenetic abnormalities (which would include contiguous gene syndromes). The overwhelming majority of genetic syndromes are caused by single gene mutations and are therefore categorized by the mode of inheritance, including autosomal dominant, autosomal recessive, X-linked recessive, and X-linked dominant. There is another category of genetic causation, polygenic and multifactorial traits, but like contiguous gene syndromes, such disorders are only hypothesized and there is no firm proof for the existence of such disorders.

As described in Chapter 2, a mutation is a "change" or alteration of a gene. Because genes can exist in multiple forms (alleles), the term mutation is typically reserved for changes that result in major alterations of gene effect considered to be abnormal for that species. Of course, the process of mutation is responsible for evolution within and between species, but, in effect, the mutations that cause the dramatic alterations necessary for one species to evolve into another are abnormal for the original species. For example, the transition from reptilian dinosaurs to birds involved the development of feathers. Although feathers are an advantage to birds, they are abnormal for reptiles.

Mutations occur frequently in all organisms, often resulting in traits incompatible with life. Such mutations often result in spontaneous abortions or stillbirths (a much larger number than result in living individuals who have multiple anomaly syndromes). When individuals with mutations survive to term, the mutant gene may be expressed as a single anomaly or multiple anomalies. For example, polydactyly, or the presence of an extra finger or toe, is a fairly common anomaly resulting from a mutation of a gene that regulates the formation of digits (a gene present in all species that have limbs). In this case, a single gene mutation can be expressed as an isolated anomaly compatible with life. Other mutations, however, result in multiple anomalies and recognizable syndromes. Because there are approximately 100,000 genes that regulate human development, there are obviously many opportunities for mutations and resulting syndromes. Furthermore, because genes may consist of many thousands of base pairs, there may be more than one type of mutation which can occur in that gene and result in different syndromes.

McKusick's compendium of genetic disorders listed over 5,000 genetic disorders categorized by mode of inheritance in its 11th edition (McKusick, 1994). This is in contrast to the first edition of the same book which listed 1,487 genetic disorders (McKusick, 1966). New genetic disorders are constantly being delineated. Even more important, many disorders not known to be of genetic causation are now having a genetic basis discovered. Other disorders known to have a genetic causation based on observed patterns of inheritance are now having the exact nature of their genetic etiology discovered.

Modes of Inheritance

At this point, a description of the modes of inheritance is important. The importance of understanding patterns of inheritance cannot be understated because genetic counseling and parental understanding of recurrence risk and their reproductive future is at stake. Although genetic counseling must be provided by a trained professional, all clinicians who deal with individuals who have genetically caused disorders must be cognizant of the consequence of both diagnosis and the importance of the patient and his or her family understanding the potential for additional individuals being born with the same disorder.

Patterns of inheritance are basically determined by the ability of the gene to be expressed. In cases of mutant genes that cause multiple anomaly syndromes, the mode of inheritance depends on the type of chromosome where the gene is located (autosome versus sex chromosome) and whether or not the gene is "switched on." If a gene is not switched on and therefore not expressed, it is not **penetrant**. Penetrance refers to the frequency with which a gene is expressed compared to how often it should be expressed given its pattern of inheritance. For example, if an autosomal dominant gene would normally be expressed in 50% of offspring, but it is observed to be expressed in only 40% of offspring (the observation being recorded in a large number of cases), then the disorder is 80% penetrant (i.e., 40% in relation to a 50% recurrence risk, which equals $^4/_5$, or 80%). Remember that all genes are half of a pair of genes, the other gene in the pair being located on the other chromosome in the pair. A gene is dominant when it is expressed even though the other gene in the pair does not code for that trait. A gene is recessive when it can only be expressed if both members of the pair have the same mutation. There is also a type of gene known as **codominant** which can be expressed in a milder form when the other gene in the pair does not have the same mutation.

Autosomal Dominant. A gene that has the ability to be expressed even when the other member of the pair does not code for the same trait is known as dominant. If that gene is located on one of the autosomes (chromosomes 1 through 22), it is known as an autosomal dominant. Autosomal domi-

nant traits, if 100% penetrance is presumed, have a recurrence risk of 50% when one parent is affected. Figure 3–8 is a schematic representation of how autosomal dominant inheritance works. One parent (in the case of the illustration, the father) has a mutant gene for a dominant trait on one of the autosomes. During meiosis, one half of the father's reproductive cells receive the autosome with the mutant gene, the other half receive the autosome with the normal gene. Both of the reproductive cells resulting from the mother's meiotic divisions have the normal gene. The possible matings of reproductive cells that would occur between these two parents are represented in Figure 3–8. Because half (two) of the father's reproduc-

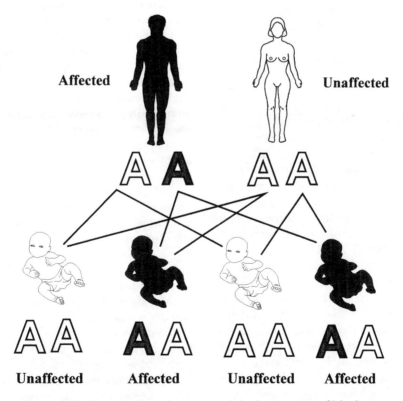

Figure 3–8. Schematic illustrating autosomal dominant pattern of inheritance resulting in a 50% recurrence risk. The white "A" represents the normal allele on one paternal chromosome, the gray "A" represents the mutant allele on the other paternal chromosome. The mother has two normal A alleles. The possible segregations of the A gene is represented by the row of affected and unaffected infants at the bottom. Because these alleles are located on autosomes, the sex of the parent and child does not affect the inheritance of the trait.

tive cells have the mutant gene, and there are four possible pairings of the four reproductive cells, 50% of the possible offspring from this mating would be affected by the mutant gene. Therefore, the recurrence risk is 50%. This does not really mean that 50% of the offspring of these parents will have the syndrome caused by this gene. This 50% figure is the probability of the syndrome occurring for each established pregnancy. In other words, for each pregnancy established, it is as if the parents flipped a coin to see if the offspring would be affected: heads affected, tails unaffected. The parents could be very lucky, and, if they established three pregnancies, get tails three times in a row. Similarly, they could be unlucky and get two heads and a tail. Therefore, the 50% probability exists for each pregnancy established. It does not mean that if they had two unaffected children, the odds increase on the third. Even with two lucky outcomes on the first two pregnancies, the probability on the third is still 50%. For autosomal dominant traits, it usually does not make any difference if the abnormal gene is located on one of the father's chromosomes or the mother's chromosomes. The recurrence risk is still 50%, usually without difference in expression if the affected child is female or male.

There are some exceptions to the role of sex in the expression of syndromes. One exception is if some of the abnormal traits are sex specific. A number of syndromes that have genital anomalies as prominent features, such as Robinow syndrome, LEOPARD syndrome, and Cowden syndrome. Robinow syndrome (Shprintzen, Goldberg, Saenger, & Sidoti, 1982) is a multiple anomaly syndrome that involves craniofacial abnormalities (orbital hypertelorism, short nose, macrocephaly, cleft lip and/or palate), limb anomalies (short fingers), and hypospadias with micropenis in males. Although females may have hypoplastic labia and clitoris, the male genital anomalies are far more obvious and make the syndrome easier to detect. The same is true for LEOPARD syndrome. Cowden syndrome is a disorder

that has hemartomas (papillomatous tumors) of the breasts in females, but no such anomaly in affected males.

Another exception that affects the expression of autosomal dominant traits in relation to sex is **imprinting**. Imprinting is the phenomenon in which the same genetic mutation results in different disease expressions based on the origin of the parental chromosome with the mutation. There are several well known examples of imprinting, some inferred by the traditional genetic technique of pedigree analysis and others determined by the newer techniques of molecular genetics, such as the process of **haplotyping**. An example of imprinting obvious from pedigree analysis is the difference in the expression of myotonic dystrophy, an autosomal dominant form of muscular dystrophy. When the mutant gene is inherited from the father, the gene may not be expressed clinically until the second decade of life. For example, I have several patients whose fathers had a mild expression of myotonic dystrophy. The affected sons or daughters were clinically normal with no evidence of the myopathy associated with the disease until the age of 14, 15, or 16 years. In several of these patients, the first expression was the late onset of hypernasal resonance caused by progressive muscle disease. In males with late onset, there can be personality change, male pattern baldness, and generalized myopathy with progressive worsening. It has been observed that, when transmitted paternally, even though the onset is late, with each successive generation, there is a slightly earlier age of onset, a phenomenon known as **anticipation**.

When myotonic dystrophy is inherited from the mother, the disease is present at birth and is more severe. Affected children have significant myopathy, which is recognized almost immediately because it may result in failure-to-thrive, obvious movement disorder, and developmental delay. Children with the congenital form of myotonic dystrophy are often cognitively impaired and developmentally delayed, which is not the case in the paternal transmission.

Perhaps the most interesting manifestation of imprinting is the expression of what appear to be two separate syndromes caused by the same genetic deletion. Prader-Willi syndrome is a disorder familiar to many speech-language pathologists because of a global developmental delay, language impairment, hypotonia, and early hypernasality. Other important findings include hypogonadism (obvious as micropenis and hypoplastic testes and scrotum in males), eventual mental retardation (usually moderate), and limited sexual development. One of the most recognizable findings is polyphagia, an uncontrolled appetite with resultant obesity. The hypotonia, which can be severe in infancy, usually improves to the point of resolving in later life, usually by the second decade. In studying the hypernasality in individuals with Prader-Willi syndrome, David Foushee (as reported by Sadewitz and Shprintzen, 1987) and Kleppe, Katayama, Shipley, and Foushee (1990) found that, even when severe in childhood, hypernasality often resolved by adolescence with the resolution of the hypotonia. This important finding points out the importance of making the proper syndromic diagnosis as described in Chapter 1 with reference to a syndrome's natural history. The clinician who understands that hypernasality is likely to resolve with age in Prader-Willi syndrome will not be in a rush to recommend surgery. If this aspect of the syndrome's natural history were not known, many patients with Prader-Willi syndrome would undergo unnecessary major operations. Prader-Willi syndrome has been linked etiologically to a small deletion of the long arm of chromosome 15 (from the 15q11 band through 15q13), which is cytogenetically visible only with high resolution karyotype. However, in Prader-Willi syndrome, the chromosome involved in the deletion is inherited from the father. Even though the father's chromosome 15 might not be deleted so that the rearrangement occurred de novo, the deleted chromosome was derived from the father (as determined by molecular techniques).

The same deletion of 15q11→q13 has also been found in Angelman syndrome, also known as *happy puppet* syndrome. In Angelman syndrome, the deleted chromosome is inherited from the mother. The syndrome is characterized by severe mental retardation, ataxia, absence of speech and language development, and often unprovoked fits of laughter. This example of what appears to be imprinting is a fascinating one because of the dramatic difference in presentation between the two syndromes. It is unclear at this time, however, if the syndromes are actually caused by deletions of 15q. Many patients with both Prader-Willi and Angelman syndromes do not have the deletions. In those who do, it has been hypothesized that the syndromes are contiguous gene disorders, although a single gene has not been ruled out.

The majority of syndromes likely to be seen in speech-language-hearing facilities have autosomal dominant patterns of inheritance. Although there are many syndromes of hearing loss with autosomal recessive patterns of inheritance, the majority of syndromes characterized by structural anomalies are autosomal dominant. This is especially true of syndromes that have craniofacial anomalies as prominent features. Examples of autosomal dominant syndromes that cause a variety of communicative disorders include Treacher Collins syndrome (conductive hearing loss, cleft palate which can cause hypernasality, choanal stenosis which can cause hyponasality, and anterior skeletal open bite which can cause articulation impairment), Waardenburg syndrome (sensorineural hearing loss and occasionally cleft palate), and Apert syndrome (mental retardation, open bite, cleft palate).

Autosomal Recessive. In autosomal recessive inheritance, both halves of the gene pair must be the same copy of the gene to be expressed. If only one copy of the gene is present and the other member of the pair is not the mutant gene, the resulting individual is phenotypically normal, but is known as a **carrier** because he or she has one copy of the mutant allele. Carriers are at risk for having children with the recessive trait only if their mate is also a carrier. Figure 3–9 illustrates autosomal recessive inheritance. When two carriers mate, the recurrence risk is 25% for expression of the trait, and 50% for resulting offspring to be carriers. There is only a 25% risk that the offspring will be neither affected nor a carrier. If one parent does not carry a copy of the mutant gene, there is a 50% probability that resulting offspring would be carriers, but there would not be any affected offspring.

Although a large number of autosomal recessive syndromes have structural anomalies as a primary component, recessive disorders often have metabolic problems as primary features. Many recessive disorders in-

volve sensorineural hearing loss as well, including Usher syndrome and Refsum syndrome. Recessive disorders are also more likely to involve degenerative processes than dominant ones.

X-Linked Disorders. X-linked disorders may be either recessive or dominant, although there are far more X-linked recessive disorders. The mechanism of gene expression (i.e., dominant versus recessive) is essentially the same, but the mode of inheritance is different because the mutant genes are on the X chromosome.

In order for a recessive trait to be expressed if the gene for the trait is located on an X chromosome, one of two conditions must be present. The individual must either be homo-

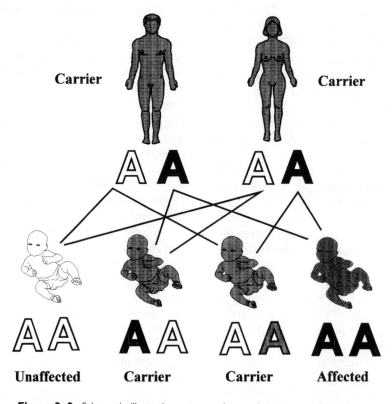

Figure 3–9. Schematic illustrating autosomal recessive pattern of inheritance when both parents are carriers of a mutant allele that is not expressed as long as the other allele is the normal one. Based on the possible segregation of the alleles, 25% of the possible offspring will inherit both mutant alleles and will be affected, 50% will be unaffected carriers, and 25% will be unaffected noncarriers.

zygous for the mutant gene (in other words, the gene must be located on both X chromosomes), or the individual must be missing the second X chromosome in the pair. There are only two circumstances that cause an individual to be missing the second X chromosome in the pair of sex chromosomes. One is if the individual has Turner syndrome (with a chromosomal compliment of 45X). The second, and far more common circumstance, is if the individual is male. The Y chromosome is not a match for the X chromosome, even though it is one of the sex chromosomes. The term "sex chromosome" is applied basically because the X and Y chromosomes are the only chromosomes that play a role in determining if the individual will be female (with two X chromosomes) or male (an X and Y chromosome). Since individuals with a single X chromosome and no Y chromosome (Turner syndrome) are phenotypically female, it is clear that the Y chromosome is responsible for providing the male phenotype.

Figure 3–10 illustrates X-linked recessive inheritance. If an unaffected male mates with a female who is a carrier of a mutant X-linked recessive gene (the carrier female, like the carrier of an autosomal recessive trait, is phenotypically normal), the probability of an affected child being born is 25%, as it is for an autosomal recessive trait. The difference is, however, that all affected children would be male, whereas in autosomal recessive traits, there is no difference in the possible expression between male and female (there is a 50–50 distribution of males and females). Therefore, the probability is that 50% of male offspring will be affected, 50% of male will be normal, 50% of female offspring will be phenotypically normal carriers, and 50% of female offspring will be normal homozygotes. Although males are the only children who will be affected, only females can be carriers (because they will have the normal allele on the other X chromosome).

An interesting phenomenon can be observed in carrier females. Females who are heterozygotes (also known as hemizygous) for X-linked recessive syndromes tend to show very minor manifestation of the disorder. For example, carrier mothers of males affected with Duschenne muscular dystrophy have slightly elevated levels of the muscle enzyme which, when expressed fully in males with the disease, proves to be fatal in early adult life. In cases where molecular genetic tests are not available to confirm that an individual is a carrier, this phenomenon may prove useful in identifying female carriers.

The only way a female can be affected by an X-linked recessive syndrome is if an affected male mates with a carrier female (Figure 3–10). In such cases, 50% of the possible offspring would be expected to be affected, one male and one female. Of the two other possible offspring, one would be an unaffected male, the other a carrier female. It is very unusual for X-linked recessive traits to be expressed in a female, transmitted by an affected male, unless there is a consanguineous mating (the mating of close blood relatives). In cases of consanguineous matings, the probability of X-linked traits being expressed in female offspring increases because the gene is so frequently found among family members.

There are fewer X-linked recessive disorders than autosomal disorders, which is to be expected even though the X chromosome is a large chromosome. The reason for this is quite simple. There are 22 times as many autosomes as X chromosomes in females and 46 times as many autosomes as X chromosomes in males. Therefore, there are proportionately fewer X-linked genes than autosomal genes. There are, however, some easily recognized X-linked disorders with communicative impairments, including X-linked mental retardation (also known as Fragile X syndrome and Martin-Bell syndrome) and otopalatodigital syndrome type I (cleft palate, cognitive impairment, micrognathia, conductive hearing loss).

X-linked Dominant Traits. Dominant genes may also be located on the X chromosome.

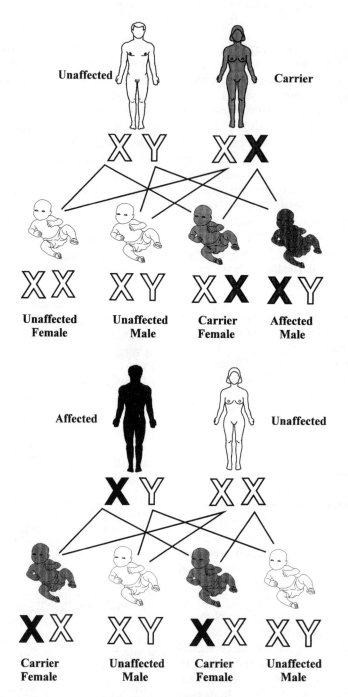

Figure 3–10. Schematic illustrating X-linked recessive pattern of inheritance resulting in a 50% recurrence risk for male offspring. In this case, the mutant allele is carried on the X chromosome. When the mother carries the X-linked recessive trait (*top*), it is not expressed in the mother because the other X chromosome has the normal allele. The trait is therefore expressed only in male offspring who have no corresponding normal allele because they do not have a matching X chromosome in their sex chromosome pair (they have a Y chromosome instead). Of the possible female offspring, there is a 50% probability they will be carriers and a 50% probability they will not. If the father is affected (*bottom*), there will be no affected males (no males inherit the X chromosome from the father), and both possible segregations resulting in females will produce carriers.

In such cases, the expected pattern of distribution of the mutant gene in potential offspring is similar to autosomal dominant traits except that there are no affected males among the children of affected males because male children can not inherit an X chromosome from a father (Figure 3–11). Therefore, 50% of the offspring of the father will be affected and both will be female (because they must inherit the father's single X chromosome). In the case where the mother is affected with the X-linked dominant syndrome, the distribution of affected offspring is exactly the same as in an autosomal dominant disorder (Figure 3–11).

Polygenic or Multifactorial Traits. In the early years of human genetics, some disorders seemed to defy the known modes of inheritance. Many anomalies and a number of syndromes, some common, did not follow dominant or recessive patterns when traced through pedigrees. A disorder might show up in a cousin or uncle or aunt of an affected individual, but seem to skip generations in a manner that would not be consistent with even recessive or X-linked traits. Probably the best example of this type of abnormality is cleft lip and/or cleft palate.

Clefting was often noted to occur in families, but did not often follow the Mendelian rules of inheritance patterns. It was often true that analysis of the pedigree of an affected individual (often referred to as the **proband**) showed that a first or second cousin, or perhaps a distant uncle or niece, was found to have a cleft, but no other individuals in the pedigree were found to be affected. In what has often been regarded as one of the most important publications in the fields of both clefting and genetics, Fraser (1970) hypothesized that clefting was most often a multifactorial trait. Additional publications followed detailing the model of multifactorial causation (Fraser, 1974, 1976, 1980). The multifactorial model hypothesized that a number of factors acting in concert could cause clefts to occur. Each individual factor by itself might not be sufficient to cause the cleft, but added together, the anomaly would occur. The term *multifactorial* has been applied because the presumption has been that both genetic and environmental factors contribute to the problem. If only genetic influences were in effect, the problem would be *polygenic* in etiology rather than multifactorial. According to Fraser (1970, 1974, 1976, 1980), the process of facial formation is a complex one dependent on the precise timing of the joining of several embryonic facial structures (Figure 3–12). The growth of these structures, known as processes, is determined by the embryo's genome. The actions of the genes cause the proliferation of cells in the maxillary processes, the median nasal processes, and the lateral nasal processes. It may be presumed that more than one gene controls these spurts in growth because several different structures are involved, and the timing of growth of each process is slightly different. It is also known that a number of environmental agents can contribute to either good or poor growth. For example, the absence of sufficient amounts of dietary folic acid can interfere with normal development of the facial processes, or the presence of known teratogenic agents (such as alcohol, phenytoins and other anticonvulsants, and retinoic acid) can interfere with normal growth. Fraser hypothesized that the medial growth of the facial processes occurs at the same time that the fetal head is expanding laterally. Therefore, there is an antagonistic "race" between the medial movement of the various processes towards each other and the outward expansion of the head, which would draw the processes away from each other. The time frame within which the medial growth of the processes have to merge is small so that any delay in growth, deficiency of growth, or excessive lateral expansion of the head would move the process of fusion away from a *threshold*, or window of opportunity, for fusion to occur. Fraser hypothesized, by both the application of mathematical models and pedigree analysis, that clefting fit this type of thresh-

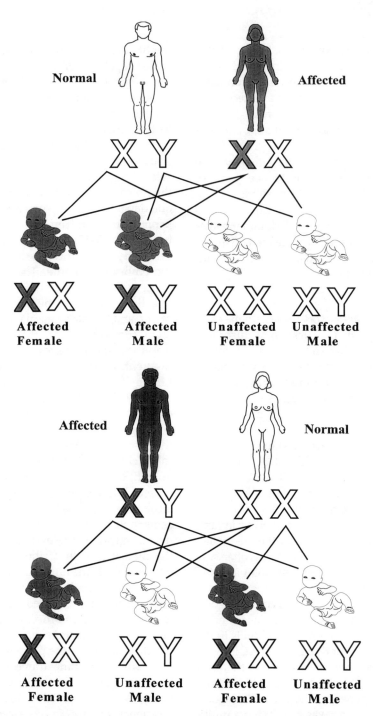

Figure 3–11. Schematic illustrating X-linked dominant pattern of inheritance. If the mother is affected (*top*), there is a 50% recurrence risk and either a male or female child inheriting the mother's X chromosome could be affected. If the father is affected (*bottom*), only female offspring could be affected because no male children inherit the father's X chromosome. In cases where the father passes on an X-linked dominant trait, all female offspring will be affected, but no male children will be affected.

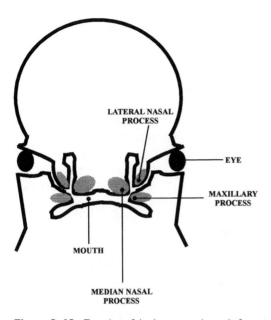

LATERAL NASAL
PROCESS

EYE

MAXILLARY
PROCESS

MOUTH

MEDIAN NASAL
PROCESS

Figure 3–12. Drawing of the human embryonic face at approximately 5 weeks postfertilization showing the various facial processes and where fusion occurs (*stippled area*). Failure for fusion to occur along these processes will result in a cleft lip.

old model, implying that both genetic and environmental agents contributed to the mechanism of fusion.

The problem with multifactorial models and presumptions of polygenic contribution is that they are hard to prove and evidence for them is purely hypothetical and based on implications of observations unrelated to specific individuals with clefts. First, very few environmental agents are known to contribute to clefting. Although a substantial number of teratogenic agents have been demonstrated to cause clefts in mouse embryos, the same agents have not been implicated in human clefting. To date, only a small handful of known teratogens contribute to clefting in humans, and even when these teratogens are confirmed, there is a broad spectrum of teratogenic effects in the resulting babies which go far beyond isolated clefts of the lip and palate. Therefore, the known teratogenic influences are seen as part of teratogenic syndromes (see below) rather

than as contributors to isolated clefts (i.e., clefts in the absence of other anomalies). Therefore, environmental contributors to clefts in the multifactorial model can only be hypothesized. Because nearly all pregnant women can be exposed to literally hundreds of environmental agents that presumably could be toxic or threatening to the fetus (everything from household cleaning items to a cold virus) and relatively few have babies with clefts, one should not be overzealous in drawing a connection between such exposures and resulting anomalies.

Similarly, polygenic contributions (when not contiguous genes on the same chromosome) have never been confirmed in playing a role in the induction of anomalies. Techniques for isolating genetic contributions to anomalies have been effective in isolating single genes as causative factors, but not multiple noncontiguous genes. Although it may be logical to assume that each individual facial process has a different genetic instigator, this is not the only possible explanation of the failure for facial processes to grow sufficiently. The cells that make up the various facial processes are derived largely from an early single cell source known as the **neural crest**. The action of a single gene may be responsible for insufficient numbers of neural crest cells migrating into the facial processes, thus inhibiting eventual mitotic growth. Another possible explanation is that some genes are known to be regulatory in nature. That is, they switch on and switch off other genes, which in turn control specific growth functions. For example, earlier in this chapter, Stickler syndrome was discussed in relation to club foot. Stickler syndrome is one of the most common syndromes associated with cleft palate, accounting for approximately 5% of all babies with clefts of the palate without cleft lip (Shprintzen, Siegel-Sadewitz, Amato, & Goldberg, 1985). Stickler syndrome is an autosomal dominant disorder caused by a mutation in a gene located on chromosome 12 which regulates the formation of a type of connective tissue in the body, collagen II. Collagen II is a connective tissue found in many parts of the body, including the joints of the long bones, the spine, the mandible, the palate, and the eyes. A flaw in this type of collagen can therefore cause anomalies of any or all of these structures, including cleft palate, micrognathia, lax joints, and myopia (caused by abnormal curvature of the eye).

Therefore, although multifactorial inheritance has been hypothesized, it has yet to be conclusively proven. As the human genome continues to be completely analyzed and new gene functions discovered, it is possible, if not likely, that most disorders will eventually be ascribed to single gene mechanisms.

Teratogenic Disorders

The term teratogen translated literally from its Greek roots means "monster maker" (**teratos** = monster; **gen** as derived from the same root for **gene** = derived from). The practical application of the term is reserved for substances that produce anomalies when the developing embryo is exposed to them. There have been a substantial number of reports in the popular press of the possible teratogenic effects of many substances. Nearly everything, from aspirin to caffeine, has been incorrectly cited as being teratogenic, but the reality is that there are very few confirmed human teratogens.

There are a number of different categories of teratogens: chemicals, therapeutic drugs, illicit drugs, viruses and other microbes, maternal metabolic disease or toxicity, and changes in the immediate maternal or embryonic environment caused by environmental change or maternal metabolic abnormalities. One must be cautioned that there can be enormous variation in the phenotype of individuals with teratogenic syndromes because the expression of the teratogenic exposure is dependent on the following factors, which are not mutually exclusive and may be additive:

1. The timing of the exposure in terms of embryonic/fetal development.
2. The time of exposure (i.e., duration).
3. The mother's metabolism and general health which intervenes between the environment and the developing conceptus.
4. The dose of the exposure (the amount or strength of the teratogen).
5. The interaction between multiple teratogens, or between potential teratogens and other anomalies or genetic traits in the developing conceptus.

Chemicals

One is immediately tempted to believe that any agent which in any way has a negative connotation for the environment, or which could cause physical injury to a person (such as an acid burn or abrasive rash), must be teratogenic. However, for an environmental agent to be injurious to an embryo or fetus, it must reach the developing baby. The only route to the conceptus is through the maternal bloodstream which communicates with the baby's via the placenta. Not all agents in the maternal bloodstream are able to cross the placenta. Therefore, not every agent that can affect the mother physically can affect the developing conceptus physically. The only other mechanism of teratogenesis would be the exposure of primary germ cells to an agent which would alter chromosome structure in either the male or female. This phenomenon is possible with radiation exposure, which will be discussed in more detail later. However, confirmation of this type of primary germ cell mutation remains elusive in nearly all cases.

Few chemicals are known to be clearly teratogenic, although suspicions run high among the lay public and environmental advocacy groups that there are many such agents. Because the issue of protecting a developing human life is such an emotionally charged one, which can be used to political advantage, people sometimes confuse reports in tabloid newspapers or public relations campaigns with scientific fact. Perhaps the best example is the furor caused by the suspicion that agent orange (dioxin) must be teratogenic. Many veterans, male soldiers who were exposed to dioxin and subsequently had babies with congenital anomalies found it natural to blame their exposure for the resulting disorders. After all, dioxin did cause a variety of physical ailments in people exposed to it. However, dioxin does not cause chromosome rearrangement, nor can a teratogen reach the maternal and fetal bloodstream through the father. Therefore, the issue of congenital anomalies being caused by paternal dioxin exposure is a spurious one, which was largely accepted as fact by the news media and the American public. In reality, the rate of congenital anomalies among the children of Viet Nam veterans exposed to dioxin was no higher than that expected in the general public. However, because a substantial number of newborns do have at least some minor anomalies (at least 14%), the relatively common occurrence of observed malformations in the veterans would be correlated with the dioxin exposure, leading to the conclusion that dioxin was the cause. However, in science, it is axiomatic that a correlation (i.e., the co-occurrence of two observed events) never implies a cause and effect relationship. Therefore, what turns out to be good news for expectant mothers regarding the relative safety of the human fetus often turns out to be politically unpopular to various advocacy groups. Scientists must be rigorous in applying careful study to issues of such important public concern.

Known teratogens that fit into the category of chemical environmental agents include methyl mercury, polychlorinated biphenyls (PCBs), and possibly toluene. Methyl mercury is usually consumed inadvertently when food or water is contaminated. Individuals born after maternal consumption of mercurial compounds are usually small, have mental retardation, neuromuscular problems, blindness, and sensorineural hearing loss. Babies exposed to PCBs in utero are usually born with "Cola-colored" skin and tend to be small. Toluene, a solvent that is often found in paint, has been reported as a teratogen in a small number of individuals from a single source (Hersh, Podruch, Rogers, & Weisskopf, 1985). Resulting anomalies include craniofacial abnormalities (micrognathia, maxillary deficiency, frontal bone narrowing, small eyes), limb anomalies (short fingernails, short distal ends of the digits), and renal anomalies. There are several good catalogues of known confirmed teratogenic agents (Hanson, 1983; Hill, 1984; Shepard, 1986).

Therapeutic Drugs

A substantial, but small, number of therapeutic drugs are known to have teratogenic effects. The most publicized and well recognized teratogenic drug, thalidomide, sensitized the general population to teratogenesis while stiffening the resolve of the Food and Drug Administration to continue to carefully monitor medications for adverse effects on developing embryos and fetuses. Although the limb reduction anomalies caused by thalidomide were largely limited to Europe (thalidomide was not an FDA-approved medication in the U.S.), the shock of a large number of children being born with absent or hypoplastic arms and legs captured the attention of the world at the time. As a result, the public has become sensitized to the possibility that any drug could be teratogenic.

Certain classes of drugs have a higher likelihood of teratogenic effect, including anticonvulsant medications and anticoagulant medications. Of the anticonvulsants, perhaps the best recognized teratogens are the phenytoins and hydantoins, such as Dilantin®. Dilantin embryopathy, depending on dosage, timing of delivery, and maternal metabolism, causes craniofacial anomalies (hypertelorism, depressed nasal root, short nose, cleft lip and/or cleft palate), limb anomalies (short distal phalanges, hypoplastic nails, abnormal thumbs, and dislocated pelvis), growth deficiency, possible mild mental retardation, small stature, occasional heart anomalies, and low anterior or posterior hairline. Although a fairly potent teratogen, it is possible to monitor blood levels of phenytoins so that placental transmission of teratogenic doses is not possible.

Anticonvulsants other than phenytoins that are known teratogens include trimethadione and structurally similar drugs known as oxazolidinediones, and valproate (valproic acid). Barbiturates (such as phenobarbital) are also suspected of being teratogens.

Anticoagulants using coumarin derivatives, such as Warfarin, result in babies with hypoplastic noses, hypoplastic fingernails, low birth weight, and mental retardation. There is a distinct time frame for the teratogenic effects of coumarin derivatives to be expressed, 6 to 9 weeks postfertilization (Hall, Pauli, & Wilson, 1980).

Another group of medicinal agents that has received some scrutiny in recent years are isoretinoins, such as retinoic acid, vitamin A, and vitamin A congeners. Facial asymmetry, external ear anomalies, heart anomalies, small eyes, and cleft palate have all been associated with retinoic acid and vitamin A (Lammer, 1985). This particular association is alarming because of the high percentage of the general population that uses vitamin A or retinoic acid in some form as a supplement (Hall, 1984), including so-called "megadoses."

A number of chemotherapeutic drugs have also been generally accepted to be teratogens. The most frequently reported teratogenic drugs used in chemotherapy are aminopterin and methotrexate. Aminopterin effects have been observed most frequently because it was often used to initiate abortions.

Psychotropic medications, such as sedatives, are known to have major teratogenic effects. Thalidomide was already mentioned as a potent teratogen. Meprobamate, also known as Milltown, is a commonly prescribed sedative that has been implicated in causing mental retardation, cleft palate, heart anomalies, and limb anomalies, although the risk is considered to be low.

Illegal Drugs and Intoxicants

Clearly, the most common teratogenic agent in humans is ethyl alcohol. The fetal alcohol syndrome has become widely recognized by both the professional community and lay public, to the point where alcoholic beverages now contain warning labels regarding the possibility of "birth defects" being caused by maternal consumption of alcohol. The pattern of anomalies caused by maternal alcohol consumption during pregnancy, although well recognized by clinicians in general, is highly variable because of the dose and timing effects, which are dependent on the mother's particular pattern of drinking. Because alcohol undergoes a number of digestive and metabolic processes, the mother's physical processing of alcohol probably plays a more significant role in the expression of alcohol teratogenesis than is found with other drugs or chemical agents.

Alcohol is teratogenic throughout pregnancy, and the effect can be quite variable depending on the pattern of consumption. Because alcohol can interfere with essentially any developmental process in the embryo or fetus, the variation in both the physical and behavioral phenotype can be quite dramatic. For example, if the mother is a persistent drinker throughout the pregnancy, especially early in the first trimester when there is a lot of activity in facial, limb, and cardiac development, the occurrence of cleft lip, congenital heart anomalies, severe brain malformations, very small stature, and severe microcephaly are likely (Figure 3–13). In cases where heavy drinking is done only in the last trimester, when facial and heart development are largely complete but brain growth is very active, facial and limb anomalies are less likely to be found, but performance can be impaired by learning disabilities, perceptual impairment, and other cognitive deficiencies (Figure 3–14).

Another problem in sorting out the teratogenic effects of alcohol is the observation that many women who abuse alcohol also use illicit drugs. Patterns of substance abuse

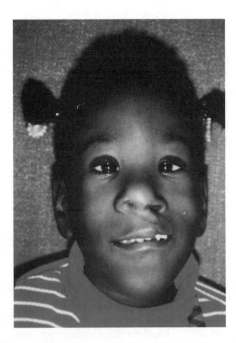

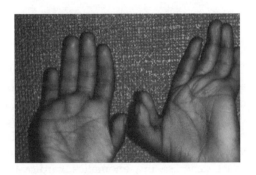

Figure 3–13. Patient with fetal alcohol syndrome. In this case, the mother drank heavily from the onset of conception. Note the cleft lip and palate, severe microcephaly, very small eyes, and limb anomalies including an extra preaxial digit.

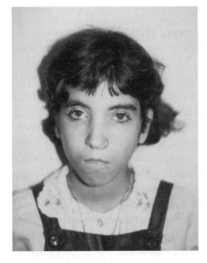

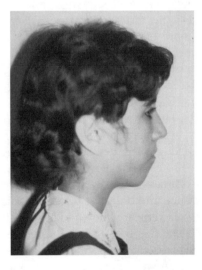

Figure 3–14. Patient with fetal alcohol effects whose mother drank heavily only during the last trimester. There are no heart or limb anomalies and the facial manifestations are very mild.

often spread to multiple substances so that women who drink may also utilize cocaine, heroin, or other illegal drugs.

Most illegal street drugs, including cocaine and heroin, have been implicated as teratogens. Most illegal drugs are thought to have teratogenic effects on the central nervous system. Facial manifestations for many teratogens include short palpebral fissures, microcephaly, and possible facial clefts.

Viruses and other Microbes

Certainly, the best known viral teratogen to specialists in the communication disorders is rubella. Rubella embryopathy is less of a common threat to pregnancy today because of widespread immunization. The rubella virus is known to cross the placenta and cause deafness, eye anomalies, cardiovascular malformations, skeletal lesions, growth deficiency, and mental retardation. The virus is known to infect the developing cochlea, resulting in the deafness commonly associated with rubella embryopathy. Although less well known as a teratogen, varicella (the virus that causes chicken pox) is a more extant virus, which can cause seizures, mental retardation, cortical atrophy, growth deficiency, limb anomalies, and scarlike skin lesions. Other viral teratogens include herpes simplex and cytomegalovirus. Herpes simplex infection can result in eye, heart, limb, and cognitive abnormalities and growth deficiency. Cytomegalovirus also causes eye and heart anomalies, plus deafness, mental retardation, growth deficiency, and digestive tract anomalies.

Few bacteria are known to act directly as teratogens (we will discuss indirect teratogenesis caused by hyperthermia later in this chapter). A well known bacteria thought to cause neural tube defects, mental retardation, and growth deficiency is mycoplasma. A parasite, toxoplasma gondii (the cause of toxoplasmosis), causes blindness, deafness, growth deficiency, and mental retardation.

Maternal Metabolic Disease or Toxicity

Because the embryo's blood supply communicates with that of the mother, metabolic abnormalities that result in toxic substances being transmitted through the maternal blood can affect embryonic and fetal development. The two best known examples of maternal metabolic disorders that can result in malformation syndromes are diabetes mellitus (not gestational diabetes) and phenylketonuria. Although women with gestational diabetes tend to have large babies, they typically are otherwise normal. However, women with diabetes mellitus that is poorly controlled during pregnancy may have children with caudal regression syndrome, a disorder characterized by limb anomalies, cleft palate, and possible heart, kidney, and spine abnormalities. In its most severe form, a severe brain anomaly known as holoprosencephaly can occur.

Severe iodine dietary deficiency during the first trimester can result in mental retardation, spasticity, and neural deafness. This deficiency is most often confined to third world countries where iodine deficiency is endemic.

Changes in the Immediate Maternal or Embryonic Environment

Changes in either the immediate intrauterine environment or the general maternal environment can have an impact on fetal development by disturbing the normal process of cell division or tissue formation. One such general maternal environment abnormality is hyperthermia, or elevated body temperature. There is substantial experimental evidence from animal studies that hyperthermia can cause major anomalies in the developing fetus, especially during the earliest stages of pregnancy. Brain formation can be impaired, and hyperthermia has been implicated as a cause of anencephaly. Excessive doses of radiation have also been implicated in causing brain maldevelopment, eye anomalies, and neoplasias (cancers). Radiation exposure can

also cause rearrangements in the chromosomes of the early embryo before the developmental process is complete, resulting in
chromosomal aneuploidies in at least some
cells of the conceptus and resulting developmental abnormalities.

Mechanically Induced Syndromes

Earlier in this chapter, amnion rupture syndrome was described and discussed (Figure
3–5). This is one of only a few mechanically
induced syndromes. Mechanical interference can cause many individual anomalies
without specifically recognized patterns of
malformation as might be seen in genetically caused syndromes.

Unknown Genesis Syndromes

In his model of syndromic delineation, Cohen
(1982) also has two other categories of syndromes which have no known cause, although
the presumption is that they represent syndromes. These two types of syndromes
both fit into a classification of **unknown genesis syndromes**. Although, by definition,
syndromes represent multiple anomalies
with a single pathogenesis, the cause may
be difficult to identify and is therefore unknown at the present time. Cohen (1982)
argues that the unknown nature of a multiple anomaly disorder's etiology does not
make it any less a syndrome. The problem
is not the syndromic association, but our
ability to isolate the cause. His logic has
proved correct because many of the disorders that were previously of unknown etiology have since been found to be genetic with
identifiable genetic mutations or deletions.

Unknown genesis syndromes were classified by Cohen into two categories: recurrent pattern unknown genesis syndromes
and provisionally unique syndromes. *Recurrent pattern unknown genesis syndromes*
are those that have patterns of malformation which the clinician or other clinicians
have seen before, but a cause for the syndrome has never been isolated. There is no
history of teratogenesis, karyotype is normal, and there is no family history of simi-

lar anomalies or patterns of anomalies. However, the grouping of anomalies could not be
anything other than a syndrome and the
pattern is a familiar one. An example of
a recurrent pattern unknown genesis syndrome is the hypoglossia-hypodactyly syndrome, a disorder comprised of a very small
or absent tongue and missing digits with
small hands. All cases reported to date have
been sporadic with no familial cases reported. Karyotypes have been normal, and no
consistent pattern of teratogenesis has been
reported. The anomalies do not fit any proposed pattern of mechanical abnormality.
However, the pattern of anomalies is well
recognized.

Provisionally unique pattern syndromes
are those that have multiple anomalies but
do not fit any pattern seen before by the
clinician. Karyotypes are normal, there is no
evidence or history of teratogenesis, and
there are no affected relatives. The pattern
of anomalies has not been reported in the
literature, the clinician consults many colleagues from many different locations and
none of them have seen the pattern before.
Therefore, as far as the clinician knows, the
individual has a unique pattern of anomalies, but because there are multiple major
anomalies, it probably represents a syndrome.
Although the pattern is unique, Cohen (1982)
prefers to label the patterns as **provisionally unique** because the individual may have
an affected child or another family member
may have an affected child, which could
reveal a mode of inheritance. This would
move the syndrome from the category of
provisionally unique unknown genesis to
recurrent pattern known genesis. The other
possibility is that a second unrelated patient
with the same pattern of anomalies will be
discovered, but is also a sporadic case with
no evidence of teratogenesis or karyotypic
abnormalities. However, even though the
cause is still unknown, the syndrome now
represents a recurrent pattern unknown genesis disorder.

As an example of the delineation of new
syndromes, the following example is offered.
The patient shown in Figure 3–15 was first
seen by me in 1975, referred with a diagno-

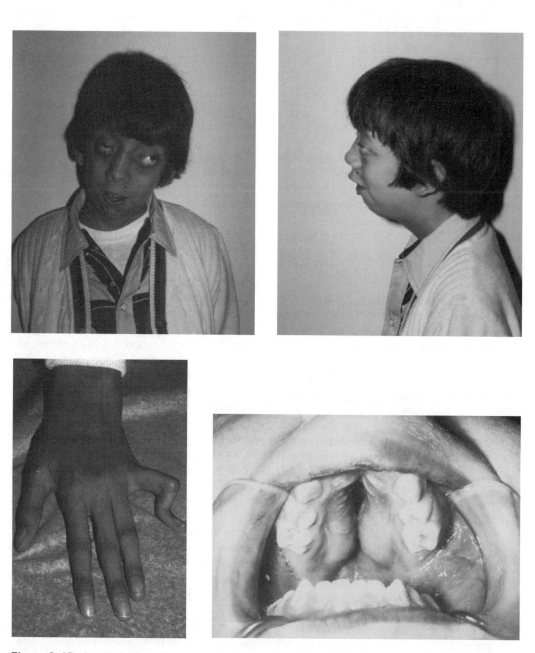

Figure 3–15. A patient seen with an unusual spectrum of anomalies, including craniosynostosis, micrognathia, exorbitism, arachnodactyly, multiple abdominal hernias, mental retardation, pectus carinatum, and spinal anomalies.

sis of Crouzon syndrome provided at another institution. Crouzon syndrome is an autosomal dominant genetic condition that has craniosynostosis as its primary feature caused by a mutation in a gene on chromosome 10 (fibroblast growth factor receptor 2 gene). Craniosynostosis is the premature fusion of the cranial bones which normally remain separated by sutures, which are spaces between the interdigitated bones of the calvarium, or cranial vault (the frontal, temporal, parietal, and occipital bones). These spaces remain between the cranial bones to allow expansion of the brain which proceeds well into the second decade of life. In Crouzon syndrome, not only are the cranial bones fused, but the bones of the skull base (such as the sphenoid and ethmoid) also are fused. Because the skull bones are fused, the brain may be compressed as it grows, causing increased intracranial pressure and very abnormal shape of the head, including eyes that bulge out of the orbits, known as exorbitism, and severe maxillary hypoplasia with marked relative prognathism (Figure 3–16).

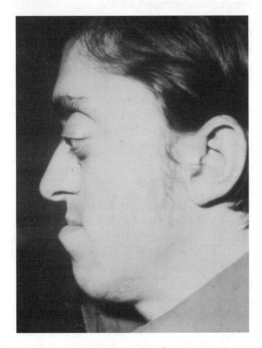

Figure 3–16. A patient with Crouzon syndrome. Note the abnormal skull shape and retruded maxilla.

There are no anomalies in Crouzon syndrome other than the craniofacial malformations. The patient shown in Figure 3–15 had many extracranial anomalies, as well as marked developmental delay and mental retardation, which is not usually found in Crouzon syndrome. The patient had micrognathia, long fingers (arachnodactyly) with contractures, multiple abdominal hernias, spinal anomalies, and very soft cartilage in the ears and nose. Other than the craniosynostosis, none of the phenotypic features in this patient are consistent with Crouzon syndrome, nor was the pattern of anomalies consistent with any that had been previously reported. Therefore, the patient was categorized as provisionally unique.

Five years later, in 1980, a patient was referred with the same pattern of anomalies (Figure 3–17). This second patient had a somewhat more severe expression of the same disorder, but the pattern was clearly the same. As a result, we reported these two patients as a new syndrome of recurrent pattern, but unknown genesis (Shprintzen & Goldberg, 1982). Since that time, an additional six cases of the same disorder have been reported so that dysmorphologists and clinical geneticists recognize this as a specific syndromic entity, the Shprintzen-Goldberg syndrome (Cohen, 1986).

SEQUENCES

Not all multiple anomaly disorders represent syndromes. The reader will recall that, in a syndrome, all of the anomalies found in the child have a single primary cause (chromosomal, genetic, teratogenic, or mechanical). It is also possible to have a multiple anomaly disorder where all of the anomalies are not directly related to a single cause. A sequence is a disorder where many of the anomalies are actually secondary disorders, caused by a single anomaly which sets off a chain reaction of changes in the developing embryo that result in other anomalies. A sequence may be defined as the presence of multiple anomalies in an indi-

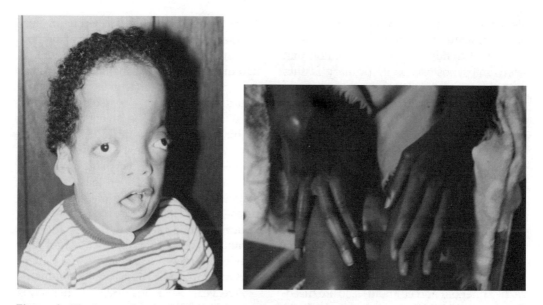

Figure 3–17. A second patient with the same pattern of anomalies as those seen in the patient shown in Figure 3–15.

vidual where most or all of the anomalies present are caused secondarily by a single known or presumed structural anomaly or error in morphogenesis (development). However, the single structural anomaly or morphogenetic error that causes the other anomalies may itself have multiple possible causes.

There are three types of sequences (Smith, 1982):

▶ malformation sequences,
▶ deformation sequences, or
▶ disruption sequences.

The difference between the three types of sequences is the causation of the anomaly that sets into motion the cascading effects that result in the sequence. In essence, the model for the disruption sequence has already been discussed in our description of the amnion rupture syndrome. Some regard this multiple anomaly disorder as a syndrome because the presumption is that the rupture in the amnion is purely accidental with no specific pathogenesis, so that the amnion rupture itself is the primary cause of the anomalies. Others regard the spectrum of anomalies caused by amnion rupture to be a sequence because of the possi-

bility (if not probability) that there is more than one possible cause of the ruptures, ranging from trauma to infection, to an intrinsic congenital anomaly of the amnion (which is part of the embryo, not part of the mother). If the amnion ruptures have multiple possible causes, then the spectrum of disorders caused by the ruptures represents a sequence.

A discussion of one of the best recognized sequences will help to clarify exactly what a sequence is and describe the difference between a malformation sequence and deformation sequence.

Robin Sequence

Many readers may be familiar with the *Pierre Robin syndrome*. Actually, there is no such thing as the Pierre Robin syndrome. This disorder, which is usually recognized as the association of a small lower jaw (*micrognathia*), a wide U-shaped cleft palate, and upper airway obstruction, is actually a sequence. Robin sequence may be further divided into the Robin deformation sequence and the Robin malformation sequence.

When first described by the French stomatologist, Pierre Robin, in 1923, cleft palate was not considered to be a part of the spectrum of anomalies in this disorder. In fact, the point of Robin's original article was to describe all of the problems that could be caused by a small mandible and its resulting airway compromise. In reality, Robin's early description is closer to the true nature of Robin sequence than what it eventually evolved into within the scientific community which studied cleft palate. It was not until a subsequent article in 1934 that Robin mentioned cleft palate anecdotally as a factor that could complicate the airway obstruction seen in infants with micrognathia. The common perception of Robin sequence as involving the triad of micrognathia, cleft palate, and airway obstruction did not become well accepted until the 1960s (Randall et al., 1965). Even today, clinicians may apply the diagnosis of "Pierre Robin" in the absence of cleft palate (i.e., micrognathia and airway obstruction only) or in the absence of airway obstruction (i.e., cleft palate and micrognathia), indicating there is significant variability of diagnostic approach to this disorder (Sadewitz & Shprintzen, 1986).

Robin Deformation Sequence

The original theory of the origin of Robin sequence postulated that the cleft and airway obstruction were caused by a mechanical obstruction of mandibular growth which resulted in both the cleft and airway obstruction, instigated by a process known as *glossoptosis*. The widely accepted hypothesis of mandibular compression leading to lingual obstruction causing the cleft is consistent with a deformation process and would progress as follows (Figure 3–18). At approximately 7 weeks of gestation, the palatal shelves are oriented in a vertical position, resting alongside the tongue which is pressed firmly against the nasal septum beneath the skull base. As the mandible begins to grow, room in the mouth is provided for the tongue to drop lower into the oral cavity so that the palatal shelves can flip into a horizontal position and begin to grow toward the midline for eventual fusion. However, if the mandible is physically prevented from growing because of some mechanical force (i.e., a deformation), the tongue will remain compressed against the roof of the nasal cavity, preventing the palatal shelves from growing toward fusion. This leaves behind a U-shaped cleft reflecting the shape of the intervening tongue. After birth, with the mandible still small and the infant an obligate nose breather (infants reflexively keep their mouths closed and breathe through their noses), the tongue cannot come forward in the oral cavity, causing a posterior obstruction of the oropharynx. The tongue falling back in the airway is known as glossoptosis and is exacerbated by any negative pressure that might occur in the airway by the posterior position of the mandible.

Thus, based on the series of cascading events described in the last paragraph, the mandibular deformation leads to the cleft and airway obstruction. However, there are multiple possible causes of mechanical compression of the mandible. They include oligohydramnios, the presence of some type of mass in the uterus, uterine compression, and a multifactorial additive process. Oligohydramnios is an abnormally small amount of amniotic fluid surrounding the embryo. With less amniotic fluid, the uterus would not expand as much and the embryonic head would not be floating as freely supported by the pressure of the fluid. At the same time the palate should be forming, the heart is also forming and the chest is very prominent in the embryo. Therefore, the chin of the embryo may become compressed against the chest, preventing it from growing forward (Figure 3–18) and leading to the cascading events of the Robin deformation sequence.

Intrauterine masses may also compress the embryo by leaving less room for the embryo within the uterus, thus crowding the mandible in against the chest. Examples would include fibroids and neoplasias (tumors). Another circumstance that could lead to intrauterine crowding would be the presence of a twin. This type of crowding is more common among dizygotic twins (Smith, 1982) because there is a separate placenta, amnion, and all other structures associated with the embryo.

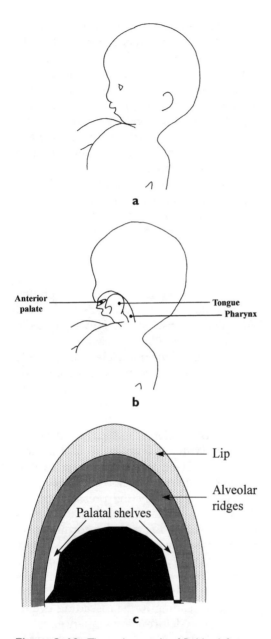

a

Anterior palate — Tongue, Pharynx

b

Lip

Alveolar ridges

Palatal shelves

c

Figure 3–18. The pathogenesis of Robin deformation sequence. In panel a, the mandible is prevented from growing forward by some type of mechanical force, in this case the chin is prevented from growing forward by the prominent chest where the heart is in the process of developing. In panel b, the tongue, which normally descends from between the developing palatal shelves so that they can grow toward the midline and fuse, fails to drop, thus physically obstructing palatal fusion. A wide U-shaped palatal cleft is therefore left behind as shown in panel c.

Uterine compression could be caused by an abnormally small uterus in the mother, uterine malformation (such as a unicornate or bicornate uterus), external compression by a growth elsewhere in the abdominal cavity, or adhesions on the uterus from previous surgery or endometriosis. Compression of the uterus could result in compression of the embryo contained within it, leading to the Robin deformation sequence.

Finally, several factors may act in concert to cause the deformation sequence. An example might be as follows. A very small mother (for argument's sake, under 5 feet tall) and a very tall father (for argument's sake, over 6 feet, 6 inches tall) establish the mother's first pregnancy so that her uterus is unstretched from previous births. Furthermore, both the father's family and mother's family tend to have fairly small lower jaws so that the baby inherits some degree of micrognathia as a separate trait. The developing baby is fairly large (because of the father's size), the mother's pelvis is small (because of her size), and there is little yield in the uterus, therefore causing some compression of the embryonic head. The developing baby already has a tendency toward micrognathia. Therefore, the jaw is small and there is intrauterine crowding, increasing the possibility of Robin deformation sequence.

In cases of Robin deformation sequence, the recurrence risk is low because it is unlikely that same set of circumstances that led to the positional deformation would exist in subsequent pregnancies. In these cases, the abnormality is extrinsic to the developing baby, although some genetic predispositions (such as the familial trait of a small mandible) might exist.

Robin Malformation Sequence

In the Robin malformation sequence, the disorder is intrinsic to the developing baby and therefore positional compression is not a factor. Therefore, any malformation that might cause the mandible to be small or cause the tongue to interfere with palatal shelf growth could cause the sequence. Because micrognathia is the instigating anomaly that sets the cascading effects of the sequence into motion, any disorder that has micrognathia as a common feature would be likely to cause a sequence. This should alert the reader to the important concept that a single individual could have both a sequence and a syndrome. Micrognathia is a common feature in many multiple anomaly syndromes. Therefore, if micrognathia occurs as a syndromic feature and the micrognathia then causes the tongue to interfere with palatal fusion and respiration, the sequence occurs as a secondary feature of the syndrome. The Robin sequence is therefore a feature associated with many syndromes and is etiologically heterogenous.

An analysis of a large sample of Robin sequence births has shown that the majority of births presenting with Robin sequence actually represent other multiple anomaly sequences that have Robin as a possible secondary sequence. One syndrome, Stickler syndrome (also mentioned earlier in this chapter) accounts for over one third, 34%, of all cases of Robin sequence (Shprintzen, 1988; Shprintzen, 1992; Shprintzen & Singer, 1992). Three additional syndromes, velo-cardio-facial syndrome, Treacher Collins syndrome, and fetal alcohol syndrome, were found to comprise 11% and 10% of Robin cases in the same sample. Therefore, over 65% of Robin sequence patients are caused by only four malformation syndromes. All four of these syndromes have some type of mandibular abnormality as a common feature, although the nature of the mandibular anomaly is different in each disorder.

Micrognathia is not the only anomaly that can lead to Robin sequence. As noted above, any syndrome that results in failure of the tongue to descend from between the developing palatal shelves can result in the Robin sequence. Therefore, syndromes in which the tongue is excessively large may also cause Robin sequence. Macroglossia is a common finding in Beckwith-Wiedemann

syndrome and cases of Robin sequence have been noted in this overgrowth disorder (Cohen, 1976). Another less common cause of Robin is the lack of mandibular exercise in the developing baby. One of the factors that allows the tongue to drop in the oral cavity is the normal up and down mandibular movements made by the fetus during growth and the swallowing of amniotic fluid. In the severe congenital form of myotonic dystrophy, such exercise may be limited or not occur at all so that the tongue does not descend. In addition, the mandible is abnormal in morphology in myotonic dystrophy, with abnormal curvature and retrognathic appearance.

Other Sequences

A number of other disorders once thought to be syndromes are also now recognized to be sequences. These include the Moebius sequence, the DiGeorge sequence, holoprosencephaly (also known as DeMyer sequence), septo-optic dysplasia, and Klippel-Feil.

The Importance of Recognizing the Difference Between Syndromes and Sequences

The clinician's goal in assessing a baby with multiple anomalies is to make an accurate diagnosis so that the phenotypic spectrum, natural history, and prognosis of the disorder become evident (see Chapter 1), and proper genetic counseling can be provided. If the sequence is mistakenly thought to be the primary or only diagnosis, so that the search for diagnosis stops with the application of "Pierre Robin," Klippel-Feil, or DiGeorge, then diagnoses such as Stickler syndrome (in Robin) or velo-cardio-facial syndrome (in both Robin and DiGeorge sequences) might not be applied and the eye and skeletal anomalies of Stickler syndrome or the learning, speech, and psychiatric disorders of velo-cardio-facial syndrome might not be anticipated. Correct counseling and clinical management are highly dependent on correct diagnosis, and although the diagnosis of a sequence is not incorrect, it is also not complete.

ASSOCIATIONS

Another category of multiple anomaly disorder that is not a syndrome is the *association*. An association is a multiple anomaly disorder that has a recurrent pattern, but for which there is no evidence of a specific etiology or sequential cascading effect. Only a few associations are currently recognized as fairly common patterns, including the VATER association and the CHARGE association. In both of these cases, the names represent acronyms. The VATER acronym represents **V**ertebral anomalies, **A**nal atresia, **T-E** Fistula, and **R**enal and **R**adial defects. The CHARGE acronym represents **C**oloboma (of the eye), **H**eart anomalies, **A**tresia choanae, **R**etarded growth and development, **G**enital anomalies, and **E**ar anomalies or deafness. It is likely that both of these disorders actually represent sequences in which the primary anomaly has not yet been identified. CHARGE has recently been linked to a deletion of the long arm of chromosome 22 in some cases, and it has been reported that some cases of velo-cardio-facial syndrome have features consistent with CHARGE as a secondary sequence (Shprintzen, 1987).

WHY SUSPECT A SYNDROME, SEQUENCE, OR ASSOCIATION?

Why should the clinician suspect that a patient has a syndrome, sequence, or association if more than one major anomaly is present? The answer to this question rests with probability theory. As an illustration, one might ask what is the probability that a child might be born with two common major malformations, such as congenital heart anomalies and an orofacial cleft, (cleft lip and/or cleft palate). Heart anomalies occur with a birth frequency of approximately 1:400 live

births. Clefting of the lip, palate, or both occurs with a frequency of 1:750 live births. What would the chance be that these two anomalies would occur in the same child unrelated to a common cause? The chance would be the same as the following probability example. Suppose there is a barrel filled with 400 ping pong balls, one of them painted red, and a second barrel with 750 ping pong balls, one of them also painted red. What would the chance be that you would be able to put one hand in one barrel and the other hand in the second barrel and pull out the two red ping pong balls at the same time? Even if you picked one red ball and one white one, you would have to replace both balls (rather than hanging on to the red one), shake the barrels, and try again. The chance of picking two red ping pong balls would be $1:400 \times 750$, or 1:300,000 live births. However, it has been well established that over 10% of all babies with clefts have congenital heart disease, which makes the actual frequency closer to 1:7500 in the general population (i.e., $.10 \times 750$), not 1:300,000. In fact, the actual frequency of clefting associated with heart anomalies is 40 times higher than predicted by chance association. Therefore, if the occurrence would not be predicted by chance association, why do clefts occur with heart anomalies? Because of syndromic association.

REFERENCES

Cohen, M. M., Jr. (1976). The Robin anomalad—its nonspecificity and associated syndromes. *Journal of Oral Surgery, 34,* 587–593.

Cohen, M. M., Jr. (1982). *The child with multiple birth defects.* New York: Raven Press.

Cohen, M. M., Jr. (1986). *Craniosynostosis: Diagnosis, evaluation, and management.* New York: Raven Press.

Down, J. L. H. (1866). Observations on an ethnic classification of idiots. *Clinical Lecture Reports, London Hospital, 3,* 259–262.

Fraser, F. C. (1970). The genetics of cleft lip and palate. *American Journal of Human Genetics, 22,* 336–352.

Fraser, F. C. (1974). Updating the genetics of cleft lip and palate. *Birth Defects Original Article Series, 10*(8), 107–111.

Fraser, F. C. (1976). The multifactorial/threshold concept—uses and misuses. *Teratology, 14,* 267–280.

Fraser, F. C. (1980). Evolution of a palatable multifactorial threshold model. *American Journal of Human Genetics, 32,* 796–813.

Hall, J. G. (1984). Vitamin A: A newly recognized human teratogen. Harbinger of things to come? *Journal of Pediatrics, 105,* 583–584.

Hall, J. G., Pauli, R. M., Wilson, K. M. (1980). Maternal and fetal sequelae of anticoagulation during pregnancy. *American Journal of Medicine, 68,* 122–129.

Hanson, J. W. (1983). Teratogenic agents. In E. H. Emory & D. L. Rimoin (Eds.), *Principals and practices of medical genetics* (pp. 127–151). Edinburgh: Churchill Livingstone.

Hersh, J. H., Podruch, P. E., Rogers, G., & Weisskopf, B. (1985). Toluene embryopathy. *Journal of Pediatrics, 106,* 922–927.

Hill, L. M. (1984). Effects of drugs and chemicals on the fetus and newborn. *Mayo Clinic Proceedings, 59,* 755–765.

Kleppe, S. A., Katayama, K. M., Shipley, K. G., & Foushee, D. R. (1990). The speech and language characteristics of children with Prader-Willi syndrome. *Journal of Speech and Hearing Disorders, 55,* 300–309.

Lammer, E. J. (1985). Retinoic acid embryopathy. *New England Journal of Medicine, 313,* 837–841.

LeJeune, J. (1959). Le mongolisme. Premier example d'aberration autosomique humaine. *Annales Génétic, 1,* 41–49.

Manning, K. P. (1977). The larynx in cri-du-chat syndrome. *Journal of Laryngology and Otology, 91,* 887–892.

McKusick, V. A. (1966). *Mendelian inheritance in man* (1st ed.). Baltimore: Johns Hopkins University Press.

McKusick, V. A. (1994). *Mendelian inheritance in man* (11th ed.). Baltimore: Johns Hopkins University Press.

Morrow, B., Goldberg, R., Carlson, C., Gupta, R. D., Sirotkin, H., Collins, J., Dunham, I., O'Donnell, H. O., Scambler, P., Shprintzen, R. J., & Kucherlapati, R. (1995). Molecular definition of the 22q11 deletions in velo–cardio-facial syndrome. *American Journal of Human Genetics, 56,* 1391–1403.

Randall, P., Krogman, W. M., & Jahina, S. (1965). Pierre Robin and the syndrome that bears his name. *Cleft Palate Journal, 2,* 237–244.

Robin, P. (1923). La chute de la base de la langue considérée comme une nouvelle cause de gene dans la respiration naso-pharyngienne. *Bulletin d'Academie National Medicine, 89,* 37–41.

Robin, P. (1934). Glossoptosis due to atresia and hypotrophy of the mandible. *American Journal of Diseases in Children, 48,* 541–547.

Sadewitz, V. L., & Shprintzen, R. J. (1986). Pierre Robin: A new look at an old disorder. Video tape produced for the March of Dimes Birth Defects Foundation.

Sadewitz, V. L. &, Shprintzen, R. J. (1987). Communication impairment in children with multiple anomaly syndromes. Video tape produced for the March of Dimes Birth Defects Foundation.

Séguin, E. (1846). *Le traitement moral, l'hygiene et l'education des idiots.* Paris: J. B. Bailliere.

Shepard, T. H. (1986). *Catalog of teratogenic agents* (5th ed.). Baltimore: Johns Hopkins University Press.

Shprintzen, R. J. (1987). Reply from Dr. Shprintzen: CHARGE vs. velo–cardio-facial syndrome. *American Journal of Medical Genetics, 28,* 753–755.

Shprintzen, R. J. (1988). Pierre Robin, micrognathia, and airway obstruction: The dependency of treatment on accurate diagnosis. *International Anesthesiology Clinics, 26,* 84–91.

Shprintzen, R. J. (1992). The implications of the diagnosis of Robin sequence. *Cleft Palate Journal, 29,* 205–209.

Shprintzen, R. J., & Goldberg, R. (1982). A recurrent pattern syndrome of craniosynostosis associated with arachnodactyly and abdominal hernias. *Journal of Craniofacial Genetics and Developmental Biology, 2,* 65–74.

Shprintzen, R. J., Goldberg, R, Saenger, P., & Sidoti, E. J. (1982). Male-to-male transmission of Robinow's syndrome. *American Journal of Diseases in Children, 136,* 594–597.

Shprintzen, R. J., Siegel-Sadewitz, V. L., Amato, J., & Goldberg, R. B. (1985). Anomalies associated with cleft lip, cleft palate, or both. *American Journal of Medical Genetics, 20,* 585–596.

Shprintzen, R. J., & Singer, L. (1992). Upper airway obstruction and the Robin sequence. *International Anesthesiology Clinics, 30,* 109–114.

Smith, D. W. (1982). *Recognizable patterns of human malformation* (3rd ed.). Philadelphia: W. B. Saunders.

CHAPTER

4

THE STARTING POINT: TAKING A DETAILED HISTORY

The process of diagnosis is, in many ways, like solving a mystery. In some caes, a presenting phenotype is so obvious that diagnosis is practically unmistakable. In other cases, laboratory tests, such as karyotypes or metabolic tests can be used to confirm a diagnosis. However, to apply laboratory tests or to formulate a list of possible diagnoses (known as the process of **differential diagnosis**), the clinician must always have a starting place, a point of origin based on some piece of information that allows a narrowing of the field of possible diagnoses. Most experienced clinicians find this starting point by obtaining a thorough history. Historical data may even provide such strong evidence of a particular diagnosis that some disorders can be ruled out completely prior to examination.

Obtaining a good quality history is dependent on both the person taking the history and the person providing the information. In the best of all possible worlds, the history taker asks all of the right questions to elicit all of the right responses from the historian. However, a poor quality history can be the result of either a failure of the history taker to ask pointed and specific questions or a historian who is vague or disinterested. In addition, a history may require more than a single session because certain information is available, but not necessarily remembered accurately by the patient or the parents. Some information can only be gleaned from records, such as hospital records or reports from various professionals, after an initial visit. However, even finding out about the existence of such records is dependent on the process of asking the right questions.

TAKING AN ACCURATE HISTORY: WHERE TO START

The starting point to a good history actually occurs prior to the time when the patient is seen. When an appointment is made, the parent or guardian of the child, or whoever is bringing the child to the appointment, should be asked to bring along any and all available medical, dental, speech pathology, psychology, educational, or other relevant records. If the parent does not have these records available, the clinician should ask for the records to be obtained prior to the visit. This process can be expedited by having the parent or guardian sign a release form so that the clinician can obtain the records directly. Also important, the clinician should try to ensure that the parent or guardian accompanying a child to the visit is the person most familiar with the individual's history. In today's society where both parents often work during the hours of typical patient visits, it is not unusual to have a grandparent, aunt or uncle, friend, or hired help bring a patient to a visit. Nonparental custodians may have little or superficial knowledge of the child's pertinent history. Therefore, clinicians should encourage parents to attend the appointment. One way to do so is to emphasize that, without an adequate history, it may be necessary to schedule an additional appointment.

It is also important to ask the parent to provide a provisional diagnosis at the time of referral. This could include diagnoses applied by other clinicians or health care providers, or a description of the problem in the parent's own words. This provisional diagnosis is important as a template for reviewing the records prior to the appointment and for researching conditions with which the clinician has little familiarity. By being prepared for an appointment, the clinician can avoid significant embarrassment which can arise from seeming ill-prepared. More important, however, is that the records and/or provisional diagnosis can focus the process of taking a history so that questions for the person providing the history can be to the point and directly aimed at obtaining the most relevant information. For example, Stickler syndrome, as described in Chapter 3, has severe myopia as a possible finding. Stickler syndrome is a common genetic form of connective tissue dysplasia and perhaps the second most common syndrome associated with cleft palate in the absence of cleft lip (Shprintzen, et al., 1985). Stickler syndrome is also the most common cause of Robin sequence, accounting for over one third of all patients with

Robin. If a patient with a cleft palate and micrognathia was referred for an evaluation, and in reviewing the records, the clinician found evidence of a club foot and eye problems (such as strabismus or the use of corrective lenses at an early age), the clinician would be able to ask pointed and specific questions about the findings associated with Stickler syndrome in the proband and immediate relatives. For example, the clinician could ask any of the following questions meant to elicit a history consistent with Stickler syndrome:

"Does your child or anyone else in your family ever complain of joint pains in the knees or ankles, or perhaps lower back pain?"

"Has anyone in your family ever lost vision in one or both eyes? Has anyone ever had a retinal detachment? Is there anyone in the family who wears very thick glasses?"

"Does anyone in your family have a hearing loss? Is it a high frequency hearing loss?"

With questions, the clinician is trying to elicit a history of the joint pains often associated with Stickler syndrome, the predisposition to retinal detachment and vitreoretinal degeneration, and the high frequency sensorineural hearing loss found in approximately 15–20% of patients with Stickler syndrome. These conditions are sufficiently unusual that a clinician would not typically ask about them in the average child with a cleft palate. Often, unless parents are asked a specific question about a condition, they might either forget or avoid responding to a more general question.

Prior to an appointment, it is also wise to advise the patient or the parent to be as familiar as possible with both the patient's history and the backgrounds of as many family members as possible. This includes knowing of any congenital anomalies in relatives, the causes of death of deceased family members, histories of learning disabilities, mental retardation, attention deficit disorder, dyslexia, and other disorders of structure or function. If there is a history of congenital anomalies, the clinician can ask the patient or the parents to bring photographs of family members who might be affected. If caretakers of the patient are not well prepared to give a detailed history, the diagnostic search is less narrowed and additional contacts may be necessary to obtain the needed historical data.

THE INTERVIEW

There are many possible starting points in the interview process designed to elicit a detailed history. The clinician can begin by asking questions about the patient, about the family, or about past history. A good opening question can relate to the reason for the patient being in your office. Questions such as, "What brings you here?" or "What problem does Johnny have that brought you here?" This question can help to show that you want to get down to business, that you want a description of the problem in the parent's own words, and that your primary interest is in the patient's disorder. After the initial description and/or provisional diagnosis is provided by the parents, the clinician can then focus on the specific problems of the child. If the clinician has had a chance to review records that have previously documented some of the problems, a list of questions can be drawn from the already available data. If, however, no records are available, the clinician must respond to the answers of the parents by asking a question designed to narrow the search for the underlying problem. Before asking any questions about other family members, it is important to first develop a good picture of the child's disorder.

It is usually a good idea to begin with the birth of the child. Ask where he or she was born, his or her birth weight, length, and the nature of the delivery (spontaneous vaginal delivery, induced labor, caesarian section). Ask how the patient's condition was immediately and shortly after birth. Were there any problems? What were the Apgar scores? How long was the hospital stay? How was his or her general health? Were any anomalies noted at or after birth? Were there any feeding or breathing problems?

A careful pregnancy history should be obtained for a number of reasons: to determine if the mother had any problems during pregnancy, to rule out any possible teratogenic or mechanically caused anomalies, and to establish a complete history of previous pregnancies and problems that may have occurred with previous or subsequent pregnancies. You should ask if the pregnancy went to full term. Then ask if there were any problems during the pregnancy. Ask what the mother's weight gain was. In obtaining the pregnancy history, it is important to be very specific about exposures to known teratogens. Questions should be aimed at specific teratogens or classes of teratogens. For example, it is not sufficient to ask if the mother took any drugs or medications. The examiner should ask specifically if the mother drank alcohol, if she used any tranquilizers, hallucinogens, amphetamines, cocaine, anticonvulsants, or blood thinners. The examiner should ask if the mother had any prolonged fevers during pregnancy. Was the mother exposed to or did she have any illnesses such as rubella, chicken pox, cytomegalovirus, and other viral or bacterial infections? Was her pregnancy monitored and did she get good prenatal care? What were the results of sonograms? Was there any bleeding or spotting? How many ultrasounds were done, when were they done, and what was the outcome? Did mother have gestational diabetes? Did mother have toxemia or high blood pressure? When did mother first feel quickening? Was the baby active throughout the pregnancy? Was the baby in a breech or transverse position? In other words, questions should be specific, but not asked in a way as to connote blame, shame, or judgment. Table 4–1 presents a list of items that should provide source material for questions regarding pregnancy.

After all questions have been exhausted, the examiner should conclude with a general question, such as, "Is there anything else you can tell me about the pregnancy that you think is important, or that I should know?" This type of question serves two purposes. First, it allows the mother to reflect back one

TABLE 4–1. A sample of questions to be asked about the mother's pregnancy and delivery during a history taking session.

Questions	Reasons for Asking
Where was Mary born?	General information.
How much did she weigh?	To compare to norms.
Do you know what her length was at birth?	To compare to norms.
Do you know what her Apgar scores were?	To determine if there was any immediate compromise at birth.
How long did she stay in the hospital after birth?	To determine if there were any problems in the neonatal period.
Was it a normal delivery?	To assess maternal problems or fetal distress.
Was labor spontaneous, or was it induced?	To determine if there were any gestational problems.
How long were you in the hospital after birth?	To determine if maternal health was good.
Was your pregnancy full term?	To check for prematurity.
Were you receiving good prenatal care from an obstetrician or family doctor?	To check for prenatal problems.
Did you have any sonograms during pregnancy? When? Were they normal?	To check for prenatal problems.
Did you have an amniocentesis or CVS (chorionic villus sampling)?	To determine if a karyotype or other diagnostic procedures were done.
Did you have any problems during pregnancy?	To check for uterine environment or teratogenic problems.
How much weight did you gain?	To assess maternal health.
Did you have any bleeding or spotting?	To check for possible intrauterine problems.
Did you have any problem establishing the pregnancy?	To determine if there were fertility problems and/or use of fertility drugs.
How many children do you have?	Pedigree information and family history.
Let me have their names and ages.	Pedigree information and family history.
How many pregnancies have you had?	Pedigree information and family history.
Did you have any miscarriages?	Pedigree information and family history.
Were any of your pregnancies terminated?	Pedigree information and family history.
Are all of your children living?	Pedigree information and family history.
I'm sorry to hear that. What happened? (*to be asked if any children have died*)	To determine if the proband's problem is familial.
When did you first feel Mary move during pregnancy?	To assess prenatal maturity and health.
Was it a normal amount of movement?	To assess prenatal maturity and health.

(continued)

Questions	Reasons for Asking
Did you take any medications of drugs during pregnancy?	To check for teratogenic influences.
Have you ever had any seizures or take anticonvulsant medications, like dilantin? Did you use any street drugs, such as cocaine, heroin, or amphetamines?	To check for teratogenic influences.
Did you drink alcohol during pregnancy?	To check for teratogenic influences.
Did you have any high fevers during pregnancy?	To check for teratogenic influences.
What was the highest fever, and how long did it last?	To check for teratogenic influences.
Did you have any rashes during pregnancy, or just before?	To check for teratogenic influences.
Did you have any illnesses during pregnancy? Did you have German measles, measles, chicken pox, or any other viral illness?	To check for teratogenic influences.
Were you treated for any infections during pregnancy?	To check for teratogenic influences.
Did you use any antibiotics or other medicines during pregnancy?	To check for teratogenic influences.

more time to make sure she did not forget something important. Second, on many occasions, mothers may secretly harbor some feelings of guilt because of things that they may believe, incorrectly, led to the problems in their child. In some cases, guilt may be bound up in folk beliefs or superstitions. Some European folk myths suggest that women who are frightened by animals during pregnancy, particularly rabbits, may give birth to a child with a cleft lip ("hare" lip). In other cases, mothers may believe that substances that they consumed were teratogenic, even though they are not. For example, although many substances have been reported to be suspected teratogens in the popular press, scientific study may not have confirmed this suspicion. Common substances such as aspirin and caffeine have been implicated as teratogens in newspapers, which may have been read by millions of people, whereas scientific publications refuting these substances as teratogens are read by relatively few professionals in scientific journals. Therefore, a mother's suspicions that she may have done

something wrong may not necessarily be ascertained during questioning because the suspicion is so off base that the history taker would not even think of asking pertinent questions.

THE PEDIGREE

Once the specifics of the pregnancy have been recorded, it is time to turn attention to other family members, other children, and pregnancies. It is at this point that genetic counselors and clinical geneticists construct a pedigree, which contains a family tree that displays anomalies and diagnoses in the proband's extended family. The pedigree is a very useful tool for the geneticist, both for diagnosis and counseling. Pedigrees help to show modes of inheritance and possible clues regarding anomalies or traits shared by more than one family member. The pedigree is constructed based on the information obtained from the history. There are standard symbols used by geneticists who construct pedigrees (Figure 4–1). Figure 4–1 shows the

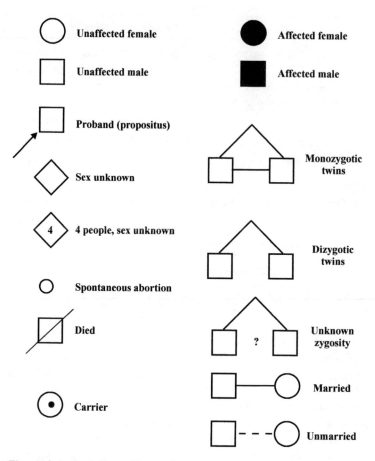

Figure 4–1. Symbols used in a pedigree.

symbols typically used in a pedigree to connote various individuals and conditions. Figure 4–2 shows a pedigree of a family with van der Woude syndrome. In this case, the pedigree is very informative, and the diagnosis can essentially be made from the pedigree information. It can be seen in the key that only three anomalies are present in this large pedigree: cleft lip, cleft palate, and lower lip pits or mounds. Each generation of the family has affected individuals so that a vertical pattern of transmission is evident in the pedigree. Because both females and males are affected and because there is male to male transmission, the trait must be autosomal dominant (see Chapter 3). Also important is the fact that within the same sibship there are individuals

who have cleft palate without cleft lip and individuals who have cleft lip with cleft palate. Mixing of cleft type within a family is essentially always indicative of a syndromic cause for the cleft. There are a number of multiple anomaly syndromes which may have either cleft lip and palate or cleft palate only as clinical features. The most common of these syndromes is van der Woude syndrome (the association of clefting with pits or mounds in the lower lip), but the same mixing of cleft type also occurs in popliteal pterygium syndrome (which may also have associated lip pits), Robinow syndrome, Rapp-Hodgkin ectodermal dysplasia, Treacher Collins syndrome, and femoral dysgenesis-unusual facies syndrome, among others. Therefore,

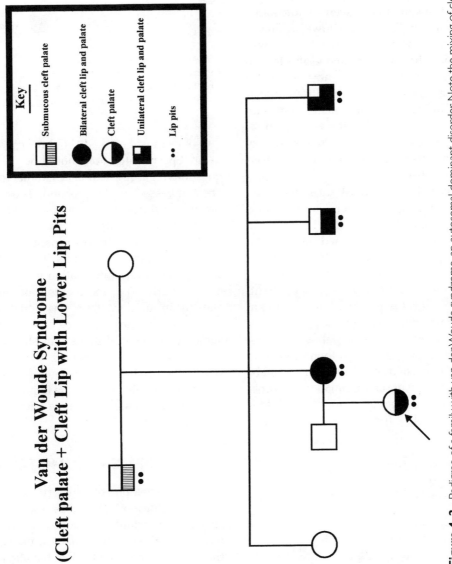

Van der Woude Syndrome
(Cleft palate + Cleft Lip with Lower Lip Pits)

Key

☐ Submucous cleft palate

● Bilateral cleft lip and palate

◑ Cleft palate

◪ Unilateral cleft lip and palate

∷ Lip pits

Figure 4–2. Pedigree of a family with van der Woude syndrome, an autosomal dominant disorder. Note the mixing of cleft type within a single sibship, something that only occurs in syndromic clefting.

the vertical pattern of transmission, the mixing of cleft type, and the presence of lip pits without other anomalies is diagnostic of van der Woude syndrome, which is caused by a mutant gene on the long arm of chromosome 1.

Pedigrees showing autosomal recessive traits will not usually show the vertical pattern of transmission as seen in autosomal dominant conditions, as shown in Figure 4–2. In autosomal recessive traits, pedigrees may show more than one affected sib with both parents being normal. Autosomal recessive traits can be differentiated from X-linked recessive traits if there is an affected female child (Figure 4–3). In X-linked recessive pedigrees, except in very rare cases, only male children will be affected (Figure 4–4).

The clinician should ask questions in an orderly sequential manner. The questions should be aimed not only at living children, but also any other established pregnancies. If either parent has had more than one mate, questions must also be asked to ascertain information about any children not currently living with the parents, but who might share genetic material with the proband. It is typical to start by asking about the first established pregnancy and then proceed to any younger children. The parent should be asked if there were any anomalies, any problems with the pregnancy, and if the child is alive and well. If the child is not alive, then

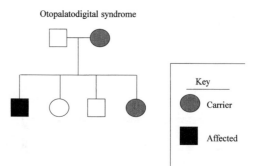

Otopalatodigital syndrome

Figure 4–4. A pedigree showing X-linked recessive inheritance of otopalatodigital syndrome, type I.

questions must be asked about the cause of death. Specific attention should be paid to questions regarding anomalies similar to the ones expressed by the proband. The same process should be carried out for each child. The number of spontaneous abortions (miscarriages) should be documented along with the length of gestation. It should be determined if any information is available on the abortus (i.e., the presence of anomalies, if an amniocentesis was done), and problems with the pregnancy. Table 4–2 lists some of the general items that should be covered in process of taking the history with reference to specific congenital anomalies which might occur in the family, especially for the speech-language pathologist or audiologist.

DEVELOPMENTAL HISTORY

A careful developmental history should be obtained. Questions should be asked about specific important milestones, including when the baby first held its head up, when the baby sat unassisted, when babbling began, the age at the production of first words, when the baby crawled, cruised, and walked, and when phrases and sentences were produced. It is obviously important for the clinician to be familiar with the range of normal development for these milestones. Depend-

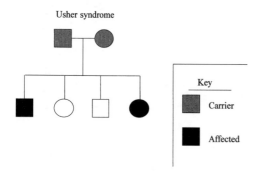

Usher syndrome

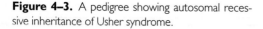

Figure 4–3. A pedigree showing autosomal recessive inheritance of Usher syndrome.

TABLE 4–2. A sample of questions to be asked about anomalies in other family members.

Questions	Reasons for Asking
Are all of your children alive and well?	Pedigree information and family history.
Tell me about Alan. What was his date of birth? Does he have any problems? Does he have any abnormalities in his structure, such as facial, hand, or heart anomalies? Is his development normal? Is he of normal growth and development? Does he have the same problem as Mary?	Pedigree information and family history and to determine if any other family members have the same problems (accounting for variable expression) as the proband.
(The same questions should be asked about all siblings and both parents)	
Is there anyone in the family with mental retardation or learning disabilities?	Pedigree information and family history.
Is there anyone in the family with any type of structural abnormality, such as abnormal ears, abnormalities of the hands, heart defects, cleft palate, or club foot?	Pedigree information and family history and to determine if any other family members have the same problems (accounting for variable expression) as the proband.
Is there anyone in the family who has trouble seeing or hearing? Is there anyone in the family with a speech disorder? What kind?	Pedigree information and family history and to determine if any other family members have the same problems (accounting for variable expression) as the proband.
Let's explore your family background. This is important because sometimes certain problems can be specific to certain population subgroups, like sickle cell anemia in African Americans, or Tay Sachs disease in people of Jewish background from Eastern Europe. Are your parents alive and well? Do they have any health problems? What are they?	To check for specific genetic disorders that known to segregate within racial or ethnic subgroups.
If the parents are not alive: What was the cause of death for your mother/father? How old was he/she when he/she died?	Pedigree information and family history and to determine if any other family members have the same problems (accounting for variable expression) as the proband.
What is your mother's ethnic background? Where was she born? Where were her parents from?	To check for specific genetic disorders which are known to segregate within racial or ethnic subgroups.
(Repeat for the father's family).	
Do you have any brothers and sisters? How many? Let's start with the oldest. When was he/she born? Does he/she have any health or developmental problems? Does he/she have children? Can you tell me who they are and how old they are? Do any of them have any health or developmental problems? Can you tell me what they are?	Pedigree information and family history and to determine if any other family members have the same problems (accounting for variable expression) as the proband.
Are there any other relatives that you know of who have any birth defects, mental retardation, developmental delay, or other health problems?	Pedigree information and family history and to determine if any other family members have the same problems (accounting for variable expression) as the proband.
Is Mary smaller (or taller) than the other members of the family?	To determine if a disorder of stature is a familial pattern or unique to the proband.
Is there anyone else in the family who looks like Mary, or who has similar problems?	To determine if there are any other affected individuals in the family.

ing on the age of the patient, the clinician should also ask about physical development, such as the age of eruption of the teeth, when handedness was expressed, the onset of puberty in males or the first menstrual period in females. Table 4–3 lists appropriate questions for this phase of the history.

A history of illnesses and hospitalizations should also be obtained. Questions regarding general health, any operations, the frequency of upper respiratory infections, ear infections, behavioral problems, learning problems, and social problems should be elicited. The clinician should be aware that parents may be reluctant to talk about some of these issues. Therefore, questions must be asked kindly, yet in a manner that is straightforward in order to elicit accurate information. Table 4–4 lists some appropriate questions regarding a health history for the patient and his or her family.

FACTORS THAT CAN CONFOUND THE HISTORY TAKING PROCESS

Even when the clinician asks all of the right questions, the history taking process can be stymied by a care provider who fails to respond appropriately to the questions. Sometimes the reason for the incorrect or incomplete answers is important to understand because it may connote problems that can interfere with good patient care. These problems may cause the parent to refuse care for the child, misdirect care, or, by inaction, cause care to be withheld.

Denial

Most parents want to have a "perfect" child. Far from being a selfish desire, it is more one of hopefulness and the normal parental motive to want a child to have a happy and healthy life. Parents have a 9-month "waiting period" during which their hopes and fears are compounded with each passing day.

When a child is born with congenital anomalies, one of the common psychological defense mechanisms for dealing with the problem is **denial**. Denial may be expressed in a number of ways, including the practice of **avoidance**. In its most benign form, parents who exercise denial minimize the severity of the child's problems, although they do attend to them properly. This type of denial can be recognized by passivity on the part of the parents during the interview and history. Important components of the history may be reported almost incidentally in this type of situation, as if they were not terribly important or worthy of attention. For example, children with Down syndrome (trisomy 21) always have some type of cognitive abnormality, ranging from severe mental retardation in the worst cases to borderline normal intellectual function in the mildest cases (which are often mosaics). The following excerpt is directly quoted from an interview conducted with the mother of a 9-year-old child with Down syndrome (the child's name has been changed):

Q: "How old was Kathy when she began speaking in sentences?"

A: "Ohhh, I'm not sure I remember, but it wasn't much different from her brother and her sisters."

Q: "Are you sure you don't remember her age? Was it before she was 3 years old?"

A: "I really don't remember exactly, but, you know, Kathy is quite bright. People are really amazed at how quickly she picks things up."

Q: "What is Kathy's current school placement?"

A: "Well, she's in a small class setting especially designed for children with communication handicaps."

Q: "Has she had a neuropsychological assessment?"

A: "What's that?"

TABLE 4–3. A sample of questions to be asked about a patient's developmental history.

Questions	Reasons for Asking
Were Mary's developmental milestones normal?	To assess developmental milestones.
How old was Mary when she was able to lift her head?	To assess motor milestones.
How old was she when she sat unsupported?	To assess motor milestones.
How old was she when she was able to stand?	To assess motor milestones.
How old was Mary when she began to cruise?	To assess motor milestones.
How old was she when she walked?	To assess motor milestones.
How old was Mary when she began to babble?	To assess speech/language milestones.
How old was Mary when she said her first word?	To assess speech/language milestones.
What was her first word? (*parents usually report the child's first word to be ma-ma. If so, ask the following question*)	To assess speech/language milestones.
When she said *ma-ma*, did she use that word specifically to signify you?	To assess speech/language milestones.
What were the next words she said?	To assess speech/language milestones.
How old was Mary when she began putting two words together?	To assess speech/language milestones.
How old was Mary when she began to speak in sentences?	To assess speech/language milestones.
How old were her siblings when they began to speak?	To assess speech/language milestones in relation to familial patterns.
How did Mary compare with her siblingss when it came to her other developmental milestones?	To assess speech/language milestones in relation to familial patterns.
How did she compare with other children and her siblings when it came to running, playing, and sports?	To assess motor milestones in relation to familial patterns.
Did anyone ever tell you that she had poor fine or gross motor control?	To assess motor milestones.
How old was Mary when she was toilet trained?	To assess motor milestones.
How old was Mary when she was able to feed herself?	To assess motor milestones.
How old was she when she could count to ten?	To assess speech/language milestones.
How old was Mary when she was able to recite the alphabet?	To assess speech/language milestones.
How is Mary with other children? Does she play well with others?	To determine if temperament is normal. To determine if social skills are age appropriate. To determine if overall development is age consistent.
What grade is Mary in at school? Is she doing well? Does she have any problems? Is she receiving any special help?	To determine if educational placement and achievement are consistent with chronological age. To determine if there are any special learning or educational deficits.

TABLE 4–4. A sample of questions to be asked about a patient's health history.

Questions	Reasons for Asking
Has Mary been in good health?	Introductory question.
Has she ever had any operations or been hospitalized since birth? What for?	To determine if illnesses are related to a genetic diagnosis.
Has she had any ear infections? How many does she get every year? Has she ever had her hearing tested? What were the results?	To determine if illness history is contributory to a communicative impairment.
Has she ever had pneumonia or bronchitis?	To determine if there is an immune deficiency which can be genetic.
Did she feed well as a baby?	To determine if there was "failure-to-thrive" in infancy.
How much did she weigh at 3 months of age? 6 months of age? One year of age?	To assess postnatal growth velocity; to determine if small stature is present and if it is consistent with prenatal or postnatal growth deficiency.
Did she sleep well as a baby?	To determine if the baby was excessively irritable, neurologically impaired, or if obstructive apnea was present.
Did she ever snore or make snorting noises during sleep, or does she snore now?	To determine if there was any evidence of obstructive respiration which might contribute to failure-to-thrive.
Has Mary ever had any seizures?	To determine if there are any signs of focal neurological lesions or neurologic disorders.
Has Mary ever had any excessively high fevers? How long did they last?	To determine if there is a history of serious illness, poor temperature control, or febrile seizures.
Has Mary had frequent middle ear infections? When? How many does she get in a year?	To determine if conductive hearing loss could contribute to speech-language disorders.
Has Mary ever had an eye examination? What were the results?	To determine if there was any indication of visual impairment.
Has Mary had all of her childhood immunizations, such as measles, mumps, rubella, and DPT?	To make sure that problems are not related to postnatal illness rather than heritable conditions.
Has Mary had a history of urinary tract infections?	Frequent urinary tract infections may be indicative of renal, urethral, or bladder anomalies.

Q: "A psychological work-up . . . such as IQ tests, perceptual tests, and so on. I would assume she has had one for school placement."

A: "I think she probably has. Is that like an IEP?"

Q: "Well, it's probable that some type of psychological assessment was done as part of the IEP. Do you remember the results?"

A: "Not really, but they did tell me that Kathy needed this special class because of her speech problem."

Q: "Before you leave, I would like you to sign a release form so we can get copies of the IEP. They're not included in the records you've given me today."

A: "OK."

Following this interview, the records indicated that Kathy had a measured IQ of 60 with significant perceptual and learning problems, as well as marked language impairment. Her class placement was in a special education setting for children with mild mental retardation. Although the mother knew this to be the case, it may have been too painful for her to admit, so she carefully choreographed her way around a direct answer, but even with her denial being obvious, she still managed to arrange all appropriate therapies for her daughter and placed her in the best possible educational setting. Therefore, she used her denial as a successful defense mechanism without letting it lead to avoidance.

When parents exercise avoidance, they not only deny the problem, they also fail to follow through on proper treatment and follow-up. An example of avoidance is illustrated by the following excerpt from an actual interview of an individual with Usher syndrome (see Chapter 3), an autosomal recessive genetic syndrome of deafness. The responses have been translated from American Sign Language:

Q: "When did you find out you had Usher syndrome?"

A: "Not until I was over 20 years old. When I was a boy, I knew my brother was deaf, and I thought that was all there was to it. My brother, who is 2 years older than me, always wore glasses, so I wasn't surprised when his vision started getting worse. I left home at 18 to go to college and while I was there, I started to notice that I wasn't seeing as well as before. I went to an eye doctor for the first time. He told me I had retinitis pigmentosa. He asked me how many of my family members had Usher syndrome. I had never heard of Usher syndrome and never knew anyone who had it. When I came home for Christmas vacation a week later, I asked my mother if she knew I had Usher syndrome, and if she knew, why she never took me to an eye doctor. She broke down and started to cry. She said she had known I had Usher syndrome ever since my brother had been diagnosed over ten years earlier. She was afraid to tell me because she didn't want me to know I might go blind, too. She also told me that she felt very guilty because it was a genetic dis-

ease and she gave it to me and my brother. She said that if she had known about it after my brother was born, she wouldn't have had any more children. That made me cry."

The intent of exercising avoidance is not the same for everyone. In some cases, the parents are seeking to defuse feelings of guilt they may have because they interpret the problems their child is having as being their fault. Feelings of guilt are not specific to the etiology of the anomalies in the child. Whether the disorder is chromosomal, genetic, teratogenic, or mechanically induced, the parents may feel that something they did or failed to do contributed to the problem. Nor is the presence of denial and avoidance necessarily related to the reality of the parental contribution to the problem. For example, many chromosomal anomalies or genetic disorders are the result of spontaneous mutations or rearrangements of genetic material. Such rearrangements are completely unpredictable and are, in fact, part of the normal process of cellular activity. Anomalies resulting from spontaneous alteration of the human genome could occur in anyone and can appropriately be regarded as chance occurrences. Therefore, there is nothing one can do to avoid such spontaneous changes, and the parent of a child who has one of these newly occurring disorders is truly blameless in every sense of the word. However, the guilt patents feel for bringing a child with a problem into the world is often difficult to manage.

Feelings of guilt are also not necessarily related to the severity of the problem. Some parents regard even minor anomalies as major catastrophes, whereas others contend with major problems extremely well. Two cases will help to illustrate this disparity in parental response. In the first case, a child was referred at 1 month of age with a mild cranial asymmetry, which was secondary to intrauterine constriction. The child was in a breech presentation for a prolonged period of time so that the head was not free to move normally and the neck muscles were not able to stretch. With the neck in a chronic flexed position to one side, there was a shortening of the muscles on one side causing the head to be pulled abnormally to the side with the shortening. This condition is known as torticollis. Because of the constant muscular force on the one side of the head, a constricting pressure is applied to the calvarium and skull base which may result in craniosynostosis, or premature fusion of the cranial sutures (which normally remain open into adult life). When detected early enough, physical therapy can be applied to the shortened muscles to stretch them out and allow a full range of motion for the head and neck and a smaller likelihood that craniosynostosis will advance and cause more severe cranial and facial asymmetry. This condition is a deformation rather than a malformation. In fact, it is a deformational **sequence**. In such cases, the torticollis and craniofacial asymmetry are secondary to the positional compression of the fetus resulting in shortening of the sternocleidomastoid muscle. The shortening of the sternocleidomastoid then causes the presentation of the torticollis and craniosynostosis. By removing the deformational force and resolving the shortening of the sternocleidomastoid, normal growth can resume and very often, the facial asymmetry will resolve within months or a year or two. The child in question was worked up by the craniofacial team and found to have a torticollis and just the beginning of a slight fibrous fusion of the coronal suture on the left side of the skull (Figure 4–5). No surgery was recommended for the cranial deformity because the fusion was not solid bone and it was anticipated that resolution of the torticollis would result in normal growth of the left side of the cranium. Physical therapy was prescribed and the infant was treated for approximately 4 months with complete resolution. The patient was seen back every 3 months and serial photographs and measurements of the cranial landmarks (anthropometrics) were taken. By 9 months of age, the child's appearance was normal and continued follow-up through 3 years of age showed continued normal growth. Although the disorder in this case was unavoidable, it was not related to anything the mother did, was not caused by a maternal or paternal genetic disorder, and did not involve surgical treatment, the parents were devastated by the problem. They initially refused to accept the diagnosis and denied that there was a problem. They resisted the scheduling of the CT scan, even though they had visited a second craniofacial center and had been given the same diagnosis. It took enormous effort to convince them of the need for physical therapy, and even after initiation of the treatment, they resisted follow-up appointments to check on the progress of craniofacial growth. The mother would become very agitated at each appointment and resist any suggestion that their child looked abnormal. It was only with the intervention of their pediatrician, who was a close personal friend of the father, that the family was convinced to come in for appointments. Genetic counseling was provided for the family. The session was contentious and the family was clearly unhappy about the fact that the child had an anomaly. During the session, they insisted that they would have no more children because of their experience with their son, even though there was an extremely low recurrence risk (just fractions of a percent because the disorder was related to a positional deformation) and even though the child's problem was resolved without the need for dangerous or long-term treat-ment. Feelings of guilt were expressed by the mother in particular, even though she was told that there was no possible fault on her part. In this case, the parent's response to a relatively minor abnormality was deemed by the clinicians to be far out of proportion with the actual problem.

At the opposite end of the spectrum is a case of a mother who had a bilateral cleft lip and palate as part of the spectrum of a single gene autosomal dominant condition known as van der Woude syndrome. Van der Woude syndrome is the association of clefting of the palate and/or lip and palate and pits or mounds of the lower lip (Figure 4–6). Van der

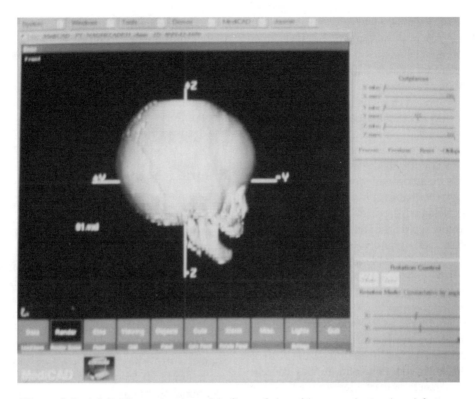

Figure 4–5. A 3-D CT scan showing a slight fibrous fusion of the coronal suture in an infant secondary to a positional deformation resulting in torticollis.

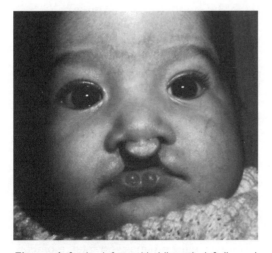

Figure 4–6. An infant with bilateral cleft lip and palate and lower lip pits (van der Woude syndrome).

Woude syndrome represents an excellent example of **variable expression** as discussed in Chapter 2. Looking at the pedigree of the patient described here, it can be seen that there are many affected individuals (Figure 4–2). However, it can also be seen that some individuals have cleft lip and palate (both unilateral and bilateral) with lip pits, some individuals have cleft palate without cleft lip in association with lip pits, and others have lip pits without a cleft of any type. Mixing of cleft type within a family (i.e., cleft lip and palate versus cleft palate without cleft lip) is only found in syndromes. This is because nonsyndromic clefting is specific to the timing of the embryonic events of lip fusion and palate fusion. Lip fusion occurs at approximately 4 weeks postfertilization while palate fusion occurs at approximately 9 weeks postfertilization. In embryonic terms, 5 weeks difference is a very long time. Much happens in embryonic development over the course of 5 weeks (actually, a lot happens in the course of a single day). Therefore, it would be unreasonable to think that the same causal agent would be present at both 4 weeks of development and 9 weeks of development. Genetic influences, however, are present for as long as the gene is active or for as long as a teratogenic influence is present (as in prolonged drinking in fetal alcohol syndrome). In the case of this particular patient, the mother received genetic counseling and was told of the diagnosis and the fact that her risk of having a child with the syndrome was 50% (as it is in autosomal dominant disorders). Although the chance of inheritance of the gene can be calculated, the degree of expression cannot. In other words, the fact that the mother had a bilateral cleft lip and palate would have no influence on the possible expression of the syndrome in the child. The mother decided to have a child, knowing of the risk. She called me from the birthing room within 30 minutes of the birth of her daughter to tell me how happy she was that "my baby only has a cleft palate."

These two disparate reactions to the birth of a child with congenital anomalies merely show that reactions to problems are as variable as people's personalities and temperaments. The clinician must not be judgmental about the reactions of parents and patients to their circumstances. Most importantly, the clinician must avoid any comments or questions that might imply fault or blame, such as, "Didn't you know you have a genetic disorder?" Probing questions regarding teratogens are also potentially laden with guilt connotations and must be asked matter-of-factly without judgmental intent or tone. Therefore, rather than asking if a mother drank to excess, drank heavily, or drank too much, the question should simply be, "Did you drink alcohol during pregnancy?" If there is a positive answer to that question, the mother should be asked, "What did you drink?" In other words, the historian is trying to determine if the mother drank beer, hard liquor, wine, or other alcohol-containing substances, such as cough syrup or mouth wash. The next question should be "how much did you drink?" If the mother is unable to answer, then the historian can ask more specific, but again nonjudgmental questions using the information obtained regarding the mother's favorite form of alcohol, such

as, "How many beers did you drink each day?" Subsequent questions can then be asked to determine if the consumption of alcohol occurred at a specific time each day, if the mother was a binge drinker (i.e., if she drank infrequently but consumed a large amount of alcohol during a single binge episode), and if she drank to the point of getting drunk.

Shame

Denial is one mechanism parents have for avoiding guilt and, as described above, may result in interference with adequate history-taking and patient care. Some people, however, cannot avoid feeling guilt and feel significant shame. In some cases, the shame is a reflection of deep sorrow over having "caused" the problems in the child. These feelings can be so strong that some parents may choose to avoid appointments because each contact with health care workers is an unpleasant reminder of the disorder, thus provoking additional shame and sorrow. Expressions of shame are usually recognized during the history session and other contacts. Parents often seem overly concerned about their child, may be weepy or sad, and may express regret that the child was born. Such regret may be a reflection of guilt, or may be an expression of humiliation or disgrace, especially in cultures where the offspring has a significance that goes beyond the simple birth of a child. Dealing with shame in most cases is easier for the professional than in dealing with denial. First, during the initial contact and history session, the health care provider should provide a positive perspective on patient care. It should be pointed out for the parent that keeping appointments and providing appropriate diagnostic and therapeutic expertise will make the child better. Negativity should be avoided in such cases, even if the prognosis for total resolution of a problem is poor. This does not mean that the clinician should lie to the family. This should never be done. However, information can be presented with a variety of accompanying explanations which help to put problems in their proper perspective. For example, during an initial visit when a comprehensive history is being taken, it is not unusual for parents to ask questions regarding their child's condition. Answers should be honest, but in situations where the parent's guilt is obviously resulting in shame and sorrow, every attempt should be made to shift answers away from enhancing their sorrow and feelings of guilt. The following conversation is an example of this type of approach in a family presenting with a child with a cleft palate:

Clinician: Are there any other people in your family who have cleft lip or cleft palate?

Mother: Not as far as I know. Does that mean that my baby has a cleft because of something that I did?

Clinician: No, it doesn't mean that at all. Is there anyone in your family who has small bumps or openings in the lower lip?

Mother: Why do you ask that?

Clinician: Sometimes there are little clues in people's faces or other body parts that help us determine genetic reasons for clefts happening.

Mother: So that if you don't find any clues, it means that I did something to cause the cleft?

Clinician: No, that's not what it means. Look, in many cases, clefts occur as brand new anomalies in families with no history of problems and without any contribution from the mother's actions during pregnancy or her general health. Based on what you've told me, your pregnancy was completely normal, you were extremely careful to maintain a good diet and avoid using drugs, and you have no family history of clefting. But perhaps what is most important is that your baby has a problem which can be fixed. Even though this will mean that he will have an operation, the large majority of these operations are successful

and his prognosis for a perfectly normal life is excellent. I would focus on that if I were you.

In this hypothetical case (although it is truly based on a composite of actual case interviews of similar content), the attention was turned away from the parent's guilt and focused on the excellent prognosis and normal life to be expected for the child. Of course, the parent's guilt will not be assuaged on a single visit, nor will he or she be convinced that everything will be fine based on a single counseling session. However, the process of breaking through feelings of shame induced by guilt must be begun as early as possible to prevent the parents from reinforcing their own sorrow over a long period of time. When the process runs unabated for years, the negative feelings will be much more difficult to reduce.

A more difficult form of shame to deal with is that prompted by cultural or social mores that are tied closely to the attributes of the child. In many societies, children are prized possessions and are seen as extensions of the parent (particularly the male children of male parents). Some cultures deem it important for men to have male children who will carry on the family name and who will be worthy of the existing family name. If the child is in any way unfit, his presence in the family may be viewed as a mark of shame, or a measure of inadequacy of the father. In some cases, fathers may spurn such children, or relegate them completely to mother's care while not participating in their lives at all. This type of response from a parent is extremely difficult to resolve because it is deeply ingrained in the parent's entire social, cultural, and possibly religious background. If nothing else, this type of parental reaction points out how sensitive genetic diagnosis and information can be. If handled insensitively, clumsily, or without regard to the family, genetic diagnosis and its sequelae can disrupt lives enormously. However, when used constructively and with care, the correct diagnosis often helps to improve patient care and provide a level of comfort to the parents because the information can help the parents come to terms with their child's problems. Although sorrow is a normal response at first, the clinician should bear in mind that if the parent's sorrow is related to anguish for the child rather than self-pity, it becomes easier to convince the parent that adequate follow-up is important for the patient so that the problem doesn't become worse.

A GUIDE FOR ASKING QUESTIONS

The tables in this chapter list a sampling of questions that can assist the clinician in initiat-ing a careful history session. They are grouped according to each phase of the history-taking session. Obviously, many questions are derived from previous responses and may be specific to an individual diagnosis. A full catalogue of such questions cannot be listed here, but many questions can be applied to nearly all people. For this list of questions, we will name the hypothetical patient Mary and her mother is the historian. Mary has two siblings, Alan and Sally. Some helpful guidelines for specific conditions are also provided in Table 4–5.

TABLE 4–5. Questions for some specific groups of disorders.

Questions	Reasons for Asking
A. HEARING LOSS	
When was her hearing loss first noticed?	To determine if the hearing loss presented at birth or later, thus providing clues to the possibility of congenital versus acquired loss.
Has her hearing gotten worse with age?	To determine if the hearing loss is progressive, which occurs in many multiple anomaly syndromes.
Were you told what caused her hearing loss?	General information.
Has Mary ever have any other abnormalities, like even minor defects of her hands, eyes, hair, or skin, like patches of different colored hair, rough and scaly skin, or different colored eyes?	The association of specific anomalies of various body structures is highly specific and may help to limit the field for diagnostic purposes, such as a white forelock or heterochromia iridium (different colored eyes) in Waardenburg syndrome, retinitis pigmentosa in Usher syndrome, or ichthyosis in Refsum syndrome.
Has Mary had a worsening in her coordination or school performance?	Some syndromes of hearing loss are associated with neurologic or central nervous system degeneration, such as Refsum syndrome or Cockayne syndrome.
Does she have any small holes or extra pieces of skin on her neck or near her ears?	Some syndromes have preauricular or cervical pits and/or tags, such as oculo-auriculo-vertebral dysplasia, BOR syndrome, and Townes-Brock syndrome.
Does Mary have any skin growths, birth marks, areas of skin discoloration, lumps, bumps, or even large freckles?	Syndromes with hamartoses (abnormalities of tissue organization often resulting in tumorlike growths) are often associated with hearing loss, such as neurofibromatosis type II (NF II), and LEOPARD syndrome.
Does Mary, or anyone in the family have any abnormalities of the kidneys?	Renal anomalies occur associated with hearing loss in a number of syndromes, such as BOR (branchio-oto-renal) syndrome.
Has Mary had an unusual increase in head size, the shape of her head, or forehead?	Bone overgrowth syndromes frequently result in hearing loss secondary to compression of the auditory nerve or temporal bone abnormalities, such as in frontometaphyseal dysplasia, craniometaphyseal dysplasia, craniodiaphyseal dysplasia, sclerosteosis, and van Buchem disease.

(continued)

B. CLEFT PALATE ± CLEFT LIP

Questions	Reasons for Asking
Does Mary have a history of cardiac abnormalities or a heart murmur? Has she ever had a chest X-ray?	Velo-cardio-facial syndrome is the most common syndrome of clefting, accounting for 8% of children with cleft palate without cleft lip and a smaller percentage of cleft lip cases. Right sided aortic arch, which can be found on chest X-ray, can occur in asymptomatic cases.
Does Mary or anyone else in the family have small bumps, mounds, or holes in the lower lip?	Van der Woude syndrome is a common syndrome associated with clefting and popliteal pterygium syndrome may also have lip pits and clefting.
Does Mary or anyone in the family have brittle hair, missing hair, abnormalities of the finger nails, or absence of sweating?	A number of syndromes with ectodermal dysplasia, such as EEC syndrome, Hay-Wells syndrome, and Rapp-Hodgkin syndrome, are associated with clefting.
Does Mary or anyone else in the family wear very thick glasses? Does she complain of joint pains, such as in her ankles, knees, or back?	Stickler syndrome accounts for nearly 5% of cases of cleft palate without cleft lip and over one third of all cases of Robin sequence.
Does Mary, or anyone else in the family have a history of learning disabilities, mental retardation, or mental illness, such as bipolar disorder (manic depressive illness)?	Over 25% of children with clefts have some cognitive deficiency. Essentially all children with velo-cardio-facial syndrome have learning disabilities, and over 70% have some form of bipolar disorder.
Does Mary or anyone else in the family have abnormalities of the fingers or toes?	Approximately 18% of children with clefts have anomalies of the limbs (mostly the fingers), such as contractures in Freeman-Sheldon syndrome, or ringlike constrictions in amnion rupture sequence.
For male children: Does he, or any male relatives, have abnormal genitals, such as a hypospadias, small penis, or undescended testicles? What about inguinal hernias?	Approximately 5% of children with clefting have syndromes which have genital anomalies, such as micropenis in Robinow syndrome, hypospadias in velo-cardio-facial syndrome, and cryptorchidism (undescended testicles) in Freeman-Sheldon syndrome. Inguinal hernias are also found in many of these syndromes.
Does Mary or anyone in the family have any missing teeth, enamel problems, or extra teeth?	Dental anomalies are common in a number of clefting syndromes, including those involving ectodermal dysplasia. Enamel hypoplasia is common in the primary dentition in children with velo-cardio-facial syndrome and several other disorders. Extra teeth are common in a few syndromes, including cleidocranial dysplasia (as is late dental eruption). A single central incisor is essentially pathognomonic for a mild form of holoprosencephaly. It should be kept in mind that nearly all children with complete clefts of the lip and palate have missing or supernumerary teeth secondary to the cleft.
Does Mary or anyone else in the family have any endocrine problems, such as pituitary abnormalities, hypocalcemia, diabetes, hyperthyroidisim, hypothyroidism, or hypoparathyroidism?	Growth deficiency occurs in over 20% of children with syndromes of clefting including both genetic and teratogenic disorders. Hypocalcemia occurs in velo-cardio-facial syndrome (as is hyperparathyroidism and hypothyroidism). Diabetes mellitus is found in several syndromes, including Turner syndrome. Hypoglycemia is common in Beckwith-Wiedemann syndrome.

(continued)

TABLE 4–5. *(continued)*

Questions	Reasons for Asking
C. COGNITIVE (LANGUAGE, LEARNING, AND INTELLECTUAL) DISORDERS	
For male children: Are his genitals of normal size?	The most common form of mental retardation in males (seen only in males because it is X-linked), the so-called Fragile X syndrome (Martin-Bell syndrome) has enlarged testes and/or enlarged penis in the majority of cases. Hypergenitalism and hypergonadism is also found in a number of other syndromes. Hypoplastic genitals (testes and/or penis) is also found in a substantial number of syndromes of cognitive impairment, such as Aarskog syndrome, CHARGE, Klinefelter syndrome, Noonan syndrome, and Prader-Willi syndrome.
Does Mary or anyone else in the family have abnormalities of the arms, legs, fingers, or toes?	Minor abnormalities of the fingers or toes are very common in many syndromes with cognitive impairment, such as hypoplastic or missing fingernails in fetal hydantoin syndrome, abnormal palmar creases in fetal alcohol or Down syndrome, contractures in Shprintzen-Goldberg syndrome, and shortening of the arms in de Lange syndrome.
Does Mary or anyone else in the family have abnormalities of the skin, such as different colored areas, birth marks, nevi, or different textured skin?	Cognitive impairment occurs in approximately 25–35% of individuals with neurofibromatosis, type I (NF I) which includes café-au-lait spots or small tumors on the skin. NF I accounts for approximately 90% of all NF cases and is one of the most common of genetic disorders. Skin anomalies with cognitive impairment also occurs in many other syndromes, such as LEOPARD syndrome, Sturge-Weber syndrome, and tuberous sclerosis.
Does Mary or anyone else in the family have any endocrine abnormalities?	Pituitary, thyroid, and parathyroid disorders are frequent findings in a large number of syndromes with cognitive impairment. Hypercalcemia is common in Williams syndrome, hypocalcemia in velo-cardio-facial syndrome. Adrenal abnormalities may also occur, as in Beckwith-Wiedemann syndrome.
Does Mary, or anyone else in the family have any eye abnormalities?	Embryologically, the eyes are formed from outpouchings of the developing brain. Structural anomalies of the eyes, such as retinal or iris colobomas or small eyes, are very frequently associated with cognitive impairments.

REFERENCES

Shprintzen, R. J., Siegel-Sadewitz, V. L., Amato, J., & Goldberg, R. B. (1985). Anomalies associated with cleft lip, cleft palate, or both. *American Journal of Medical Genetics, 20,* 585–596.

CHAPTER

5

THE DIAGNOSTIC PROCESS

It is very important to assign a diagnosis to the child or adult with multiple anomalies, but clinicians must walk a slender tightrope in the process, being careful not to make a slip that will ultimately result in poor or ineffective care for the patient. The danger of assigning an incorrect diagnosis is a major potential pitfall. Clinicians may be reluctant to provide a diagnosis if they have any degree of uncertainty. This reluctance may be spurred by concerns over medicolegal issues, concern that inappropriate treatments may be applied to the patient, or concern over influences on the family's long-term reproductive decisions. However, if this reluctance results in failure to provide accurate diagnosis to the patient, the potential for treatment errors or inadequate patient care may loom as large as if the wrong diagnosis had been applied. Therefore, clinicians should regard the process of diagnosis as a flexible and open-ended one. It then becomes easier to avoid some of the dangers associated with the precarious stroll across the decision-making tightrope.

ELEMENTS IMPORTANT TO ASSIGNING THE CORRECT DIAGNOSIS

As discussed in Chapter 1, the benefits of correct diagnosis accrue to both the patient and the clinician. The goal is better patient care, both to the individual patient under care by the particular clinician as well as to all patients with the same condition being treated by other clinicians. In other words, as more is known and understood about the condition by a larger number of professionals, the better patient care will be for all patients. By keeping the diagnostic process open-ended, as new information is gleaned by studying the patient, it can be reported and applied to other patients by other clinicians. Therefore, although a correct diagnosis may be reached, sometimes almost instantaneously, there is often more to learn about both the individual patient and the condition. The steps in the process of diagnosis and continuing research follow.

A Careful History

Because the process of obtaining a careful history is so important, an entire chapter was devoted to it in this book. The reason for the importance of the history is that it is the launching point for the diagnostic process. Because there are thousands of possible genetic and syndromic diagnoses, it is important to narrow the search as early as possible in the diagnostic process. The history session during the initial contacts with the patient is the first opportunity to reduce the field of possible diagnoses and may actually be the point in the process where the greatest percentage of narrowing of the search takes place. The history can often establish a mode of inheritance, a phenotypic spectrum, a natural history, and suggested diagnoses from other professionals. All of these factors become useful in the process of ruling out certain disorders while suggesting others as possible diagnoses.

Mode of Inheritance

For disorders of known genetic causation, establishing the mode of inheritance from the history can narrow the field of possible diagnoses significantly. This is especially true if the disorder can be established to have an X-linked mode of inheritance because of the relatively small number of X-linked disorders. However, even if an autosomal dominant mode of inheritance is established, the clinician is able to eliminate syndromes and disorders of autosomal recessive and X-linked inheritance.

Other Etiologies

For disorders of suspected teratogenic origin, diagnosis is actually completely dependent on historical information. Although the clinician may suspect a teratogenic disorder based on the patient's phenotype, there is a great deal of phenotypic overlap between genetically caused and teratogenically caused syndromes. For example, patients with velo-cardio-facial syndrome have an expansive phenotype with over 160 clinical findings. Among the clinical features associated with velo-cardio-facial syndrome are congenital heart anomalies (including, but not restricted to tetralogy of Fallot, aortic arch anomalies, and septal defects), cleft palate, learning disabilities, attention deficit disorder with hyperactivity, immune deficiency, relatively small stature, umbilical and inguinal hernias, a thin upper lip, retrognathia, and, in some cases, Robin sequence. Patients with fetal alcohol syndrome also may have any or all of these anomalies. Therefore, the phenotypes of velo-cardio-facial syndrome and fetal alcohol syndrome show a significant degree of phenotypic overlap so that diagnosis based solely on examination may be difficult for clinicians with limited experience with either disorder. However, if a history of ethanol teratogenesis is obtained, either from parental report or from medical records, the diagnosis of fetal alcohol syndrome is easily established. Without confirmation of alcohol use during pregnancy, the diagnosis of teratogenesis cannot be confirmed, even though the phenotype may be highly suspicious.

Historical reports of exposure to teratogenic agents may be difficult to obtain for a number of reasons. For one thing, there may be the perception of responsibility on the part of the patient's mother. For example, a mother who drinks ethanol during pregnancy even though she knows that alcohol is a teratogen may feel significant guilt because of her actions, regarding herself personally responsible for her child's anomalies. The perception of guilt might be very different, however, for a mother exposed to mercury by consuming tainted water or eating tainted fish. Because she did not consume the mercury voluntarily, she may feel anger, rather than guilt, because others may have been responsible for her consumption of the teratogen. She would therefore be likely to volunteer the information without hesitation, whereas a mother who drank large amounts of alcohol during pregnancy might be reluctant to implicate herself in behavior that carries a distinct implication of personal responsibility.

Sometimes the person providing the history will make a difference in the provision of information. In cases where teratogenesis is related to the consumption of alcohol or illegal drugs, biological mothers may not necessarily be the child's primary caregiver. On occasion, foster mothers, grandmothers, or other relatives may be the historians because mothers have abrogated their caregiving responsibilities because of addiction or illness. In such cases, it is usually easier to extract information regarding teratogenesis from a third party who does not feel personal responsibility for the child's condition. However, because people who use illicit drugs or drink alcohol to excess are often secretive about their consumption of these substances, third parties may not have the best quality of information regarding the pattern of use.

Unless the right questions are asked during the history session, the mother may not be aware of her exposure to a teratogen. It is therefore important for the clinician to be thorough and direct in questioning the mother, as described in Chapter 4.

Historical clues to causation by mechanical factors are much more difficult to ascertain. In general, indications of mechanically induced anomalies, whether deformations or disruptions, are based on clues that require the clinician's interpretation because the opportunity to observe mechanically induced events is rare. One exception is the observation or history of abnormal fetal position, such as a breech presentation. Both clinical examination by the obstetrician or ultrasound can document fetal constriction in breech presentation. Resulting anomalies, such as club foot, can be directly linked to this type of constriction. The presence of a twin within a constricted space can also be seen with ultrasound studies. Other deformations, such as amnion rupture sequence (see Chapter 3, Figure 3–5), can only be inferred from the specific dysmorphic features associated with the amniotic adhesions. In some cases, remnants of amniotic tissue can be found adhering to

the clefts, ringlike constrictions, or amputations. However, in the majority of instances, mechanically induced anomalies are diagnosed based on a combination of factors, including the absence of familial history; the absence of a recognizable syndromic pattern of genetic, chromosomal, or teratogenic etiology; and the probability that the observed anomaly is related to physical compression or distortion.

In the majority of cases, chromosomally caused disorders will not be revealed by historical data, usually because they will have been detected prior to referral, most often in the newborn period. Because the large majority of chromosomal syndromes involve major and severe malformations, pediatricians, neonatologists, or clinical geneticists will have been consulted in the neonatal period and a karyotype will have been ordered. This is true for the syndromes caused by large chromosomal rearrangements, such as trisomies, monosomies, and other aneuploidies involving large segments of chromosomes. However, a number of syndromes with less severe presentations are now known to have very small deletions or other chromosome rearrangements, which can, on occasion, be detected by high resolution karyotypes (see Chapters 2, 3, and 7). High resolution karyotypes are relatively new procedures for chromosome analysis and must be specifically requested if a clinician suspects that the patient has a disorder that might be caused by one of the very small chromosome rearrangements and would not be visible using standard karyotypic procedures. (See Chapter 7 for additional discussion of high resolution chromosome analysis.) A number of syndromes have recently been found to be associated with very tiny chromosome abnormalities, such as velo-cardio-facial syndrome (the long arm of chromosome 22 at the 22q11 band) and Prader-Willi syndrome (the long arm of chromosome 15 at 15q11 through 15q13 band). Standard karyotypes will not reveal the 22q11 deletions associated with velo-cardio-facial syndrome, and even high resolution karyotypes will detect these deletions only approximately 15% of the time. In addition, clinicians must suspect the diagnosis in order to request that the karyotype be done. A careful history can potentially yield information that might lead to the suspicion of the diagnosis, both in terms of information about the patient and, in familial cases, information about other family members. In general, certain parameters lead to the suspicion of a chromosomal rearrangement:

1. A history of frequent spontaneous abortions (miscarriages) or neonatal deaths.
2. The association of multiple major anomalies that do not fit a pattern of a known syndrome of genetic causation (i.e., not related to a chromosomal aneuploidy), especially if mental retardation, developmental delay, and/or short stature are a part of the phenotype.
3. The association of certain types of major anomalies, especially heart, limb, brain, and craniofacial.

A potential problem related to requesting karyotypes is that the cost of the procedure often is not covered by medical insurance policies. Insurance companies, particularly managed care systems, are denying payment for high resolution karyotypes costing hundreds of dollars (which may be out of the reach of many patients) because they regard them as being "medically unnecessary"). This problem undoubtedly will increase in the frequency of occurrence over time.

Informed Patient Families

As discussed in Chapter 4, it is extremely important for the people providing the historical data to know as much as possible about the patient and as many family members as possible. Of course, the corollary to this point is that the clinician taking the history must be interested in these data. It is the responsibility of the clinician to impress

on the family both the necessity for the information and the honest reporting of it. The clinician must also understand that the process of gathering information may be a continuing one. New members with anomalies may be born into the family after the initial contact with the patient. Another possibility is that other members may develop disorders consistent with a particular diagnosis. For example, in velo-cardio-facial syndrome, psychiatric problems tend to develop in adolescence or early adult life. There may be affected individuals in the family who did not display these symptoms at the time of the initial history session, but developed them a year or two later.

The Transdisciplinary Approach

It has been stated by many authors on many occasions that patients with complicated problems are best served when evaluated and treated by teams of professionals made up of individuals from multiple disciplines. This type of model has been used in the management of patients with clefting disorders and craniofacial anomalies for over 50 years and is held as the gold standard for case management. However, as pointed out recently (LeBlanc & Cisneros, 1995; Shprintzen, 1995), there are differences in the types of interactions among members of teams. It can even be argued that not everyone defines **team** in the same way. Interactions between professionals working in the same "team" may be divided into three types: multidisciplinary, interdisciplinary, and transdisciplinary (LeBlanc & Cisneros, 1995; Shprintzen, 1995).

Multidisciplinary means that a team is constituted of a number of different individuals each of whom performs an assessment and formulates an opinion that is passed on to the patient for consideration. The patient supposedly benefits from getting many different opinions from a variety of professional perspectives. The **interdisciplinary** approach takes the team concept one step further. Not only does the patient benefit from multiple opinions, but on interdisciplinary teams, the team members interact in a way implying that they allow opinions from other team members to influence their decisions. Thus, interdisciplinary teams have a higher degree of cooperation than those that simply provide a variety of practitioners. Rather than passing on multiple opinions to the patient, on interdisciplinary teams, a single recommendation is provided, representing a distillation of the opinions of all of the professionals involved in the assessment. It is usually the practice of interdisciplinary teams to meet face-to-face to discuss their opinions openly which serves as the core of the decision-making process. The third approach, **transdisciplinary**, takes the concept of interaction one additional step further.

A transdisciplinary approach implies that individuals representing a variety of different fields of expertise go beyond interacting. They actually go to the trouble of learning as much as possible about other disciplines. Surgeons learn about dentistry, dentists learn about speech pathology, and,

in what is really the substance of this text, speech pathologists learn about genetics. In this way, professionals can make decisions based on a broader field of knowledge. The transdisciplinary approach is vitally important to the field of diagnosis in clinical genetics because the expression of most syndromes affects multiple organ systems and functions.

As an example, a look at one syndrome may illustrate why it may be difficult for one professional to make a diagnosis in an individual with multiple anomalies. Opitz syndrome is a disorder of genetic causation affecting multiple systems and functions (Figure 5–1). Clinical features may include any of the following anomalies: hypertelorism, hypospadias, cryptorchidism, abdominal hernias, cleft palate with or without cleft lip, heart anomalies, cleft larynx, tracheoesophageal fistula, kidney anomalies, imperforate anus, mild cognitive deficiency, dysphagia, and early respiratory difficulty. Each of these anomalies must be confirmed by an appropriate examination and cannot be presumed based on symp-

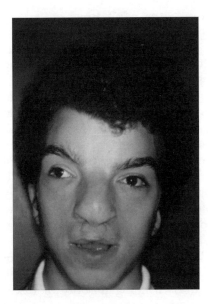
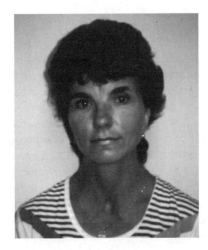

Figure 5–1. Opitz syndrome, X-linked type, in a boy with bilateral cleft lip and palate and orbital hypertelorism (left). His mother, the carrier of the X-linked gene, shows minor manifestations including mild hypertelorism (right).

toms or inferences. A number of anomalies could be assessed by most professionals with an interest in dysmorphology, including speech-language pathologists and audiologists. Hypertelorism is easily assessed by anthropometric measurement of the distances between the inner canthi (the inner corner of the eyes), the outer canthi (the outer corner of the eyes), and the pupils. Cleft lip and/or cleft palate is also easily assessed by facial and peroral examination. However, the other anomalies associated with Opitz syndrome require special expertise, sophisticated tests, or extensive experience. Speech-language pathologists and audiologists do not have the experience nor proper credentials for assessing either genital or rectal anomalies. It is clearly inappropriate for a patient seeking diagnosis for a speech or hearing disorder to have their genitals examined by a nonmedical practitioner. Although some individuals have crossed disciplinary lines, it is always prudent for clinicians to confine their examinations to areas in which they feel confident they can serve their patients well.

Similarly, pediatricians and geneticists typically are not capable of providing accurate data regarding speech, language, voice, resonance, and hearing disorders. Therefore, assessments of possible impairments of voice or resonance should be made with the same attention to detail as physical anomalies. A cleft of the larynx or tracheo-esophageal fistula must be diagnosed by endoscopic and/or radiographic investigation, making the participation of a radiologist and otolaryngologist necessary. Kidney anomalies require ultrasound examinations; cognitive assessments require a neuropsychologist; and respiratory disorders might require an otolaryngologist or pulmonologist. Therefore, a team of professionals becomes essential to establish the specific anomalies indicative of Opitz syndrome. Because establishing the diagnosis is so important, presumptions about the presence or absence of anomalies cannot be tolerated.

The need for several or many professionals from a diverse representation of disciplines to both delineate features of syndromes and diagnose individual patients points out the imperative for the participation of speech-language pathologists and audiologists in the process of genetic investigation. The more transdisciplinary knowledge is shared by the professionals, the better equipped each individual clinician is to participate in the process. In other words, the more knowledge that is shared, the more receptive each specialist is to the data provided from a less familiar field of science. It is easier for the cardiologist to accept the input of the speech-language pathologist if he or she understands the difference between a developmental articulatory impairment and an obligatory placement problem related to a skeletal openbite. In the case of Opitz syndrome, if the speech pathologist understands the structural significance of a laryngeal cleft as imparted by an otolaryngologist, it becomes easier to predict or explain both the voice and swallowing difficulties that would result.

Knowledge of Other Fields of Study

Although individual fields of expertise must be applied to successfully accomplish both syndromic delineation and diagnosis, it is very important for each professional to know something of other specialties. Otherwise, successful triage through other services and disciplines could not possibly be accomplished. It is difficult to request a diagnostic service or special laboratory test if its existence or import is not known or understood. For example, in velo-cardio-facial syndrome, hypernasal speech is one of the most common findings, and is usually severe. The recommended treatment in the overwhelming majority of cases is a very wide pharyngeal flap, which requires dissection of a flap of tissue from the posterior pharyngeal wall. It is has been found, however, that individuals with velo-cardio-facial syndrome have anomalies of the major arteries of the pharynx, including the internal carotid arteries and the vertebral arteries (Mackenzie-Stepner et al., 1987; Mitnick, Bello, Golding-Kushner, Argamaso, & Shprintzen, 1996). Speech-language pathologists and audiologists are very likely to encounter velo-cardio-facial syndrome in their clinical practices because nearly all children with this disorder have hypernasality, severe articulatory impairment (usually glottal stop substitutions), language impairment, high-pitched voice, conductive hearing loss, and occasionally sensorineural hearing loss. Faced with severe hypernasality, speech-language pathologists often refer such cases to surgeons for pharyngeal flap surgery. If the surgeon is unaware of the diagnosis and is also unaware that the internal carotid arteries may be medially dislocated and close to the mucosal surface of the pharynx, a potentially fatal surgical complication could occur if the arteries were severed. Therefore, it is important for the speech pathologist who is involved in the triage of the patient to know something about the anomalies found in the patient (the phenotypic spectrum) and the nature of pharyngeal flap surgery as a possible treatment option for the patient. In this particular case, without the knowledge of how pharyngeal flap is implemented, where incisions are made, and the role of the internal carotid arteries in supplying blood to the brain, the simple act of patient referral may play a major role in the future well-being of the patient. The need for fairly sophisticated transdisciplinary knowledge is not isolated to this single syndrome or specific anomaly. Many such examples exist which clearly demonstrate the need for the speech-language pathologist or audiologist to have knowledge of other fields of clinical practice with which they may have frequent or even occasional contact.

Knowledge of Available Diagnostic Tests

Essential to the transdisciplinary evaluation of patients with multiple anomalies is a comprehensive understanding of the diagnostic tests available to other disciplines that would help to decipher the diagnostic dilemma presented by complex cases. For example, molecular genetics has provided a long list of new sophisticated molecular probes and procedures that can determine if genetic deletions or mutations are present in the DNA of an affected patient. Referring clinicians should be aware that such tests exist to provide the impetus for referral to the proper facilities or geneticists who can implement them. Knowledge of the full range of radiographic, electrophysiologic, biochemical, and structural assessments must also be available to effect proper triage.

As an example, a patient is referred to a speech-language pathologist with developmental delay, language impairment, dyspraxia, and a variety of perceptual impairments. On peroral examination, the patient has a submucous cleft palate and a single central incisor. Facial examination shows that the eyes appear to be close together (hypotelorism), and in one eye, the iris appears to be cleft (Figure 5–2), called an ocular coloboma. Maxillary hypoplasia is also obvious. The head circumference is small by measurement (microcephaly).

None of the structural anomalies is necessarily dramatic or even significantly abnormal in that it would not by itself cause any major dysfunction in the child. However, together they point to a possible diagnosis that has major implications. A knowledge of dysmorphology and the associations between certain facial anomalies and underlying brain malformations would lead the clinician to suspect a possible maldevelopment of the portions of the brain derived from the embryonic component known as the prosencephalon, or forebrain. The maxillary hypoplasia, submucous cleft palate, and single central incisor represent midline

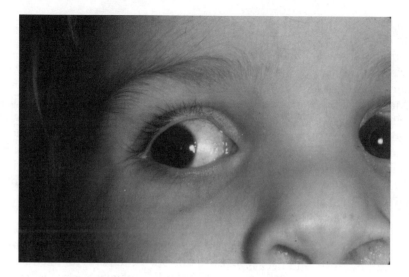

Figure 5–2. An ocular coloboma in a patient with holoprosencephaly (also known as DeMyer sequence). The cleft in the iris is often accompanied by a cleft of the retina and optic nerve.

anomalies of the face. Single central incisor is an unusual anomaly in humans. Although congenitally missing teeth are quite common, a central incisor is rarely absent. Lateral incisors, premolars (bicuspids), and third molars (wisdom teeth) are the most frequently congenitally missing teeth in humans. In many cases, absence of the central incisor is indicative of a disorder of prosencephalic development.

The coloboma of the iris is also of major importance because, embryologically, the eye is formed from the forebrain as an out-pouching of the prosencephalon early during the process of facial formation (Figure 5–3). Anomalies of the eye often reflect underlying anomalies of the brain. Anomalies of the iris, the pupil, the retina, the optic disk, and the optic nerve may all be secondary to an underlying disorder associated with brain integrity. If the substrate of the brain is not intact, the eye may not form normally as a result of that deficiency.

The patient's microcephaly would also be an indication of deficiency in the brain. There are two type of microcephaly: prima-

ry microcephaly and secondary microcephaly. Primary microcephaly is a small head circumference caused by lack of normal brain development. Head growth is driven primarily by brain growth. The skull is not a single solid bone. It is actually comprised of many bones intertwined with each other in a complex network of components including the facial bones, the skull base, and the calvarium. The skull base makes up the floor of the skull on which the brain sits. The calvarium is the dome of the skull and is made up of six separate bones (Figure 5–4), which have spaces between them to allow for expansion. The calvarial bones are the frontal bone, the occipital bone (at the rear of the skull), two squamosal (temporal) bones (one on each side), and two parietal bones (one on each side). As the brain grows, the spaces between the calvarial bones allow the head to expand in all directions, thus increasing the head circumference. The spaces between the calvarial bones, which interdigitate loosely with each other, are known as sutures. These sutures remain patent throughout the period of

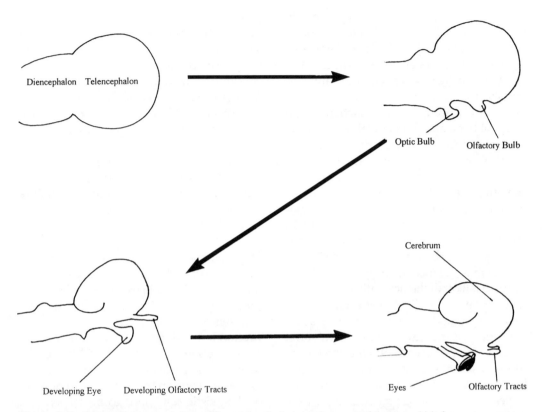

Figure 5–3. Schematic representation of the embryological development of the eye which forms as an extension from the prosencephalon.

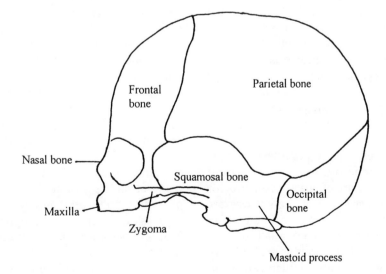

Figure 5–4. The bones of the calvarium.

time when the brain is growing (late into the second decade of life). Where the frontal and parietal bones join, there is a large area several centimeters across at birth that has no bone covering called the anterior fontanel (often referred to as the "soft spot" on a baby's head). At the junction of the occipital bone and the parietal bones at the posterior aspect of the calvarium is the posterior fontanel, a slightly smaller "soft spot." The posterior fontanel typically closes within the first few months of life while the anterior fontanel remains patent, getting gradually smaller, until about 9 to 12 month of age in most children. If the brain is not growing adequately, the head circumference may not increase normally and may begin to fall off of the normative charts. The anterior and posterior fontanels may close prematurely and there may even be some overriding of the sutures with the calvarial bones overlapping each other. If the failure for head size to increase normally is caused by inadequate brain growth pushing the bones outward, this is known as a primary microcephaly.

Secondary microcephaly occurs when the head circumference is small even though the brain is growing at a normal rate. The head circumference fails to grow because the cranial bones are fused together so that the cranium can not be expanded by the internal forces of brain growth. Premature fusion of the cranial sutures is known as craniosynostosis and may occur in a single suture, multiple sutures, or essentially all of the cranial sutures (pansynostosis). If only one or several sutures are fused, the skull tends to adopt an abnormal and asymmetric shape (called plagiocephaly) because the brain will expand out to the open sutures following the path of least resistance for growth. If most or all of the sutures are synostotic, the head shape will be regular, but the head circumference small. In such cases, there is often a dangerous build-up of intracranial pressure, which can result in headaches, neurologic symptoms, and, if

prolonged, brain damage. It is therefore vital to differentiate between primary and secondary microcephaly. This can usually be done by plotting head growth over time, checking skull radiographs and CT scans for evidence of synostosis, and assessing for a history of headaches or other indications consistent with increased intracranial pressure.

In this case, a primary microcephaly in association with hypotelorism is strongly indicative of a small forebrain. The failure for the forebrain to develop normally prevents the normal lateral movement of the orbits, thus keeping the eyes close together (hypotelorism). All of these findings raise a suspicion of a developmental anomaly of the brain and facial structures called holoprosencephaly, or DeMyer sequence. This disorder is a sequence caused by an interruption in the differentiation of the various brain components contained within the prosencephalon, particularly the cerebral hemispheres. To confirm this diagnosis, a number of diagnostic tests need to be carried out, which requires knowledge of both the disorder and the procedures available to assess the anomalies expected within the phenotypic spectrum.

In holoprosencephaly, there are varying degrees of abnormal septation of the cerebral hemispheres. In the worst cases (Figure 5–5), there is no septation with a single "holosphere" and single abnormal ventricle rather than two cerebral hemispheres with a normal ventricular system. This form of holoprosencephaly with a single large ventricle and no evidence of septation is known as alobar holoprosencephaly (Figure 5–5). The faces of babies with this type of brain are almost always severely abnormal. In the worst facial expression, there is true cyclopia with a single orbit and eye. Other facial expressions include cebocephaly (Figure 5–6) with severe hypotelorism and a rudimentary nose with a single nostril and premaxillary agenesis holoprosencephaly with a true midline cleft of the lip, and absent

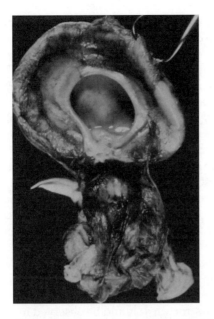

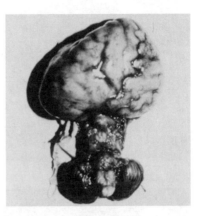

Figure 5–5. The brain of a baby with alobar holoprosencephaly showing no cerebral hemisphere differentiation. The holoprosencephalic brain has a single central ventricle instead of the normal ventricular system found in a normal brain.

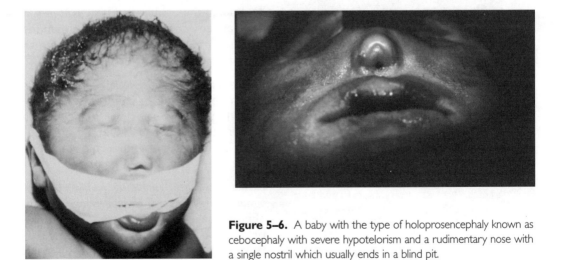

Figure 5–6. A baby with the type of holoprosencephaly known as cebocephaly with severe hypotelorism and a rudimentary nose with a single nostril which usually ends in a blind pit.

premaxilla, severe hypotelorism, and severe midfacial deficiency (Figure 5–7). Babies with alobar holoprosencephaly rarely survive the newborn period. They may have associated anomalies, including heart malformations. They also typically have central apneas (stoppages of breathing caused by an anomalous brain) or obstructive apneas related to their craniofacial anomalies. They also have absent pituitary glands resulting

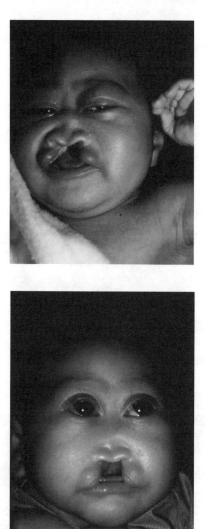

Figure 5-7: Two babies with the type of holoprosencephaly known as premaxillary agenesis. There is a true midline lip and maxillary cleft, with or without clefting of the secondary palate. The maxilla is severely hypoplastic and the eyes are hypoteloric.

in a variety of growth and endocrine disorders, including diabetes insipidus. Regulation of many bodily functions is also abnormal and there are often wild fluctuations of body temperature. Babies with alobar holoprosencephaly usually expire within the first month or two of life.

In milder forms of holoprosencephaly, the brain may have partial septation yet still have communication between the lateral ventricles. This is known as partially lobar holoprosencephaly (Figure 5–8). In partially lobar holoprosencephaly, the facies are usually not as severely abnormal as in alobar holoprosencephaly. Cleft lip and/or palate, mild hypotelorism, maxillary deficiency, eye anomalies, and single central incisor (as described in the case presented here) may be found in such cases. Therefore, clinicians who detect these anomalies need to request the following diagnostic procedures:

Magnetic resonance imaging (MRI): MRI is the best method for imaging the brain. The presence and structure of the brain's midline structures should be observed in detail, including the corpus callosum and the pituitary gland. The presence and size of the olfactory bulbs should also be assessed because they are often absent or small in holoprosencephaly. Careful attention should be paid to the ventricular system to see if there are any communications between the lateral ventricles, which is a clear sign of holoprosencephaly.

Endocrine assessment: Diabetes insipidus is a common finding in children with holoprosencephaly who survive infancy. In the milder forms, such as lobar holoprosencephaly, the first presenting symptom may be diabetes insipidus.

Dental assessment including panoramic radiograph: Single central incisor is an anomaly almost exclusively associated with holoprosencephaly. It is possible for both primary central incisors to be present, but with only a single secondary central incisor. Prior to eruption of the permanent teeth, a panoramic radiograph is necessary to determine which secondary teeth are present.

Ophthalmology consult: Although a coloboma of the iris is easily detected by any clinician, it is possible for the iris to be intact, but for the retina and/or optic nerve to be

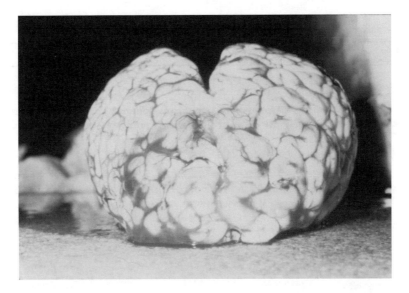

Figure 5–8. A brain showing a partially lobar holoprosencephaly. Note the hemispheric differentiation in the posterior portion, but absence of a central sulcus anteriorly.

cleft. Colobomas of the retina and optic nerve are also strong indication of holoprosencephaly because the eye and optic nerve are embryologically closely associated with the forebrain.

Assessment of the sense of smell: Another portion of the brain that is anomalous in holoprosencephaly is the olfactory system, including the olfactory tracts and olfactory bulbs. Anosmia (lack of a sense of smell) is a clinical finding in holoprosencephaly that is not found often in other disorders, although lack of a sense of smell can be caused by a number of other factors, such as chronic nasal congestion or a deviated septum. However, because MR imaging of the brain will also be obtained in these patients, the association between brain anomalies and anosmia will be strongly suggestive of the diagnosis.

Without the knowledge of the kinds of tests that should be done to confirm the presence of holoprosencephaly, the diagnosis might not be made at all. With appropriate knowl-edge of data that can be provided by other disciplines, the clinician is able to triage the patient properly and also provide clinical and molecular geneticists with the information necessary to determine if the condition is heritable in the individual case. Genes responsible for causing holoprosencephaly have been linked to several chromosomal regions, including the short arm of chromosome 2.

Table 5–1 lists a sample of diagnostic procedures that may be applied by medical and dental colleagues that provide information which could be potentially useful in providing information applicable to the diagnosis of multiple anomaly syndromes. The list of such tests will, of necessity, not be all-inclusive. First, there are too many tests to be listed within the confines of this text. Second, new tests and diagnostic procedures are being developed all of the time, many which will undoubtedly first appear after this text is published. Therefore, it becomes very important for clinicians to pursue sources of knowledge, especially by maintaining close contact

TABLE 5–1. A listing of frequently used diagnostic procedures and the information they might yield that would be of value in establishing a syndromic diagnosis.

Diagnostic Test	*Information Provided*
CT scan of cranium	Presence or absence of craniosynostosis which may be diagnostic of Crouzon, Pfeiffer, or other syndromes of craniosynostosis. CT scan can also show evidence of bony sclerosis (as in Van Buchem syndrome or Robinow syndrome), anomalies of the foramen magnum (as in achondroplasia or Apert syndrome), and other abnormalities of skeletal landmarks. In general, CT is the procedure of choice for skeletal assessments of the head.
MR of brain	Presence of structural brain anomalies, including: communication between the ventricles possibly indicative of holoprosencephaly; absence of the corpus callosum which is seen in many syndromes; the presence of cysts, masses, or structural anomalies. In general, MR is the imaging procedure of choice for soft tissue or brain assessments or for angiography.
Angiography	Assessments of abnormal vasculature may be important for syndromes with abnormal blood vessels (as in Fabry syndrome or velo-cardio-facial syndrome) or hypervascularization (as in Sturge-Weber syndrome). Angiography may be done with standard angiograms, CT angiography, or MR angiography, with MR procedures being the least invasive.
Cranial ultrasound	May be used in infancy prior to closure of the anterior fontanel to assess the status of the ventricles so that hydrocephalus or holoprosencephaly may be detected.
Radiographs (X-rays)	Skeletal structural anomalies of the limbs, digits, spine, and other osseous structures which often accompany skeletal dysplasias, syndromes of short stature, and other genetic conditions, as in epiphyseal dysplasia in Stickler syndrome or thin ribs in oto-palato-digital syndrome.
Cephalometric radiographs	Cranial measurements and angular relationships of the craniofacial structures, such as an obtuse cranial base angle in velo-cardio-facial syndrome, an acute cranial base angle in Treacher Collins syndrome, short anterior cranial base in Crouzon syndrome, or steep mandibular plane angle in Steinert syndrome.
Panoramic radiographs	Presence or absence of permanent teeth or tooth buds and the shape of individual teeth or their roots which might reveal missing teeth, as in EEC syndrome, or conical teeth in Hay-Wells syndrome.
Echocardiogram	Structural or functional heart anomalies, such as mitral valve prolapse or aortic regurgitation in Marfan syndrome, right sided aortic arch in velo-cardio-facial syndrome, or ventriculoseptal defect in Noonan syndrome.
Renal ultrasound	Kidney anomalies or masses, such as cystic kidneys which are common in many syndromes, or missing or hypoplastic kidneys, which are also common syndromic features.
Enzyme or hormone assays	Specific metabolic disorders are often detectable by blood tests designed to detect the presence or absence of specific hormones or enzymes, such as β Glucuronidase deficiency in Sly syndrome, thymic hormone deficiency in velo-cardio-facial syndrome, or excess serum calcium in Williams syndrome (hypercalcemia).
Tissue biopsy	For abnormal masses, the type of tissue found may be diagnostic of specific types of syndromes, such as congenital teratoma, syndromes with hamartomas (such as acanthosis nigracans, Cowden syndrome, and basal cell nevus syndrome), neurocutaneous syndromes (such as neurofibromatosis), and syndromes with malignant neoplasias (such as Bloom syndrome and hemihypertrophy).

(continued)

Diagnostic Test	Information Provided
Nuclear medicine techniques	Nuclear medicine procedures allow assessments of growth activity by determining the uptake of radioactive isotopes into certain tissue types. For skeletal growth activity, scintigraphy or SPECT scanning (**S**ingle **P**hoton **E**mission **C**omputed **T**omography) may be used to determine how active growth is in the skeleton which may help to predict when surgery is best performed for reconstructions, as in hemihypertrophy, oculo-auriculo-vertebral spectrum, and hemimaxillofacial dysplasia.

with the professionals with whom they work. This will serve the dual purposes of providing information for the clinician while also demonstrating to colleagues from other professions that transdisciplinary interaction is being encouraged and fostered by someone from the communicative sciences.

Recall: An Important Part of the Diagnostic Process

Diagnosis is not always instantaneous. As mentioned at the beginning of the chapter, the process of diagnosis must be open-ended. For one thing, not all anomalies are expressed at birth. Phenotypes often develop with time and not all components of a syndrome are recognizable until later in childhood or, in some cases, adolescence or adulthood. For example, Figure 5–9 shows a child born with Apert syndrome shortly after birth, at 1 year, 3 years, and 5 years of age. At birth, the child does not express the severe degree of dysmorphic appearance that is present at age 5. This progression of the facial phenotype in Apert syndrome is typical of craniofacial syndromes. The progression of phenotypes occurs in other types of syndromes, as well. In lysosomal storage disorders, syndromes that have a genetic metabolic disorder and typically are inherited in an autosomal recessive manner (see Chapter 2), the children appear fairly normal at birth. Depending on the disorder, the eventual expression may result in severe growth disturbance, or even death within the first few years of life. For example, in Tay-Sachs disease, Hunter syndrome, or

Hurler syndrome, the absence of obvious clinical manifestations is the rule in newborns. These diseases become expressed as the metabolic abnormalities caused by their recessive genetic errors that cause various cellular waste products to be stored in the tissues of the body. The gradually coarsening facial features, distortion of the spine, enlargement of internal organs, respiratory obstruction or failure, and neurologic degeneration begin in infancy and progress until death occurs in childhood from the various complications of the metabolic disorder. Because these disorders are autosomal recessive in etiology, cases may present as de novo presentations in families with no history of similar problems. Initial presentations in these syndromes may be chronic otitis media because of copious buildup of mucus in the upper airway, or delayed speech and language development as the worsening effects of the metabolic error interrupt cognitive and motor function. Clinicians must therefore be able to know when it is appropriate to schedule follow-up visits for infants, toddlers, and children in order to determine how a phenotype is becoming expressed over time (the natural history of the disorder).

The need for this type of follow-up is even important in adolescents and adults. A vivid example is presented by velo-cardio-facial syndrome (VCFS), which has been described elsewhere on a number of occasions in this text. A number of anomalies in VCFS that have late onset and may be completely overlooked if early management of the patient is successful.

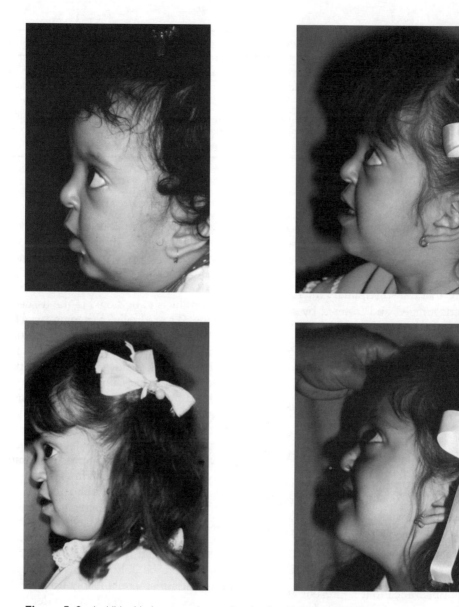

Figure 5–9. A child with Apert syndrome shortly after birth (upper left), at 1 year of age (upper right), 3 years of age (lower left), and 5 years of age (lower right). Note the progression of the facial phenotype with increasing relative prognathism, exorbitism, and hypertelorism.

Late Onset Findings in Velo-Cardio-Facial Syndrome

Velo-cardio-facial syndrome (VCFS) was first described and delineated in 1978, in large part because of a characteristic pattern of communicative impairments associated with a characteristic facial appearance, cardiac anomalies, cleft palate, and learning disabil-

ities. A brief description of the delineation of this syndrome and subsequent findings will help to illustrate the importance of frequent follow-up.

Serendipitously, in 1975, I saw six patients within weeks of each other, all of whom had severe hypernasality associated with ventriculoseptal defects, a very common heart anomaly. All of these patients also had mild language impairments. Even more interesting, all had a characteristic articulation pattern, characterized by glottal stop substitution for essentially all consonants except for the nasal consonants /m/, /n/, and /ŋ/. Although glottal stop substitutions are common in children with cleft palate or cleft lip and palate, they are not typically substituted for all consonants, and often there are other compensatory substitutions in response to both velopharyngeal insufficiency and oral anomalies (Golding-Kushner, 1995; Witzel, 1995). Unlike other children with clefts, children with VCFS typically do not develop pharyngeal fricatives, pharyngeal stops, mid-dorsal stops, and other abnormal substitutions.

In the years that followed, several more patients were found to have the same pattern of anomalies and a more thorough assessment of the anomalies was undertaken. In 1978, a dozen cases were published and the term velo-cardio-facial syndrome was introduced (Shprintzen et al., 1978). A dozen anomalies were described, including a characteristic facial appearance, heart anomalies, cleft palate, learning disabilities, hypernasal speech, hypotonia, retrognathia, hearing loss (both conductive and sensorineural), laryngeal web, inguinal and umbilical hernias, and hypospadias. One of the patients had Robin sequence. In that earliest report delineating VCFS, a single case of dominant transmission was reported (an affected mother and daughter). The next report on the syndrome was in 1980 when Young, Shprintzen, and Goldberg described the range of cardiac anomalies in the syndrome, from ventriculoseptal defect to tetralogy of Fallot to interrupted aortic arch. In that 1980 report, it was discovered that a high percentage of patients with VCFS (approximately 40%) had a right-sided aortic arch, which does not occur as frequently in the general population. In 1981, Shprintzen, Goldberg, Young, and Wolford described 39 patients with the syndrome, expanding the phenotype to over 20 anomalies, including the new findings of scoliosis, slender,

tapering fingers, and relative short stature. In 1984, abnormal angulation of the skull base was found based on cephalometric data (Arvystas & Shprintzen, 1984), a feature which was found to cause deepening of the pharynx which contributed to the severe velopharyngeal insufficiency usually associated with this syndrome. In 1985, Golding-Kushner, Weller, and Shprintzen reported on the nature of the learning disabilities, the language impairment, and typical personality associated with VCFS. Also in 1985, it was found that DiGeorge sequence was also caused by VCFS (Goldberg, Marion, Borderon, Wiznia, & Shprintzen, 1985). In that same year, the inheritance of VCFS was confirmed to be autosomal dominant (Williams, Shprintzen, & Goldberg, 1985). In 1987, it was determined that many patients with VCFS have congenitally missing or hypoplastic adenoids (Williams, Shprintzen, & Rakoff, 1987), abnormal retinal blood vessels (Mansour, Wang, Goldberg, & Shprintzen, 1987), and abnormal location of the internal carotid arteries (MacKenzie-Stepner Witzel, Stringer, Lindsay, Munro, & Hughes, 1987).

Thus, it can be seen that, over a relatively short period of time, the phenotype of this common genetic syndrome expanded considerably. But the most significant phenotypic finding was not reported until 1992 when psychosis was recognized to be a frequent clinical feature of VCFS (Shprintzen, Goldberg, Golding-Kushner, & Marion, 1992). The reason this was not detected until 1992 was that the initial patients studied were all young children, the majority being 4 or 5 years of age. In their initial work-ups, the obvious physical anomalies were found, and there was no evidence at that point of progression of the physical phenotype. The behavioral disorders noted in the young children included learning disabilities and typical affect and temperament. Golding-Kushner, Weller, and Shprintzen (1985) described the temperament in this way:

Social interaction was typically poor with respect to both quantity and quality. The children were described as demonstrating extremes of behavior, being disinhibited and impulsive or serious and shy. (p. 264)

This early description of the behavioral profile in VCFS was actually highly predictive of the more significant adult psychiatric disorders, which would become expressed later in life in this syndrome. It is now known that a very high percentage of patients with VCFS have bipolar affective disorder ("extremes of behavior"), with many of them developing psychotic episodes, in its worst form manifested by schizoaffective disorder (Papolos et al.,1996). Based on the earlier descriptions of Golding-Kushner et al. (1985) and our longitudinal observations of several hundred patients with this syndrome, we now understand that the earlier description of the temperament of children with VCFS was really a description of the earliest manifestations of bipolar disorder. However, bipolar disorder is extremely difficult to diagnose in children, and early manifestations are often confused with other less ominous diagnoses, such as attention deficit disorder, depression, and generalized anxiety disorder. Therefore, although a syndrome may be delineated with a broad spectrum of anomalies described, without observing the syndrome longitudinally through adult life, the complete natural history may not be defined, nor will the prognosis be completely understood.

There are many examples of late onset findings that will cause the natural history and prognosis to represent less optimistic outcomes than might be expected from the initial phenotype. For example, in Refsum syndrome, the initial presentation is sensorineural hearing loss, but in adult life, a gradual, but major deterioration in neurologic function begins. In Down syndrome, infants and children benefit initially from various forms of treatment, such as physical therapy, speech therapy, and occupa-

tional therapy, but as they grow older, they perform more poorly and premature senility and Alzheimer's disease cause additional deterioration in young adulthood. They are also prone to neoplasias (testicular cancer, retinoblastoma, lymphoma) and other forms of cancer (leukemia) at a rate much higher than the general population. Life expectancy is usually between 30 and 40 years of age.

New Syndrome Delineation

The number of new syndromes that have been delineated recently is really quite astonishing. As mentioned in Chapter 3, thousands of new genetic syndromes were delineated in a relatively short period of time with the burgeoning growth of both clinical and molecular genetics in the 1980s. The growth in the delineation of new syndromes is accounted for by two factors:

1. the clinical recognition of new disorders that had not previously been determined to be syndromic associations of anomalies.
2. the isolation by cytogeneticists and molecular geneticists of tiny aneuploidies, individual genes or genetic polymorphisms that give rise to a number of similar groups of anomalies which had all previously been thought to be a single syndrome, but now are recognized as separate and distinct disorders based on different etiologies.

The Delineation of New Disorders

New syndrome delineation continues at a rapid pace. There were probably more new syndromes recognized in the 1980s relative to the number of already recognized syndromes. In other words, the percentage of new syndromes being delineated compared to those already known was very high. Although new syndromes continue to be discovered at a rate comparable to the 1980s, there is now a compendium of many thousands of recognized genetic, chromosomal, and teratogenic disorders so that the relative rate of growth is somewhat slower. This can be explained by the fact that the field of human genetics underwent a rapid expansion in the 1980s, taking it from a relatively new medical discipline to one which now is at the core of the future of clinical and research efforts for understanding and treating human disease. There are now many more clinical and molecular geneticists who have been trained and taken their place in the workplace. Therefore, with so many new and better trained personnel seeing patients, it is easy to understand why so many new genetic disorders are being recognized.

Because the largest growth in clinical genetics occurred in the late 1980s, probably the most significant expansion of clinical delineation of new syndromes occurred at that time. It is also true that scientists who have become interested in clinical genetics have come from a larger variety of disciplines, such as ophthalmology, endocrinology, otolaryngology, psychiatry, dentistry, and other clinical subspecialties. Therefore, syndromes that present with symptoms requiring special expertise to assess previously might have gone unnoticed. For example, Levin and Jorgenson (1972) described an autosomal dominant genetic syndrome with dental anomalies and sensorineural hearing loss. Called otodental syndrome, the disorder was initially identified by unusually malformed teeth. Dr. Jorgenson and the late Dr. Levin, both trained as dentists, described enlargement of the posterior teeth with bulbous projections of the enamel, particularly of the molars. Furthermore, Dr. Levin had a particular interest in hearing loss. The combined expertise of these two prominent contributors to the genetics literature allowed the delineation of a new syndrome, which otherwise might have gone unrecognized.

The contribution of cytogeneticists has not only made the delineation of new syndromes easier, but has also helped to establish causes for syndromes that previously were of unknown etiology. Over the years, karyotypes have become more sophisticated with improved techniques, allowing cytogeneticists to see smaller and smaller segments of chromosomes. Standard karyotypes (those which are not high resolution) when G banded (see Chapter 2) allow the cytogeneticist to see segments of chromosome approximately 2 million base pairs (2 megabases, or mb) in length, whereas high resolution karyotypes provide visible data on segments as small as 350,000 base pairs (3.5 kilobases, or kb). Therefore, high resolution karyotypes will permit cytogeneticists to see evidence of chromosome rearrangement in some contiguous gene syndromes caused by small deletion of chromosome material that previously were not visible. Such deletions are not always visible because the size of the deletion may be variable. Examples include velo-cardio-facial syndrome (22q11.2 deletion which is visible approximately 10–15% of the time) and Prader-Willi syndrome and Angelman syndromes (15q11→15q13 deletions) as described in Chapter 2.

Molecular geneticists have had an even more profound impact on the delineation of new syndromes and the discovery of etiologies of syndromes with previously unknown causes. The use of techniques for mapping genes, defining the DNA structure of the gene, and then determining the action of the gene has led to extraordinary findings that will help clinicians to understand why anomalies develop. For example, the gene that causes Stickler syndrome has been mapped to the long arm of chromosome 12. The gene is involved in the formation of collagen II, a necessary component of cartilage, bone, and connective tissue. Individuals with Stickler syndrome have micrognathia, cleft palate, upper airway obstruction (the Robin sequence triad), myopia, vitreoretinal degeneration, epiphyseal dysplasia, lax joints, talipes equinovarus (club foot), and occasionally, slightly short stature (see Chapter 3). Stickler syndrome constitutes approximately 35% of all cases of Robin sequence. A specific point mutation in the collagen II gene causes Stickler syndrome. However, a different mutation in the same gene causes another autosomal dominantly inherited syndrome, which also is associated with cleft palate and Robin sequence, called spondyloepiphyseal dysplasia congenita, or SED. Individuals with SED have a more severe skeletal dysplasia than those with Stickler syndrome. The facies is somewhat similar and includes micrognathia and cleft palate. However, unlike Stickler syndrome, SED is a syndrome of very short stature. Molecular geneticists were able to demonstrate the etiological basis for both of these syndromes, revealing the similarity between them, both in terms of their common genetic bond and the mechanism that results in the anomalies caused by collagen II anomalies.

Another example of this type of discovery by molecular geneticists is the specific etiology of the easily recognized syndromes of craniosynostosis, Crouzon syndrome and Apert syndrome. Mutations in a single gene located on the long arm of chromosome 10, FGFR2 (**F**ibroblast **G**rowth **F**actor **R**eceptor-2) are now known to cause these rare, but well-known syndromes. Crouzon syndrome (Figure 5–10) has anomalies essentially isolated to the head and face. Craniosynostosis of multiple sutures resulting in abnormal head shape, increased intracranial pressure, and shallow orbits (causing the eyes to bulge) are the common anomalies related to the synostosis of the cranial sutures. There is also severe maxillary hypoplasia resulting in a class III malocclusion when combined with normal mandibular growth. The nasal airway is small with choanal stenosis or atresia a common finding. There are no extracranial anomalies in Crouzon syndrome and the limbs are normal. Furthermore, if the craniosynostosis and increasing intracranial pressure are managed properly (with early cranial reconstruction), intellect and cognitive function typically are normal. Apert syndrome (see Figure 5–9) has many more anomalies in its phenotype, including cognitive, limb, skin, and extracranial skeletal

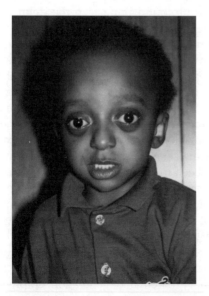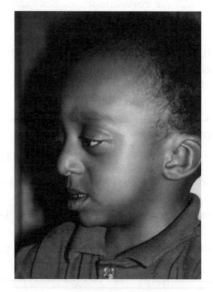

Figure 5–10. A child with Crouzon syndrome in frontal (left) and profile (right) views.

anomalies. Besides craniosynostosis and syndactyly (fusion of the fingers and toes as shown in Figure 5–9), individuals with Apert syndrome may have progressive fusion of the bones in the arms, spine, hands, and feet. Acne vulgaris (severe, large, prominent acne lesions) is found in over half of affected individuals. Cognitive function is usually impaired, ranging from learning disabilities to significant mental retardation. The skull anomalies in Crouzon syndrome and Apert syndrome, although similar, are different enough to be distinctive. In the very early years of the study of these two syndromes, clinicians regarded Apert syndrome to be essentially the same as Crouzon syndrome except for the hand findings. However, as dysmorphology became more fine tuned and the tools used to assess the anomalies became more sophisticated, the differences in skull shape, the extracranial anomalies in Apert syndrome, and the differences in cognitive function caused researchers and clinicians to conclude that these were actually very different syndromes, probably with very different types of genetic etiologies. However, the finding that both syndromes are caused by a different mutation in the same gene has brought researchers full cycle, now understanding that these syndromes may be more closely related than previously thought.

Open-Ended Diagnosis

As mentioned earlier, the diagnostic process must be kept open-ended for a number of reasons:

1. Not all anomalies are expressed at birth. Therefore, a patient may have no diagnosis applied in the neonatal period or infancy, but as more anomalies (especially behavioral disorders) become expressed in childhood, a diagnosis may become more obvious and therefore diagnosed at a later date.

2. Even if the correct diagnosis is applied early, the syndrome may be incompletely delineated and new anomalies may be added to the phenotypic spectrum over time. Fur-

thermore, the natural history of the syndrome may not be completely understood, as demonstrated by the description of velo-cardiofacial syndrome earlier in this chapter.

3. Not all syndromes have been discovered or delineated. Therefore, it is possible that earlier diagnoses are either incorrect or incomplete. They may be incorrect if the syndrome has not yet been described or delineated, but has a phenotype that has some overlapping features with other syndromes. For example, oculo-auriculovertebral spectrum (also known as hemifacial microsomia, Goldenhar syndrome, and first and second branchial arch syndrome) was first recognized as a specific pattern of malformation in 1952 (Goldenhar, 1952), but the full phenotype and spectrum of anomalies was not really well understood until the 1960s and after. Prior to Goldenhar's report and the subsequent delineation of the oculo-auriculo-vertebral spectrum (OAVS) phenotype, the disorder was considered to be a unilateral expression of Treacher Collins syndrome. In an exhaustive publication of cases with Treacher Collins syndrome (also referred to as mandibulofacial dysostosis), Franceschetti and Klein (1949) described many cases presumed to have Treacher Collins syndrome, but over half actually had OAVS. It was not until years later that it became clear that OAVS and Treacher Collins syndrome were distinct and separate disorders.

Diagnoses may be incomplete if no specific syndromic diagnosis is attached to the patient (i.e., the patient is categorized as provisionally unique. as described in Chapter 3), but some time after the patient has been seen, the syndrome becomes delineated. For example, Figure 5–11 shows a child seen by the author in 1975 who had been referred with the diagnosis of Crouzon syndrome because he had craniosynostosis of multiple cranial sutures along with marked exorbitism (bulging eyes secondary to shallow orbits). However, examination showed too many features inconsistent with the diagnosis of Crouzon syndrome, including arach-

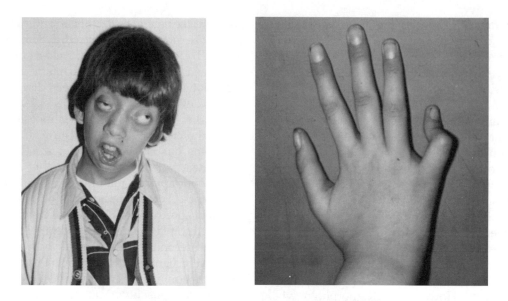

Figure 5–11. A child with craniosynostosis, exorbitism (left), arachnodactyly with joint contractures (right), spinal anomalies, developmental impairment, and multiple abdominal hernias.

nodactyly (very long fingers in relation to palmar length), camptodactyly of the fifth fingers (joint contractures of the fingers), multiple abdominal hernias, cervical spine anomalies, cognitive impairment, mandibular retrognathia, and soft, pliable ears. This pattern of malformations had never been reported previously and clearly did not represent a variant of Crouzon syndrome or any other known syndrome of craniosynostosis that had been reported previously. Therefore, the patient was classified as "provisionally unique" as described in Chapter 3. However, in 1980, a second patient with the same pattern of malformations was seen by the author after referral for craniosynostosis (Figure 5–12). With two cases sharing the same phenotype, it became obvious that this pattern was a recurrent one and represented a new syndrome of unknown causation. Therefore, a paper was published in 1982 (Shprintzen & Goldberg, 1982), and the syndrome has subsequently been referred to as Shprintzen-Goldberg syndrome (Ades et al., 1995; Saal et al., 1995). With the syndrome delineated, it then became possible

to observe the natural history of the disorder; which included worsening of the craniofacial anomalies and mental retardation with severe language impairment (Figure 5–13). It is now thought that Shprintzen-Goldberg syndrome is caused by a mutation in the fibrillin-1 gene (FBN1), which has also been linked to Marfan syndrome (Sood, Eldadah, Krause, McIntosh, & Dietz, 1996). Crouzon syndrome is caused by mutations in the fibroblast growth factor receptor-2 (FGFR2) gene located on the long arm of chromosome 10, at the 10q25 band. Thus, it can be seen that over a fairly short period of time, a patient's status may change from a unique, or undiagnosed syndrome to a syndrome that has been identified and therefore has a known natural history and prognosis.

4. With the rapid growth of molecular genetics, the specific causes of many syndromes are becoming known, which has major implications for genetic counseling, and, possibly, more effective treatments. Over the past several years, the specific genetic causes of many syndromes have

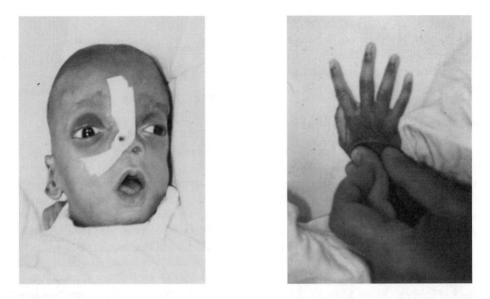

Figure 5–12. A second child, shown here as an infant, with craniosynostosis, exorbitism (left), arachnodactyly with joint contractures (right), spinal anomalies, developmental impairment, and multiple abdominal hernias seen several years after the case shown in Figure 5-11. With two cases showing the same phenotype, a new syndrome has been delineated (Shprintzen-Goldberg syndrome).

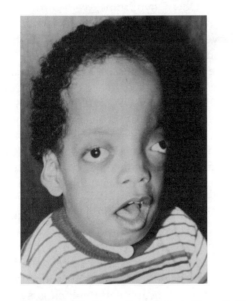
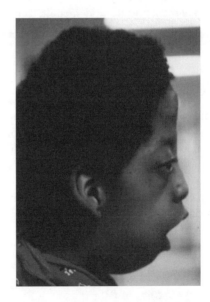

Figure 5–13. The patient shown in Figure 5-12 at 4 years of age (left) and 10 years of age (right). Other than a craniectomy in infancy, no other craniofacial surgery has been done.

been identified, such as the fibrillin and fibroblast growth factor receptor mutations mentioned above, or the role of the elastin gene in Williams syndrome, or the collagen II gene in Stickler syndrome. Gene identification has implications for prenatal diagnosis, as well as counseling for recurrence risk. Hopefully, the eventual future of molecular genetics will be the application of better treatments once the pathway for gene activity is understood fully.

Logic Versus Gestalt

The process of diagnosis is not easily taught. In essence, diagnostic skill is as individual as athletic ability or artistic aptitude. Diagnosis must be approached as a type of problem solving or, even more specifically, solving a mystery. How one goes about solving a mystery is as individual as personality, and there may not be only one successful approach. After all, literary detectives as successful as Sherlock Holmes, Miss Marple, Hercule Poirot, Nancy Drew, and the Hardy Boys all solved mysteries, although their approaches could hardly be called similar.

Two basic elements involved in the diagnostic process are often discussed by clinical geneticists: logic and gestalt. Both are important in the diagnostic process and neither is sufficient alone.

Logic

Some clinicians value logic above all in the diagnostic process. In using a purely logical approach, the clinician essentially faces a diagnostic dilemma as an issue of statistical probability. The list of anomalies found in the patient is compared to lists of anomalies associated with known syndromic diagnoses. In fact, there are several computer programs which function in just that manner. It might work this way:

Clinical Findings in Patient

Tetralogy of Fallot

Cleft palate

Small Ears

Small eyes

Hypospadias

Slightly small stature

Failure-to-thrive

Immune deficiency

Developmental delay

These findings, when seen listed on paper, represent a varied, yet clearly syndromic phenotype. In looking for syndromes that include these features, the clinician would encounter several possibilities, including velo-cardio-facial syndrome, fetal alcohol syndrome, fetal hydantoin syndrome, Down syndrome, and a number of others. The problems with this probability approach, especially when computer assisted are as follows:

1. A complete description of the syndrome on paper may not fully capture the appearance or specific qualitative (rather than quantitative) features of the disorder. As in the list of features above, children with Down syndrome, velo-cardio-facial syndrome, and fetal alcohol syndrome all have distinctive appearance, but these syndromes certainly do not resemble each other at all. It is difficult to characterize the true appearance of the child with Down syndrome in words, but once seen, the phenotypic appearance is unforgettable.

2. It is not known if the anomalies present in a particular child are high- or low-frequency anomalies associated with the particular syndrome expressed in the child. The lists of findings in known syndromes, like Down or VCFS, are typically rank ordered in relation to how commonly they are expressed in that syndrome. Therefore, the presence of an anomaly in the patient which is a low frequency finding in the syndrome, but which is a major and distinctive anomaly and therefore considered to be important in that patient, may undermine the logical approach to syndrome identification. Therefore, in the listing above, tetralogy of Fallot (TOF), a major heart anomaly, is impossible to ignore in the child because of its life-threatening potential. The TOF becomes the focus of attention in the care of the child, but may be misleading in terms of diagnosing a syndrome. When presented with TOF as a finding, the computer or the clinician would immediately think of a number of syndromes where conotruncal heart anomalies such as TOF are common. But, if the patient has a disorder in which TOF is a rare or uncommon finding, this type of logical approach will lead the clinician down the wrong path.

3. The larger the number of anomalies in a particular syndrome, the larger the number of possible permutations that would result in overlapping features with other disorders.

4. The fewer the number of anomalies in a particular syndrome, the less opportunity there is for creating a probability scale for potential diagnoses.

5. Clinical judgment, while hardly a quantifiable entity, should not be discounted as an important, if not the most important, component of the diagnostic process. The clinician contains his or her own computer (called *the brain*), which processes information in ways not analogous to a PC or main frame. Using a system of pure logic, clinical judgment is bypassed in favor of pure probability analysis.

Conversely, logic can not be eliminated from the diagnostic process. Some components of probability analysis must be used to avoid obvious mistakes. If a clinical finding or group of findings are inconsistent with a particular diagnosis, even though other features are suggestive of that diagnosis, then logic would dictate that the probability of that diagnosis being correct is very low. For example, the patients cited above with Shprintzen-Goldberg syndrome had first been thought to have Crouzon syndrome. Consistent with the diagnosis of Crouzon syndrome was craniosynostosis of multiple sutures and exorbitism. However, the patient also had arachnodactyly, multiple abdominal hernias, cervical spine anomalies, mandibular retrognathia, and cognitive impairment. Because these features are not known to be found in any reported cases of Crouzon syndrome, unless the clinician can offer an alternative explanation as to why they might appear in this patient, logic would dictate that their presence would mitigate against the diagnosis. In this particular example, the facial similarity between the patient with Shprintzen-Goldberg syndrome and patients with Crouzon syndrome who have exorbitism was the factor which led to an incorrect clinical judgment. Clinical judgments can be influenced by a number of factors, including the number of cases of a particular syndrome the clinician has seen, the area of expertise of the clinician (some clinicians have a lot of experience with craniofacial anomalies, some with metabolic disorders, some with syndromes of deafness, some with syndromes of short stature, etc.). It is difficult for even the busiest of clinical geneticists to have had extensive experience with all types of congenital malformations and deformations because of the sheer number of possible anomalies.

Gestalt

Gestalt is a term usually applied to the process by which people utilize their perceptions and judgment to develop an overall impression of something, often needing to fill in gaps where information might be missing to develop a firm decision. Put another way, gestalt is the process by which something can be identified even though all of its parts are not present for analysis (an object may not necessarily equal the sum of its parts). People use this type of perception all of the time in recognizing other people even when only parts of their face are visible. This represents our ability to use the computer which sits between our ears to fill in gaps in such a way that the total picture makes sense. This process is particularly useful in syndromic diagnosis because clinicians depend heavily on visual input to provide initial diagnostic clues. However, beyond the physical appearance of the patient, there is also a type of gestalt that occurs in putting groups of anomalies together in a way that makes some sense biologically. This process reflects both experience and an understanding of morphogenesis and embryogenesis, which predicts how certain types of anomalies might occur in groups. For example, the presence of ear tags or ear pits in an individual prompts experienced clinicians to look for a number of other anomalies that might help to confirm the diagnosis of oculo-auriculo-vertebral spectrum (OAVS). A complete audiometric assessment is certainly indicated to look for a unilateral conductive hearing loss. The eyes should be examined for small whitish growths on the conjunctiva (Figure 5–14), often referred to as *epibulbar dermoids*. The spine, especially the cervical spine, may show anomalies such as fusions or hemivertebrae (Figure 5–15). The process by which a clinician would suspect the presence of

these anomalies and therefore search for them reflects an understanding of the phenotypic spectrum of OAVS and the knowledge that tags of abnormally formed tissues found in inappropriate places are often found in several locations in the same patient because they are derivatives of the same error in morphogenesis. Known as *choristomas*, ear tags and dermoids in the eye are actually symptomatic of the same error of morphogenesis. Knowing the gestalt of OAVS and the gestalt of the embryonic process, the clinician develops a possible diagnostic pattern based on the presence of sometimes only a single key anomaly.

Therefore, it becomes essential for the clinician to be able to take the best parts of both the logical approach and the gestalt approach while avoiding the pitfalls of both in order to reach the correct diagnosis. Experience is obviously a great teacher and experience can be obtained even without applying diagnoses to patients. It is sufficient to be a careful observer of the patient and to follow the development of the patient over time while reviewing the diagnoses applied by

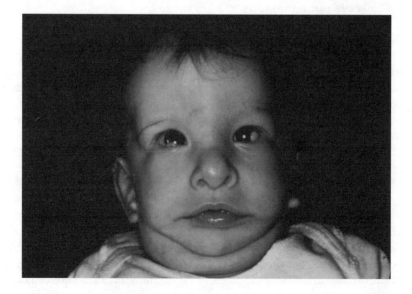

Figure 5–14. An epibulbar dermoid, or choristoma, in a patient with oculo-auriculo-vertebral spectrum.

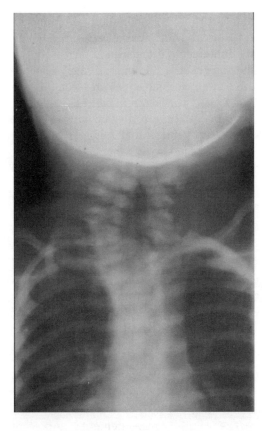

Figure 5–15. Hemivertebrae (spina bifida occulta) in the cervical spine of a patient with oculo-auriculo-vertebral spectrum.

ears, the teeth, the hair, the hands, the skin, and overall height and weight (somatic size). Even casual examination of the craniofacial complex (i.e., head, face, eyes, ears, and hair) and the limbs (i.e., the hands) will result in the detection of many possible diagnoses because these structures are affected in the large majority of multiple anomaly disorders (Cohen, 1982). For additional accuracy, it is possible to take surface measurements of the anatomy, a process known as *anthropometrics.*

Anthropometrics

Anthropometrics is the process by which individual parts of the body can be measured and compared to established norms. Norms are available for a wide range of facial and somatic features, such as height, weight, head circumference, hand and finger length, ear length, the distance between the eyes, span, foot size, genital size, chest circumference, the length of the philtrum, and nearly any other structure that can be measured with a tape measure, caliper, or ruler. For an excellent guide to the process of anthropometric measurement of the craniofacial complex, the reader is referred to the works of Farkas (Farkas, 1981; Farkas & Munro, 1987; Farkas & Posnick, 1992; Farkas, Posnick, & Hreczko, 1992a-c; Farkas, Posnick, Hreczko, & Pron, 1992a, 1992b) or to the appendixes in *Syndromes of the Head and Neck* (Gorlin, Cohen, & Levin, 1990) and *Smith's Recognizable Patterns of Human Malformation* (Jones, 1992). Some anthropometric charts are included in Appendix 2.

Measurement of easily accessible body parts is a simple noninvasive procedure, and may yield vital information in the diagnostic process. It is difficult to rely on visual impressions because the relationships of various structures may present as optical illusions, which lead to mistaken diagnostic conclusions. For example, assessing the distance between the eyes is a very important diagnostic component in children with sus-

others and determining if they make logical and clinical sense. Is there anything in particular that specialists in the communicative disorders can observe without resorting to thorough physical examinations? Absolutely.

Structures That Give Clues

During the process of either a speech-language evaluation or audiometric assessment, clinicians certainly have the opportunity to observe many characteristics of the patient's physical appearance without performing an in-depth physical examination. Clinicians can easily notice portions of the child's anatomy that are clearly visible so that even minor anomalies can be detected. They include the head, face, the eyes, the

pected craniofacial syndromes. By definition, orbital hypertelorism is an increased separation of the entire orbit, including its contents (i.e., the eye) and is a common finding in a large number of syndromes, such as Crouzon syndrome. Hypotelorism is a decreased space between the eyes and is a less common, but important, finding in a number of disorders, such as holoprosencephaly. It is important to obtain three different measurements to confirm the presence or absence of hypertelorism or hypotelorism, namely, the inner canthal distance, the outer canthal distance, and the interpupillary distance (Figure 5–16). True orbital hypertelorism may be diagnosed if the inner canthal distance, outer canthal distance, and interpupillary distance are all increased,

indicating that the entire bony orbit and its contents are wider apart than normal. If only the inner canthal distance is increased, but the outer canthal and interpupillary distance are within normal limits, this condition is known as *dystopia canthorum,* or *telecanthus.* Dystopia canthorum may be caused by the presence of epicanthal folds or by small orbits that are widely separated at the inner edge. Dystopia canthorum is a common finding in a number of syndromes, such as Waardenburg syndrome. An additional measurement, the palpebral fissure length (Figure 5–16), should be taken to confirm this. Reduced palpebral fissure length may indicate small orbits, and therefore small eyes. Small eyes are a diagnostic feature of a number of syndromes and may have serious ramifications for underlying development of the forebrain because, as mentioned earlier in relation to holoprosencephaly, the eyes are embryologically closely related to forebrain development. A more detailed explanation of ocular measurements will follow later in this chapter.

The process of measurement is important because the clinician can be misled by relative sizes or distances. For example, if the body is relatively small, but the head circumference is normal, it may give the incorrect impression of an increased head circumference. If the nasal root is very wide, it may present the illusion of widely spaced eyes, even though the distances may be normal. Because the process of measurement is completely noninvasive and requires minimal skill and training, there is no contraindication to any clinician performing these tasks. Measurement of height, weight, span, head circumference, ocular distances, ear length, and hand and finger length are valuable diagnostic indicators of the presence of anomalies. If a milliner can measure your hat size, or a haberdasher your span, there is certainly no contraindication to a clinician in the communicative disorders doing the same with a modicum of training by an experienced anthropometrist.

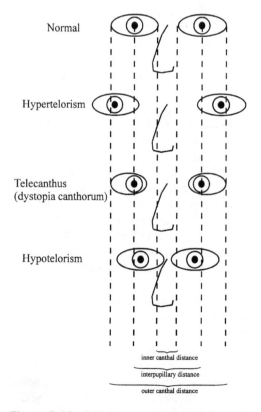

Figure 5–16. Orbital measurements and diagnostic terms applied to abnormalities of orbital distances.

The Head

The cranium may express a variety of anomalies, including abnormalities of size, shape, and symmetry. As discussed earlier in this chapter, abnormalities of cranial size are most often related to abnormalities of brain size. If the brain is too small, the skull will be too small (a condition known as primary microcephaly). If the brain is too large, or if the ventricles are dilated excessively (hydrocephalus), the skull will be excessively large (a condition known as macrencephaly). Although a normal sized skull does not imply a normal underlying brain, the correlation between either a small or large cranium and cognitive disorders is strong. A small cranium can also indicate the possibility of craniosynostosis (secondary microcephaly, implying that the brain is of normal size and being constricted by the failure for the cranium to expand) and a large cranium could indicate excessive bone growth (macrocephaly), but these anomalies also represent cause for concern and the need for further diagnostic efforts. Although it is not possible to "eyeball" a skull to determine its size, skulls that are unusually large or small may be suspected by even casual observation. Anthropometric measurement is the best method for assessing head size and should certainly be performed on every child. It is customary for pediatricians to follow head circumference in their patients throughout childhood. Therefore, even if a measurement is not obtained at the time of examination (although it should be), it may be possible to obtain serial head circumference measurements from past medical records. Primary microcephaly is a common feature of many syndromes with brain anomalies and often is a prognostic indicator for subnormal cognitive development and/or mental retardation. It is therefore important to distinguish between primary and secondary microcephaly to determine if the abnormality is seated in the brain or in the cranium. Serial head circumferences will be helpful, especially if early developmental milestones are within normal limits. In primary microcephaly, the head circumference is often small at birth and cranial expansion follows the normal growth curve, but falls consistently below age norms (Figure 5–17). In secondary microcephaly, the growth curve almost always continues to fall away from the normal growth curve, often at a rapid pace (Figure 5–17). Although there are many exceptions to these patterns of growth, a small head circumference discovered at any point in time should be explored carefully to determine risk factors and to apply a primary diagnosis. Diagnoses associated with microcephaly are listed in Appendix I.

Abnormalities of cranial shape may be primary features of certain syndromes, reflect underlying brain anomalies, indicate anomalies of the skull base, or represent craniosynostosis. Cranial anomalies might include frontal bossing, a prominent occiput, temporal bulging, posteriorly sloping forehead, flattening of the occiput, or temporal depressions. Craniosynostosis of individual sutures results in fairly characteristic cranial shapes, as shown in Figure 5–18.

Skull base anomalies are common in a number of well-defined syndromes, including the syndromes of craniosynostosis, and other syndromes with craniofacial manifestations, such as velo-cardio-facial syndrome and Stickler syndrome (Shprintzen, 1982). In some of the syndromes of craniosynostosis, including Apert syndrome, Crouzon syndrome, Pfeiffer syndrome, and Jackson-Weiss syndrome, the anterior cranial base (the area anterior to the sella turcica, extending forward to the naso-frontal junction) is very short and the angulation of the skull base is very acute (a condition commonly referred to as cranial base kyphosis). The normal cranial base angle, measured from the nasion (junction of the nasal bones and the forehead) to the sella turcica to the basion (at the clivus), or B-S-N, is usually about 129°, plus or minus 3°. In syndromes of craniosynostosis, the angle may be as

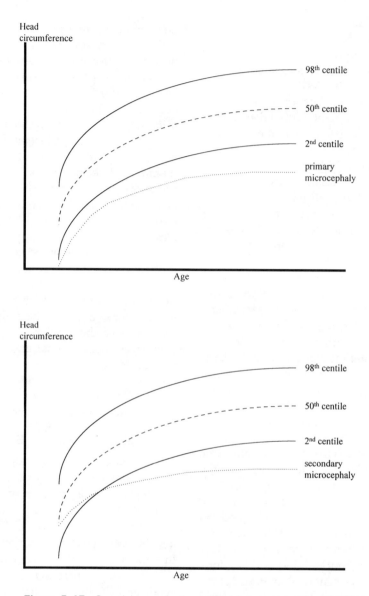

Figure 5–17. Growth curves for head circumference in a child with primary microcephaly (top) and a child with secondary microcephaly (bottom). Note that, in the case of the primary microcephaly, the head circumference is small at birth, whereas in the child with secondary microcephaly, the head circumference becomes proportionately smaller over time.

small as 110° (Figure 5–19). The short anterior cranial base is reflected in failure for the facial bones to be positioned in their normal forward position so that the midface is retruded, and when the mandible is normal, the patient has a relative mandibular prognathism because the midface is so deficient (see Figures 5–9 and 5–10). The acute cranial base angle, or kyphosis, results from the posterior cranial base (the portion posterior

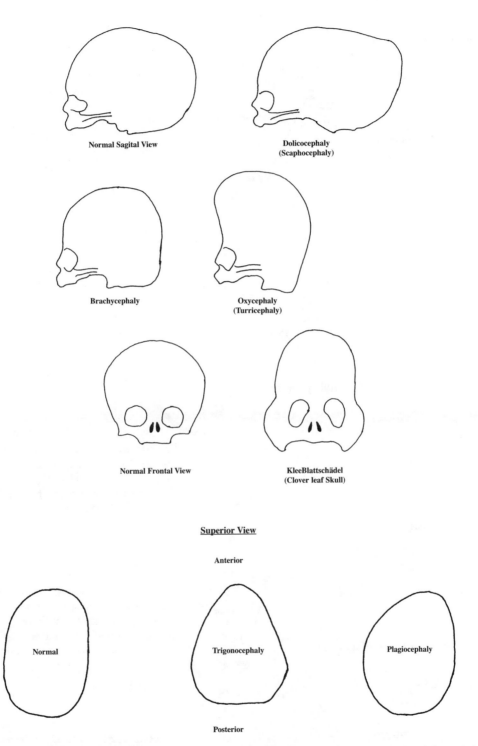

Figure 5–18. Characteristic skull shapes related to synostosis of individual cranial sutures, including dolicocephaly or scaphocephaly (sagittal synostosis), brachycephaly (bilateral coronal synostosis), oxycephaly or turricephaly, klee-blattschädel (cloverleaf skull), trigonocephaly (metopic synostosis), and plagiocephaly (unilateral coronal synostosis).

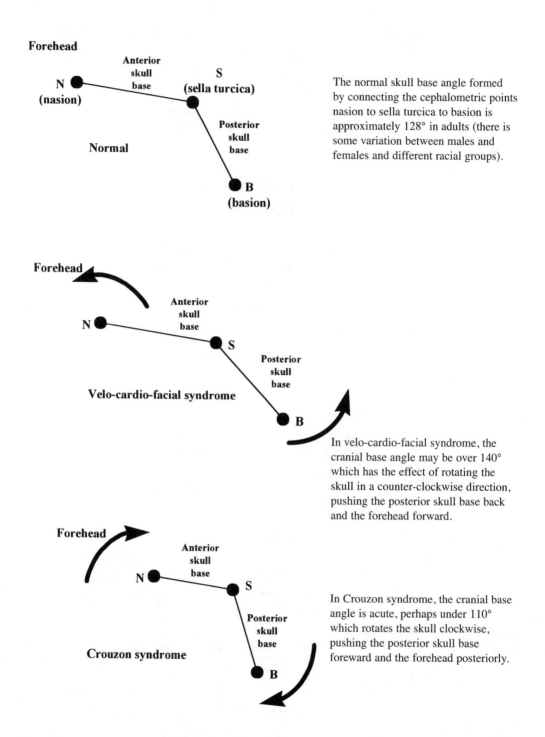

The normal skull base angle formed by connecting the cephalometric points nasion to sella turcica to basion is approximately 128° in adults (there is some variation between males and females and different racial groups).

In velo-cardio-facial syndrome, the cranial base angle may be over 140° which has the effect of rotating the skull in a counter-clockwise direction, pushing the posterior skull base back and the forehead forward.

In Crouzon syndrome, the cranial base angle is acute, perhaps under 110° which rotates the skull clockwise, pushing the posterior skull base foreward and the forehead posteriorly.

Figure 5–19. Cranial base angles in a patient with Crouzon syndrome (bottom) and velo-cardio- facial syndrome (middle) as measured from a lateral cephalometric radiograph. The arrows connote the response of skull growth to the flexion of the skull base. The bottom half of the posterior skull base is flexed anteriorly, which has the effect of rotating the top half of the skull posteriorly resulting in a posterior sloping of the forehead.

to the sella turcica) being flexed forward, which has the effect of narrowing the nasal and pharyngeal airway. Therefore, airway obstruction and/or hyponasal speech are common complications of this type of skull base anomaly. The forehead in individuals with a short anterior cranial base and kyphosis is often sloped posteriorly, which has the effect of making the brow appear very prominent (see Figure 5-10). The posterior sloping of the forehead is related to the posterior rotation of the top half of the cranial complex caused by the bottom half being flexed forward (Figure 5–19).

In velo-cardio-facial syndrome, the skull base is flexed in the opposite direction so that the angle is obtuse. Patients with VCFS may have cranial base angles as large as 148° (Figure 5–19). On the average, these angles are larger in patients with VCFS than in the general population (Arvystas & Shprintzen, 1984). The rotation of the posterior skull base away from the anterior basicranium has the effect of enlarging the pharynx, which increases the likelihood of velopharyngeal insufficiency. It also has the effect of rotating the top half of the cranium in the anterior direction, opposite to the effect seen in Crouzon syndrome (Figure 5–19) with the effect of making the forehead appear more prominent.

Not all syndromes with a short anterior cranial base are related to craniosynostosis. In Stickler syndrome, which does not have craniosynostosis as a clinical feature, the anterior skull base is slightly short and the posterior basicranium is kyphotic.

An asymmetric cranium may be indicative of a unilateral craniosynostosis, or it may be an indicator of one of the syndromes that has craniofacial asymmetry as a common feature, including oculo-auriculo-vertebral spectrum, Carpenter syndrome, Saethre-Chotzen syndrome, Townes syndrome, or Wildervanck syndrome.

Because of the strong links between easily observed cranial anomalies and the presence of multiple anomaly syndromes, observations of cranial anomalies should not be treated lightly or ignored. They should spur the clinician on to utilize the curiosity over these anomalies in the process of diagnosis. There are hundreds of syndromes that have cranial anomalies as a part of the phenotypic spectrum, and although this number is large, the finding of one or more cranial anomalies will help to narrow the search significantly. Cranial findings are also strong prognostic indicators and therefore are of major value in recommending treatment plans.

The Face

The face, although a component of the cranium, has separate importance in many respects. The face is derived from different embryologic components and begins to form somewhat later than the brain. Although there is a strong relationship between facial structure and the integrity of the central nervous system, this relation is not absolute. Many children with abnormal brains have normal faces, and many children with abnormal faces have normal brains. In general, if there is a very early embryologic insult to the brain (i.e., of chromosomal, genetic, or teratogenic influence), it is likely that the face will also be abnormal. However, if the abnormal developmental process occurs after the initial substrate of the brain is formed, it is very likely that the face will be affected, but not the brain.

The face is constituted from a number of structures, including the frontal bone of the anterior calvarium (the forehead), the orbits (the eyes), the maxilla (the region from the base of the orbits to the mouth), the nasal bones, and the mandible (the lower part of the face). Each component has a somewhat different, yet interrelated embryologic origin. Immediately posterior to the facial bones is the skeletal framework of the skull base, including the sphenoid and ethmoid bones. In other words, there is a delicate relationship between the brain, the bones of the skull and skull base, and the facial bones. Overlying the facial bones are the facial soft tissues which are derived from the median nasal process, the maxillary process, and the 1st and 2nd branchial arches. If the underlying skeleton is abnormal, the soft tissues will reflect that abnormality, such as the downslanting eyes seen in Treacher Collins syndrome (see Figure 2–1). The lateral canthi slant downward because of skeletal defects in the orbits and zygomas underneath the soft tissues. Because the face is a somewhat more complex structure than the calvarium, the number of possible anomalies is larger and the implications not so distinct as disorders of skull size, shape, and symmetry. However, anomalies of the face can be broken down into several different types, including hypoplasias, hyperplasias, clefts, asymmetries, and structural abnormalities or redundancies.

Hypoplasias

Hypoplasia, in its broadest sense, means underdevelopment of a structure. More specifically, it means that there are fewer cells making up the structure. Although hypoplasias can be caused secondarily by a lack of vascular supply during development, they usually represent an intrinsic developmental disorder caused by a chromosomal, genetic, or teratogenic influence. In cases of mechanical deformations, structures may appear to be small because of constriction (as in the isolated Robin sequence), but the cell structure and number is normal so that growth after birth proceeds normally after removal of the mechanical constriction.

Hypoplasias of the various facial components have different implications. Maxillary hypoplasia is a common anomaly in craniofacial syndromes. In some cases, it is related to craniosynostosis, as in Crouzon syndrome,

Apert syndrome, and Pfeiffer syndrome. Maxillary hypoplasia may also occur, as discussed above, if the anterior cranial base is short, as in Stickler syndrome. In such cases, the maxillary hypoplasia is a structural anomaly unrelated to brain malformation. However, in many cases, brain anomalies can also be closely associated with maxillary deficiency.

Much of the face is derived from cells that originated in a region of the early embryo known as the neural crest. The neural crest is a region above the developing neural tube, which contains a layer of cells that eventually migrate to other regions of the developing embryo, including the branchial arches and pouches, and then subsequently to the developing face (Figure 5–20). If there is an early deficiency in the neural crest, the structures that are derived from its cells will be hypoplastic. Deficiency of the neural crest cells can be caused by underdevelopment or abnormal development of the neural tube (the structure which eventually becomes the central nervous system). For example, in holoprosencephaly, severe deficiency of the midface is part of the phenotypic spectrum (see Figure 5–7). The primary defect in holoprosencephaly is the abnormal development of the neural tube and brain. When maxillary hypoplasia is accompanied by hypotelorism, the suspicion of some type of brain anomaly is heightened. If, in addition, the eyes are small (i.e., the palpebral fissure length is small), then there is another indication that there may an underlying brain anomaly. The association of maxillary hypoplasia, small eyes, and hypotelorism might be found in fetal alcohol syndrome, holoprosencephaly, and a number of chromosomal syndromes, including 18p- deletion syndrome.

Of course, as with any anomaly, maxillary hypoplasia can occur as an isolated finding. Some people simply have a smaller maxillary complex than others. In fact, it is understood that there are even ethnic and racial differences in facial features. The

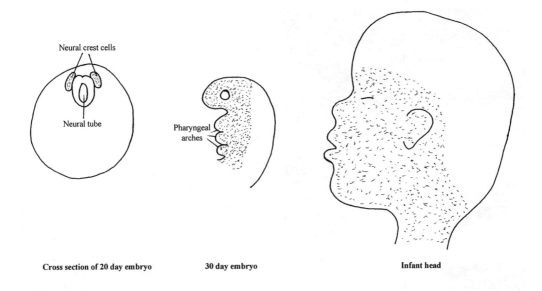

Neural crest cells

Neural tube

Pharyngeal arches

Cross section of 20 day embryo   30 day embryo   Infant head

Figure 5–20. Drawing of the early neural crest (left) and the eventual distribution of cells from the neural crest to the facial bones (stipled area).

negroid face, for example, is known to have a larger and broader midface and maxilla than the caucasian face, which in turn has a larger midface than the oriental face. Much of the difference in these racial subtypes can be appreciated by measuring the width of the nose, especially at the alar base. This variation in facial form for different racial subgroups points out the necessity for the clinician to understand the full range of variation in normal facial structure and development. Isolated maxillary hypoplasia, resulting in a Class III malocclusion (relative mandibular prognathism), may be inherited as a distinct familial trait, just like a large nose or small mandible.

Abnormal brain development may also result in secondary anomalies of the various cranial bones, which will affect facial appearance. For example, in primary microcephaly, the small brain may not exert sufficient downward force on the developing bones of the cranial base. As a result, the sphenoid bone tends to be angled differently than normal, with the wings of the sphenoid flaring upward (Figure 5–21). The facial effect of this cranial base anomaly would be upward slanting palpebral fissures and a somewhat narrow appearing cranium.

Mandibular hypoplasia has different implications than maxillary hypoplasia. The mandible, although part of the skull, is a separate bone not attached to the cranium by any other bone. The mandible has a joint with the cranial base in the glenoid fossa in a joint known as the temporomandibular joint (because of the location of this joint at the base of the temporal bone). The mandible has two larger portions of bone: the body and the ascending ramus (Figure 5–22). At the top of the ramus are the condyle (the ball-like portion which fits into the temporomandibular joint) and the coronoid process (which serves as a place for muscle attachment). The mandible may be hypoplastic as a unit, or separate components may be hypoplastic. The genetic implications for the varying types of hypoplasia are important because they relate to both specific syndromes, as well as types of anomalies related to specific tissue types and gene effects.

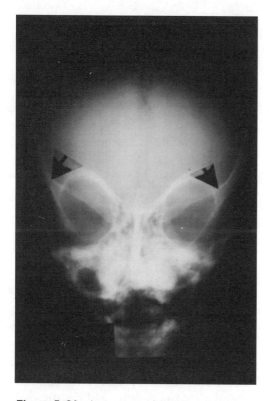

Figure 5–21. Appearance of the sphenoid bone as seen in a P-A (posterior to anterior) radiograph showing upward flaring of the sphenoid wings (arrows).

Hypoplasia of the mandibular body when the morphology of the rest of the mandible is normal tends to be a separate familial trait and not syndrome-specific. This is particularly true if the body of the mandible is small but of normal configuration. Genetic disorders, if they have an effect on the body of the mandible, tend to cause not only abnormal size, but also abnormal configuration. For example, in Treacher Collins syndrome, the body of the mandible is small and it is also malformed in that there is a deep concave depression in the base of the mandible known as an *antegonial notch* (Figure 5–23). Antegonial notching is also seen in other syndromes, including Stickler syndrome, Nager syndrome, frontometaphyseal dysplasia, Ehlers-Danlos syndrome, myotonic dystrophy, and many other syndromes with connective tissue dysplasia or muscle hypotonia.

Micrognathia is often caused by shortening of the mandibular ramus, a common finding in many syndromes where mandibular deficiency is common. In most cases, shortening of the ramus is not accompanied

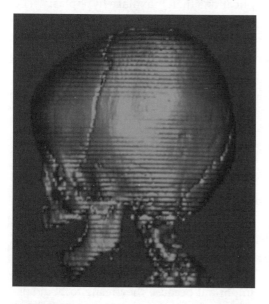

Figure 5–22. A 3-D reconstruction of the mandible from a CT scan showing the ramus, body, condyle, and coronoid process.

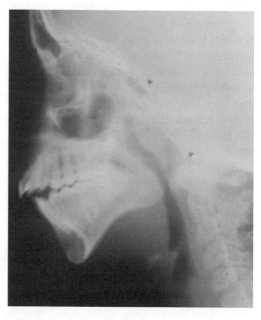

Figure 5–23. Antegonial notching of the mandible (arrow) in a patient with Treacher Collins syndrome.

by abnormalities of the condyle or coronoid process. Shortening of the ramus is common in Treacher Collins syndrome, Nager syndrome, Stickler syndrome, spondyloepiphyseal dysplasia congenita, diastrophic dysplasia, Williams syndrome, fetal alcohol syndrome, fetal hydantoin syndrome, Freeman-Sheldon syndrome, Wildervanck syndrome, Moebius syndrome, and over 100 other genetic, chromosomal, and teratogenic disorders.

Condylar hypoplasia or aplasia is commonly seen in oculo-auriculo-vertebral spectrum, but it is commonly believed that this multiple anomaly disorder is caused by a vascular disruption of the embryonic stapedial artery. As a result, there is no blood supply to the developing mandible resulting in hypoplasia or aplasia of the condyle and/or coronoid. Condylar and coronoid aplasia is accompanied by corresponding muscle deficiency and abnormality of the glenoid fossa and temporomandibular joint. This type of abnormality is not a common syndromic finding and is limited to OAVS and several lysosomal storage diseases. However, gradual condylar erosion can occur in syndromes with autoimmune disorders, such as rheumatoid changes in adolescence or early adult life. In velo-cardio-facial syndrome, which has rheumatoid disease as a late onset finding, the condyle may progressively wear and flatten so that it becomes abnormal in configuration even though it had been normal earlier in life.

On occasion, the mandible can appear retruded so that it looks like micrognathia, but in reality, the mandible is of normal size, but displaced posteriorly so that its relationship with the maxilla is retrusive. This is known as *retrognathia* rather than micrognathia. Retrognathia is caused by a flattened skull base, which has the effect of placing the glenoid fossa and temporomandibular joint more posterior than normal. Therefore, the mandible is placed more posterior so that, even if its size is normal, it appears to be small in relation to the maxilla. Retrogna-

thia is common in velo-cardio-facial syndrome, Robinow syndrome, and Weaver syndrome.

Hyperplasias

Hyperplasias are much less common than hypoplasias and tend to represent active disease processes rather than static malformations. There are relatively few syndromes with significant hyperplasia and they fall into several distinct categories: hyperplasia caused by neoplasias and hamartomas, hyperplasia caused by skeletal overgrowth, and hyperplasias caused by vascular lesions.

The majority of overgrowth syndromes are those involving neoplasias and hamartomas. One of the most common genetic diseases in humans is neurofibromatosis, actually now known to be multiple diseases, each with its own genetic etiology (see Chapter 4). The most common type, NF I, or von Recklinghausen disease, begins as multiple café-au-lait spots on the skin, especially near the axillary region (the arm pits). The natural history of NF I is that small benign tumors begin to develop on the skin which then tend to enlarge with age. NF II is probably familiar to many audiologists. NF II involves the development of acoustic neuromas. There are seven other types of NF, each with a distinctive genetic etiology and all thought to be autosomal dominant.

Other hamartomatous syndromes with facial effects include Maffucci syndrome, tuberous sclerosis, Gorlin syndrome, Cowden syndrome, Klippel-Trénauney-Weber syndrome, and Proteus syndrome. Hamartomas, usually benign congenital tumors of irregular shape and often quite large, can severely distort facial features and adversely affect speech and hearing depending on their location. The best known case of a hamartomatous syndrome is that of the so-called "elephant man," Joseph Merrick, on whose life the motion picture *The Elephant Man* was based. As pointed out by Cohen (1987), many people mistakenly believe that Joseph Merrick had neurofibromatosis, but he actually had the Proteus syndrome.

Skeletal overgrowth (other than somatic overgrowth, which will be discussed later) is found in many syndromes, but each syndrome displaying this problem is relatively rare. Skeletal overgrowth often involves the cranium and/or facial bones, as in craniometaphyseal dysplasia, frontometaphyseal dysplasia, craniodiaphyseal dysplasia (the disorder at the center of the movie *Mask*), van Buchem syndrome, sclerosteosis, and Robinow syndrome (Figure 5–24). In some cases, skeletal overgrowth occurs early in life, with major changes in appearnace shortly after birth or in early childhood, as in craniometaphyseal dysplasia, frontometaphyseal dysplasia, or craniodiaphyseal dysplasia. In other syndromes, the skeletal overgrowth does not become evident until later in life, perhaps the second or third decade of life, as in van Buchem syndrome, sclerosteosis, and Robinow syndrome. However, in all of these syndromes, the skeletal overgrowth is part of the phenotypic spectrum and directly related to gene action (autosomal dominant in the case of Robinow syndrome; autosomal recessive in the case of craniodiaphyseal dysplasia; X-linked recessive in the case of frontometaphyseal dysplasia).

Other syndromes involving hyperplasias, including Sturge-Weber syndrome, are caused by hypervascularization of the craniofacial complex. With increased blood flow to the affected region of the body, there is overgrowth of all of the tissues, including the skeleton. In Sturge-Weber syndrome, there are multiple vascular anomalies, but the primary cause for concern is the angiomatosis of the leptomeninges overlying the temporal, parietal, and occipital regions. Seizures, mental retardation, and language impairment are common in this syndrome, which is easily recognized by the large nevus flammeus (sometimes referred to as a "port wine stain") which usually covers one side of the face.

Hemihyperplasia (also known as hemihypertrophy) is a syndrome of unknown etiology (all cases have been sporadic) that presents with one side of the face being larger than the other. The hyperplasia involves the skeleton (both the mandible and maxilla) and the soft tissues, including the tongue. Although the face is asymmetric, it is easily distinguishable from oculo-auriculo-vertebral dysplasia (OAVS, which also is often called hemifacial microsomia) because the skeletal structures are normal in mor-

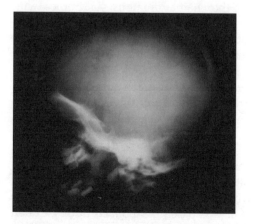 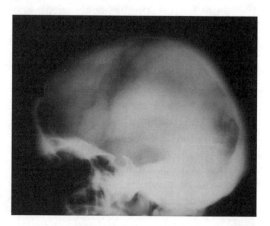

Figure 5–24. A skull radiographs of a child with Robinow syndrome (left) and an adult with Robinow syndrome (right). Note the thickening of the adult skull representing significant sclerosteosis.

phology, but unilaterally enlarged. There tends to be excessive vertical and horizontal growth of the maxilla and the teeth on the larger side tend also to be larger. The mandible shows a longer ramus, a larger condyle, and more prominent coronoid process. The diagnosis of hemihyperplasia becomes important to differentiate it from other syndromes associated with facial asymmetry because approximately 5% of affected individuals develop neoplasias, including Wilms tumor (a kidney tumor), carcinomas of the adrenal cortex, and hepatoblastoma (a liver tumor of embryonic origin). The etiology is unknown with the majority of cases being sporadic. Similar tumors may be found in Beckwith-Wiedemann syndrome, a syndrome of overgrowth, which also has mandibular prognathism, hypotonia, developmental delay, and omphalocele (herniation of the gut through the abdominal wall) or umbilical hernia. Autosomal dominant inheritance has been hypothesized, but the majority of cases have been sporadic.

Other overgrowth syndromes have facial manifestations, usually involving alterations or overgrowth of certain facial features, as well as other skeletal structures in the body. Sotos syndrome, also called cerebral gigantism, is a syndrome of excess stature, advanced bone age, early maturation, hypotonia, developmental delay, and cognitive impairment. The head is large with macrencephaly and a tall forehead with hypertelorism. Although growth slows in early adolescence, many individuals with this syndrome are very tall, and some reach exceptional heights. The facial features are distinctive because of the prominent forehead and large facial features, including the mandible, mouth, nose, and ears. Weaver syndrome, another syndrome of generalized overgrowth associated with hypotonia and developmental delay, also has a broad and prominent forehead, but the mandible tends to be retrusive. The etiology is unclear, although autosomal dominant inheritance has been suggested in some cases.

Facial Clefts

Facial clefts can occur anywhere along normal embryonic fusion lines, or may also be caused by disruptions, as with amniotic bands, and neoplasias that physically interfere with fusion. A widely accepted classification system for facial clefts was proposed by Tessier (1976), as shown in Figure 5–25. Each of the 14 clefting lines described by Tessier may have different implications with respect to etiology, and some of the more rare cleft types are strongly suggestive of specific syndromic diagnoses. For example, a lateral oral commisure cleft, classified by Tessier as the number 7 soft tissue facial cleft (Figure 5–25), occurs in relatively few conditions including oculo-auriculo-vertebral spectrum and Townes syndrome. Table 5–2 lists some of the syndromes associated with each of the Tessier cleft types.

Facial clefts can occur as isolated events, but several studies have shown that a high percentage, if not the majority, of children with facial clefts have multiple anomaly syndromes. In other words, clefts are most often symptoms (or clinical features) of multiple anomaly syndromes. However, because clefts are so obvious, especially if they involve the lip or other facial soft tissues, that they are often regarded as the primary anomaly, although in reality they are merely symptomatic of a more generalized pattern of malformation.

In the earliest studies of anomalies associated with clefts, it was reported that fewer than 3% of all children with clefts had multiple anomaly syndromes (Fraser, 1970). However, in 1981, reviewing 2,512 cases at the Center for Craniofacial Anomalies at the University of Illinois Medical Center in Chicago, Rollnick and Pruzansky reported that 44% had multiple anomaly syndromes in association with their clefts. Several years later, Shprintzen, Siegel-Sadewitz, Amato, & Goldberg (1985) reviewed 1,000 consecutive patients with clefts from The Center for Craniofacial Disorders of Montefiore Medical Center in New York, all of whom were

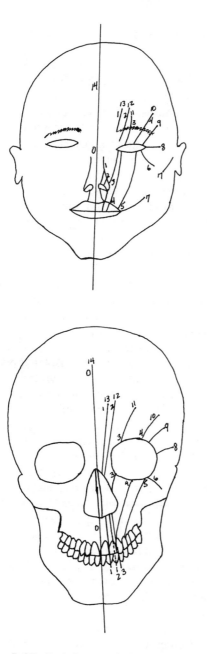

Figure 5–25. Tessier's categorization system for soft tissue (top) and skeletal (bottom) clefts.

prospectively assessed for the presence of multiple anomalies and possible syndromic associations. Shprintzen et al. (1985) found that 53% of their sample had multiple anomaly syndromes, and over 60% had multiple anomalies (i.e., not all cases with

multiple anomalies were given syndromic diagnoses). In a smaller sample of 428 consecutive cases from the Cleft Palate Program at Children's Hospital in San Diego, Jones (1988) reported that over 30% had multiple anomaly syndromes. In all three studies, the highest percentage of associated anomalies occurred in individuals with cleft palate, but no cleft lip, and individuals with submucous clefts were found to have an even higher rate of syndromic associations than those with overt clefts. Although the percentage of syndromes associated with clefts in these three studies ranged from 30% to 53%, all had far higher percentages than originally reported by Fraser (1970). It may therefore be concluded that children with clefts have a high risk for the presence of associated anomalies or syndromes. Therefore, when a child who has a cleft is seen, rather than assuming that the child is otherwise normal, clinicians should be suspicious that the child has other malformations that might require assessment. All types of syndromes (chromosomal, genetic, teratogenic, and mechanically induced) have clefts of the lip, palate, or other facial components as clinical features.

Cleft lip occurs in chromosomal syndromes, such as trisomy 13, 4p- (Wolf-Hirschhorn syndrome), 5p- (cri-du-chat syndrome), and 18p- syndrome. Van der Woude syndrome, EEC syndrome (Ectrodactyly, Ectodermal dysplasia, and Clefting), Rapp-Hodgkin ectodermal dysplasia syndrome, and Robinow syndrome are all examples of autosomal dominant genetic disorders with cleft lip as a common finding. Teratogenic syndromes with cleft lip include fetal alcohol syndrome and fetal hydantoin syndrome. Amnion rupture sequence represents a mechanically induced syndrome that often has cleft lip as a finding.

Cleft palate occurs in many chromosomal syndromes including all of the chromosomal syndromes listed above (trisomy 13, 4p-, 5p-, and 18p-), as well as many others, including Turner syndrome (45XO), 6q-, tri-

TABLE 5–2. Syndromes and common disorders associated with the facial cleft types described by Tessier (1976).

Cleft Type	Associated Syndromes
0	Holoprosencephaly sequence (premaxillary agenesis type) and all associated syndromes; oral-facial digital syndrome, types I, V, and VIII (soft tissue only); dermoid cysts; Meckel-Gruber syndrome; hydrolethalis syndrome; short rib-polydactyly syndrome, type II (Majewski type); Mohr syndrome; frontonasal dysplasia sequence; Pallister-Hall syndrome
1	Amnion rupture sequence; encephalocele
2	Amnion rupture sequence; cleft lip-cleft palate and all associated syndromes (hundreds have been delineated and will not be listed here but many are referenced in Appendix 1)
3	Amnion rupture sequence; cleft lip-cleft palate and all associated syndromes (hundreds have been delineated and will not be listed here but many are referenced in Appendix 1)
4	Amnion rupture sequence; oculo-auriculo-vertebral spectrum; nasopalpebral lipoma-coloboma syndrome
5	Amnion rupture sequence; oculo-auriculo-vertebral spectrum
6	Treacher Collins syndrome; Nager syndrome; oculo-auriculo-vertebral spectrum; Townes syndrome; Miller syndrome
7	Treacher Collins syndrome; Nager syndrome; oculo-auriculo-vertebral spectrum; Townes syndrome; Miller syndrome
8	Treacher Collins syndrome; Nager syndrome; oculo-auriculo-vertebral spectrum; Miller syndrome
9	Encephalocele; amnion rupture sequence; oculo-auriculo-vertebral spectrum
10	Encephalocele; amnion rupture sequence; oculo-auriculo-vertebral spectrum
11	Encephalocele; amnion rupture sequence
12	Encephalocele; amnion rupture sequence
13	Encephalocele; amnion rupture sequence
14	Craniofrontonasal dysplasia syndrome; amnion rupture sequence; frontal encephaloceles; dermoid cysts

somy 21 (Down syndrome), penta-X syndrome (49XXXXX), and triploidy. There are literally hundreds of syndromes with cleft palate as a finding. The most common, by far, is velo-cardio-facial syndrome (Shprintzen et al., 1985), which accounts for approximately 8% of all children with clefts of the palate without cleft lip. Other common genetic syndromes associated with cleft palate (in descending order of frequency according to the 1985 study of Shprintzen et al.) include Stickler syndrome, van der Woude syndrome, fetal alcohol syndrome, holoprosencephaly, Treacher Collins syndrome, and oculo-auriculo-vertebral spectrum, to name just a few. The majority of the syndromes with cleft palate as a feature are autosomal dominant, with just a small smattering of autosomal recessive and X-linked recessive syndromes. Teratogenic syndromes frequently associated with cleft palate are fetal alcohol syndrome and fetal hydantoin syndrome. Amnion rupture sequence can cause cleft palate without cleft lip, although it is more commonly seen in association with cleft lip or facial clefting. Another cause of disruptions leading to cleft palate are congenital tumors or defects of the skull base that

intrude into the oral cavity and prevent the palatal shelves from fusing, such as in oral teratomas, encephaloceles, or dermoid cysts.

Asymmetries

Asymmetries may be isolated to a single part of the face and occur without other anomalies, or may be found in multiple craniofacial structures and be associated with other anomalies. When associated with other anomalies, the malformations may be craniofacial and/or extracranial.

When asymmetries are isolated to a single part of the craniofacial complex, the likelihood is that the asymmetry is caused by a mechanical factor. Most syndromes that cause craniofacial asymmetry tend to affect multiple craniofacial structures and often have other anomalies in association. For example, Wildervanck syndrome is a multiple anomaly disorder that has facial asymmetry, sensorineural hearing loss, spinal anomalies (a Klippel-Feil type cervical vertebrae fusion), eye muscle abnormalities and may involve cognitive impairment (varying from mild to severe). The facial asymmetry in Wildervanck syndrome occurs in the mandible, the maxilla, the orbits, and the ears. In many cases, the entire cranium may be asymmetric. Furthermore, extracranial anomalies are common, such as the spine malformations, asymmetric shoulder (called Sprengel shoulder), and rib anomalies.

Asymmetries isolated to a single region or structure of the face are often related to fetal compression and are more common among babies in breech position, in twins (because intrauterine compression is more common in twin pregnancies), and in other instances where external mechanical forces are present. In some cases, an extracranial anomaly might be present, such as a club foot, which might also be caused by external compression, but in most instances, mechanical deformations are regional. Conversely, in cases of mild expressions of syndromes with asymmetric facies, it may appear that the anomaly is isolated to a single region of the face. However, in most multiple anomaly syndromes, the asymmetry is detectable in multiple craniofacial structures (such as the eyes, ears, and mandible), and other anomalies are usually detectable if the phenotypic spectrum is properly explored, such as ocular dermoids in oculo-auriculo-vertebral spectrum, thumb anomalies in Townes syndrome, or Wilms tumor in hemihyperplasia. It would be unusual to find a multiple anomaly syndrome with only a single affected region or body part.

Because positional deformations are often associated with a detectable problem during pregnancy (such as breech presentation, twinning, or oligohydramnios), the absence of any intrauterine disorders in pregnancy may help to convince the clinician that the anomalies present in the child are intrinsic and therefore not related to extrinsic factors. As mentioned earlier in this chapter, a careful history is very helpful in trying to sort out this dilemma.

Structural Abnormalities or Redundancies

Aberrant or redundant structures in the craniofacial complex are not as common as hypoplasias, hyperplasias, clefts, and asymmetries. Structural abnormalities (excluding hypoplasias, hyperplasias, clefts, and asymmetries) imply a completely aberrant pattern of development and very often represent severe anomalies that are either incompatible with life or result in very severe impairment. For example, otocephaly (Figure 5–26) is a pattern of malformation that has no correlate to normal human development. The infant shown in Figure 5–26 has no lower jaw, a rudimentary mouth opening placed between ears which are fused at the base of the head, abnormal orbits, and an abnormal proboscis, which is in an abnormal position with nostrils facing upward rather than downward. Although one

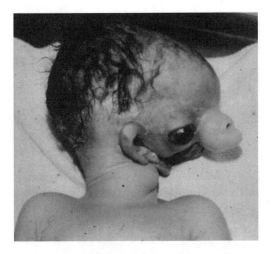

Figure 5–26. A baby with otocephaly, a severe pattern of malformation incompatible with life.

could try to explain this pattern of malformation based on possible errors of the embryonic process, in reality, it is difficult to relate otocephaly to normal embryogenesis as one might relate a cleft palate to failure of the maxillary processes to fuse. There are other such craniofacial anomalies, but they are relatively rare and of unknown causation. Because many of these anomalies are incompatible with life, there is little opportunity to determine if they are genetic (i.e., people with these anomalies can not reproduce). Other anomalies that are very aberrant include holoprosencephaly associated with cyclopia, and absence of the nose.

Craniofacial redundancies are also rare. Oral duplication (Figure 5–27) may involve either the maxilla or mandible with only the internal skeletal structures being involved. Duplication of the tongue has also been noted. Nasal duplication is extremely rare and many cases of presumed nasal duplication have actually involved a midline facial cleft with a single bifid nose. The most common form of redundancy is the presence of ear tags, which usually are found in a region between the lateral oral commissure and the tragus on the same side (Figure 5–28). Accessory ear tags are quite common

and are often found in association with a multiple anomaly syndrome, such as oculo-auriculo-vertebral spectrum, Townes syndrome, and a number of chromosomal syndromes. Ear tags may also occur in isolation, and when this is the case, they are often inherited as a separate autosomal dominant trait without associated anomalies. In general, the presence of accessory tissues on the face or head is an indication of a possible syndromic association with one of the syndromes involving a developmental interruption of the normal migration of tissues from one part of the embryo to another.

The Eyes

The old aphorism, "the eyes are the windows of the soul," may be a romantic and quaint notion, but it is true that the eyes may often be a window to a diagnosis. Because the eyes are so easily observed and often focused on by an examiner (because it is important to make good eye contact), it is possible for even casual observers to assess eye size, position, structure, color, orientation, and function.

Size

The size of the eyes is both diagnostic, and an indicator of possible developmental errors indicative of underlying brain anomalies. As discussed earlier in this chapter, the eyes are embryologic outpouchings of the brain. As such, underlying anomalies of the prosencephalon, the portion of the brain that is the substrate for eye formation (see Figure 5–3), may give rise to size or structural anomalies of the eye. Small eye size is a feature of many syndromes of chromosomal, genetic, and teratogenic causation. In almost all cases, small eyes are bilateral. Although unilateral microphthalmia (small eye) or anophthalmia (absent eye) may occur in oculo-auriculo-vertebral spectrum, in the large majority of syndromes with microphthalmia, the effect is bilateral.

In the majority of syndromes where the eyes are small, there is associated develop-

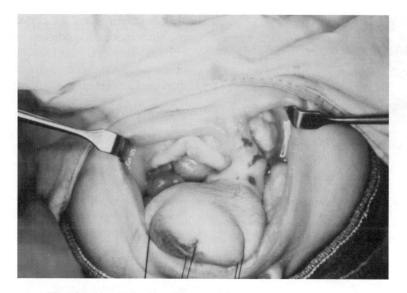

Figure 5–27. Duplication of the oral skeletal structures and the tongue in a 6-month-old infant.

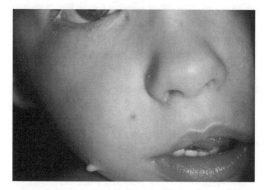

Figure 5–28. Accessory ear tags found on a line between the oral commissure and the tragus.

mental delay and/or cognitive impairment. For example, small eyes are commonly found in chromosomal disorders (which almost always have cognitive impairment as a finding) and teratogenic syndromes, such as fetal alcohol syndrome and fetal hydantoin syndrome, which also have cognitive dysfunction as a near consistent feature. Genetic syndromes with microphthalmia often have some form of cognitive impairment, such as in velo-cardio-facial syndrome, although this is not always so. Small eyes, for example, are common in Hallerman-Streiff syndrome and may be found in oculo- dento-

osseous syndrome, but mental retardation is not a consistent finding in these disorders.

Anthropometric measurements help to confirm that the eyes are small. Palpebral fissure length may be measured with a tape measure or ruler and compared to established norms. A reduced palpebral fissure length is most often indicative of structurally small eyes, but only a comprehensive ophthalmic examination can confirm that the globes are actually small.

Large eyes are not really a clinical feature of any syndrome, although prominent or bulging eyes may be found in a number of disorders. Bulging eyes may be caused by a number of factors, which may occur individually or in combination. Bulging eyes are typically labeled **exorbitism** or **exophthalmus.** Both of these terms apply to the appearance of the globe of the eye extending out from the socket of the orbit so that a substantial amount of sclera is typically showing (Figure 5–29). Exorbitism or exophthalmus may be caused by a shallow orbit, maxillary hypoplasia, posterior sloping of the forehead (frontal bone retrusion), or growths behind the globe that push forward on the eye, making it protrude from the orbit.

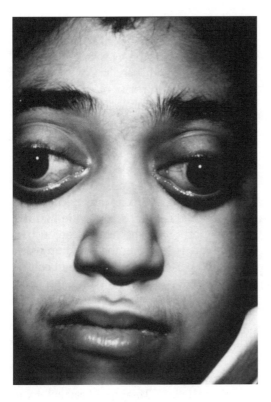

Figure 5–29. Exorbitism in Crouzon syndrome. Note the amount of sclera (the white portion of the eye) that shows because of the amount of eye exposed outside of the orbit.

Shallow orbits are seen frequently in syndromes of craniosynostosis, such as Crouzon, Apert, Pfeiffer, and Jackson-Weiss syndromes. Because pansynostosis is common in these syndromes, there is increased intracranial pressure with the brain growing inside of the cranium against a closed and locked cranial bony matrix. Therefore, the brain exerts pressure against any opening which might expand with the increasing intracranial pressure. In some cases (see Figure 5–10), when the anterior fontanel is still open even though the remaining sutures are closed, the fontanel bulges outward causing a large bump on the top of the head (sometimes referred to as a **bregmatic bump** because of its location at the bregma). Another location that provides less resistance to the expansion of the brain

is the orbit because of the opening in the back of the orbit for the optic nerve (the optic foramen). The forward pressure of the brain pushes the posterior segments of the orbital bones forward, thus reducing the depth of the orbits and forcing the eye to extend further beyond the rims of the orbits than normal. Because the syndromes of craniosynostosis also tend to have maxillary deficiency, the exorbitism is exaggerated by retrusion of the upper part of the maxilla which contains the inferior orbital rims. Furthermore, the forehead is also frequently retrusive in these syndromes because of fusion of the coronal sutures, which also tends to draw the superior orbital rim posteriorly. Shallow orbits may be found in other syndromes where there are skull base anomalies that might result in an alteration of the relationship of the depth of the orbit. Stickler syndrome may often have mild exophthalmus related to slight reduction in the orbital depth because of the acute angle of the posterior skull base. Conversely, syndromes with an obtuse angulation of the skull base, such as velo-cardio-facial syndrome, often have eyes that appear sunken or deep set. Therefore, if a patient's eyes appear to be bulging, the clinician should be aware of the possible contributions to the problem and make appropriate referrals for assessment of possible craniosynostosis or increased intracranial pressure, possibly secondary to one of the easily identified syndromes of pansynostosis. Other syndromes have bulging eyes as a feature unrelated to craniosynostosis, (related rather to maxillary hypoplasia, small orbits, or cranial base anomalies), but these syndromes, with the exception of Stickler syndrome, are relatively rare.

Position

Assessing eye position requires attention to the distance between the eyes, the symmetry of eye placement, and the vertical and horizontal placement of the eyes in relation to each other. Distances between the eyes were discussed earlier in this chapter. Figure 5–16 shows the measurements that can be applied to ocular distances. In brief summary, hypotelorism should alert the clinician to the possibility of an underlying brain anomaly in a patient and the several syndromic diagnoses that include hypotelorism as a clinical feature. Hypertelorism, a more common clinical finding in craniofacial syndromes, does not have the same implications as hypotelorism. Although both abnormalities of eye position may be associated with cognitive dysfunction and mental retardation, hypotelorism is both a more ominous and limited finding. The presumption in hypotelorism is that there was not sufficient growth in the anterior portion of the brain, the prosencephalon, to drive the eyes apart during the embryonic process. Therefore, hypotelorism is correctly associated with underlying brain malformation. Hyper-telorism, on the other hand, may have multiple developmental causes. Although certain brain anomalies might contribute to the wide spacing of the eyes, skeletal anomalies, neural crest migration abnormalities, neoplasias, encephaloceles (rupturing of the brain through the frontal bone between the eyes), and facial clefts caused by either fusion failure or amniotic adhesions can all contribute to hypertelorism. Not all of these problems will necessarily give rise to cognitive impairment.

Dystopia canthorum, also described earlier in this chapter, is caused by a lateral displacement of the inner canthus without abnormality of the skeletal orbit so that the outer canthus is normally positioned. Because dystopia canthorum can be caused by something as simple as epicanthal folds, it may not be an indicator of cognitive impairment. Because the positioning of the eyes is judged relative to other facial structures, abnormalities of position may not always be obvious. Optical illusions may interfere with judgments of ocular distances. For example, if the eyes are widely spaced, but the nose is very broad, it may

lead to the impression that eye position is normal. If, however, the nasal root is narrow or depressed, the eyes might seem to be abnormally wide-set.

Although the majority of eye anomalies are related to abnormal position of the inner canthus, one syndrome has abnormal position of the outer canthus as its primarily recognized feature (Figure 5–30). Kabuki make-up syndrome received this particular appelation because, even though the orbital and eye sizes are normal, the outer canthus is often set so wide that the reddish portion of the lateral conjunctiva can be seen, resembling the make-up worn by Kabuki performers in Japan. Not coincidentally, the syndrome was first described by Japanese clinicians.

In the majority of syndromes with eye position anomalies, orbital location is symmetrical around the facial midline. However, there are some disorders in which eye placement may be asymmetric in either the vertical or horizontal plane. This type of asymmetry is

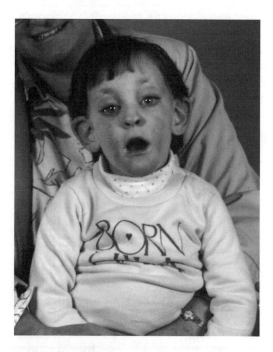

Figure 5–30. A child with Kabuki make-up syndrome.

known as dystopia. The majority of dystopias are caused by nonsyndromic disorders, such as plagiocephaly caused by unilateral coronal suture fusion, especially if the fusion is close to the skull base. If the coronal suture is fused, the orbit on the synostosed side cannot be driven into its normal position by brain growth. Horizontal and/or vertical displacement of the orbit are common in plagiocephaly, especially if left untreated beyond infancy. Unilateral orbital asymmetry can also be caused by positional deformations, torticollis (see Chapter 3), neoplasias, facial clefts, and amnion rupture sequence. There are, however, several multiple anomaly syndromes in which dystopia is an occasional or common finding. Velo-cardio-facial syndrome, Wildervanck syndrome, CHARGE association, oculo-auriculo-vertebral spectrum, Dubowitz syndrome, Saethre-Chotzen syndrome, and several other disorders all may have orbital dystopia as part of the phenotypic spectrum.

Orientation

Eye orientation refers to the angle of the palpebral fissures in relation to the rest of the facial structures. It is normal for the palpebral fissures to be oriented horizontally, essentially parallel to the ground. In other words, if one were to draw an imaginary line connecting the inner canthus to the outer canthus, this line would be close to a perfect horizontal line. Similarly, if the eyes are symmetrical and normally placed and positioned, the same line intersecting the inner and outer canthus of the left eye will intersect the inner and outer canthus of the right eye (Figure 5–31). If not normally oriented, the eyes may be upslanting or downslanting (Figure 5–31).

Upslanting eyes are often found in children with primary microcephaly. When the brain is small, during the growth and development of the skull in utero, there is insufficient expansion and pressure of the bones at the cranial base, specifically the sphenoid and ethmoid bones. As a result, the sphenoid wings may be upslanting, which then causes the orbits to be oriented in an upslanting direction. Therefore, upslanting eyes may often be indicative of a smaller than normal brain. Astute clinicians should recognize that upslanting eyes must be assessed based on the line connecting the inner and outer canthi as shown in Figure

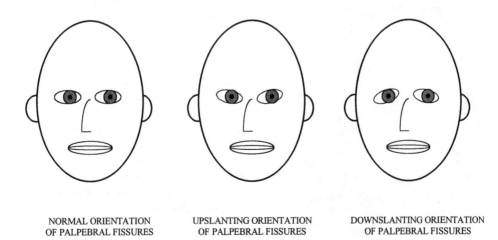

NORMAL ORIENTATION
OF PALPEBRAL FISSURES

UPSLANTING ORIENTATION
OF PALPEBRAL FISSURES

DOWNSLANTING ORIENTATION
OF PALPEBRAL FISSURES

Figure 5–31. Normal orientation of the palpebral fissures (left), upslanting eyes (middle), and downslanting eyes (right).

5–31. Otherwise, the same types of optical illusions mentioned previosuly may result in misleading interpretations of eye orientation. For example, many people mistakenly believe that people of oriental background have upslanting (i.e., "slanted" eyes). This is not at all true. Eye orientation in all races is normally horizontal. Oriental eyes are characterized by epicanthal folds, which is related to the fact that most east Asians have smaller and lower nasal roots causing some redundancy of skin at the inner canthus. The epicanthal fold makes the inner canthus look somewhat lower than in an eye without epicanthi, thus giving the impression of an upslanting eye.

Downslanting eyes are usually caused by abnormal pressure against the lateral edges of the cranium, as one might see in syndromes of craniosynostosis, especially if the skull has a *kleeblattschädel*, or clover leaf anomaly (Figure 5–32). When multiple sutures are involved, there is often bulging of the cranium in the temporal region which exerts downward pressure at the outer canthi. Downslanting eyes are also found in Treacher Collins syndrome because of abnormal ligament attachments at the outer canthi (see Figure 2–1).

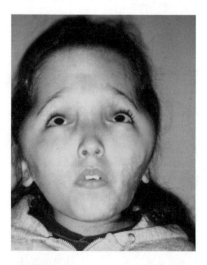

Figure 5–32. Clover leaf skull anomaly, often referred to as kleeblattschädel.

Eye Structure

Structural eye anomalies are among the most common of congenital malformations and many have strong associations with specific syndromes so that they have strong diagnostic impact. For example, dermoid cysts on the eye (epibulbar dermoids, choristomas, and conjunctival dermoids) are so commonly associated with oculo-auriculo-vertenral spectrum that, if one is detected in a patient, there is a very high probablility that the patient has OAVS (see Figure 5–14). Because the eyes are so easily visible on even cursory observation of a patient, anomalies of the eye, the lid, the eye lashes, the iris, and pupil should be noted; and the clinician should assume that they are symptomatic of the presence of a multiple anomaly syndrome. This assumption will prove to be correct the large majority of the time. Structural eye anomalies occur in isolation relatively infrequently.

Ocular colobomas, as noted earlier in this chapter, may be symptomatic of an underlying brain malformation. Colobomas of the iris occur in a small number of syndromes, including holoprosencephaly, CHARGE association, cat eye syndrome (caused by trisomy of the long arm of chromosome 22), and Rieger syndrome, which also has dental anomalies including congenital absence of some of the teeth.

Other structural eye anomalies include microphthalmia (small eyes which may be unilateral or bilateral), anophthalmia (a missing eye), an absent iris (aniridia), an acentric pupil, a small iris and pupil (usually symptomatic of microphthalmia), congenital cataracts, a dislocated lens, clefts of the eye lid, absent lashes on the bottom lid, or very thick curly lashes on the upper lid. All of these findings are known to occur in association with specific syndromic entities, which may be easily checked by any clinician who has access to a computer data base or to any of the excellent compendiums that list multiple anomaly syndromes. These associations will have both diagnostic importance as well as direct implications for patient care that may impact general health and may even expose life-threatening conditions. For example, a dislocation of the lens is a feature of only several syndromes, the most common of which is Marfan syndrome. Marfan syndrome, a common autosomal dominant genetic condition that is caused by a mutation in a fibrillin gene, has several findings that are potentially life-threatening, including dilatation of the aortic root and aortic aneurysm, which may rupture spontaneously causing sudden death. Therefore, in previously undiagnosed cases where a dislocated lens is detected or suspected, the suspicion of Marfan syndrrome becomes important to overall patient care. Anophthalmia is often associated with OAVS, cataracts with amnion rupture sequence and over 20 other syndromes, absent lashes on the lower lid in Treacher Collins syndrome and Nager syndrome, and thick lashes with several of the lysosomal storage diseases. Aniridia is most often associated with a small interstitial deletion of chromosome 11 (11p13-), which also causes mental retardation and Wilms tumor.

Eye Color

Eye color peculiarities associated with syndromes may present as heterochromia (two different colored eyes in the same patient), a predilection for a syndrome to present with a particular colored eye, an unusual pattern of colors in the iris, or abnormalities in the color of the sclera, the part of the eye that is normally white. Abnormalities of eye color are not among the most common of eye anomalies, but may provide important clues to diagnosis. Heterochromia iridium is one of the important diagnostic signs of Waardenburg syndrome, a common syndrome of sensorineural hearing loss. It is not unusual to find individuals with Waardenburg syndrome who have one blue eye and one brown eye, along with other pigmentary abnormalities, including a white forelock and depigmented areas of skin. A predisposition for hazel or blue eyes is demonstrated by Williams syndrome. Over 60% of individuals with Williams syndrome have blue or hazel eyes. Distinctive patterns of color in the iris are also common in both Williams syndrome and Down syndrome. A so-called "stellate" iris in Williams syndrome and Brushfield spots in the iris in Down syndrome (Figure 5–33) are distinctive findings that are also present in a number of other syndromes.

Eye Function

The function of the eyes may be affected by a number of factors, including eye muscle anatomy and physiology, central nervous system anomalies, eye-lid function, cranio-

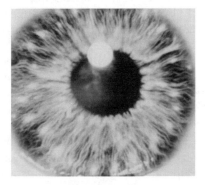

Figure 5–33. Iris pattern in an individual with Williams syndrome showing stellate pattern (left) and an individual with Down syndrome showing the Brushfield spot pattern common in trisomy 21 (right).

facial structure, retinal anatomy, and visual acuity. These factors may affect the ability of the eyes to converge, impair the light focusing capacity of the eyes, or impair the ability of the retina to receive an image and pass it along to the brain via the optic nerve.

Abnormalities of the muscles attached to the eyes within the orbits (the muscles responsible for the mobility of the eyes from side to side and up and down) can impair the two eyes' ability to converge on an object. The most common term used to describe the failure of the eye muscles to allow this type of convergence is **strabismus.** If the problem is that one eye turns out, this is labeled **exotropia.** If the problem is that one eye turns in, the problem is labelled **esotropia.** Strabismus is correctable by a number of methods, depending on the severity and duration of the problem. Lenses may be helpful when the problem is detected early and is not too severe. In other cases, eye muscle surgery is necessary. Strabismus is associated with over 50 syndromes, including the syndromes of craniosynostosis (usually exotropia), Down syndrome (usually esotropia), and Stickler syndrome (usually esotropia). Another variation of this type of problem is known as **amblyopia.** Some people refer to this problem as a "lazy eye." In amblyopia, one eye may chronically wander, so that each eye presents competing images to the brain. Rather than see double, the brain suppresses vision in the wandering eye. Therefore, unless treated early by patching, lenses, or surgery, children with amblyopia may lose vision permanently in one eye.

Some children with central nervous system impairments show another type of eye movement abnormality called **nystagmus.** There are several types of nystagmus, characterized by the types of movements that the eyes make. Nystagmus may be prompted by central nervous system anomalies, very poor vision (sometimes called "search nystagmus"), or retinal and macular anomalies. Most common is a rapid side-to-side movement, which is often rhythmic, although sometimes intermittent. Nystagmus is associated with over 50 syndromes, including various forms of albinism, Hallermann-Streiff syndrome (secondary to microphthalmia, cataracts, and poor vision), Down syndrome (secondary to neurologic anomalies), Pena-Shokeir syndrome (secondary to brain anomalies), holoprosencephaly, and Cockayne syndrome (secondary to central and peripheral nervous system degeneration).

Other eye motility disorders may be caused by agenesis or hypoplasia of the cranial nerves, such as Duane anomaly, which is associated with a number of multiple anomaly syndromes. The Duane anomaly is a disorder of both eye and eyelid movement thought to be caused by hypoplasia or aplasia of the VIth cranial nerve nucleii. Lateral or up-and-down movements of the globe may be impaired, as well as narrowing of the palpebral fissures by the eyelids.

Craniofacial structure may also contribute to abnormal eye function. The most direct effects on the eye can be caused by craniofacial anomalies that contact the eye and can cause changes in the curvature of some or all of the eye, thus resulting in astigmatism, abrasions, cataracts, or amblyopia. In Treacher Collins syndrome, the lashes of the lower lid are often turned in against the eye because of structural anomalies of the lid and its attached muscles. The constant rubbing of the lower lashes against the eye can result in astigmatism and abrasions. Astigmatism is also a likely outcome in oculo-auriculo-vertebral spectrum because of dermoid cysts and choristomas (see Figure 5–14). Eyelid anomalies caused by amnion adhesions may also cause similar problems.

Dystopia (see above) may also cause alteration of visual function, especially if the problem is severe. If the eyes are at different vertical levels, the natural tendency is for the patient to try to accommodate by positioning the head tilted to one side to keep the eyes level. If the dystopia is severe in the horizontal direction, so that one eye is shadowed by the nose or other facial structures, lateral gaze may be affected and result in amblyopia.

Structural anomalies that block vision in one eye are also likely to result in amblyopia. For example, tumors, eyelid anomalies, cataracts, or choristomas may cover part or all of the pupil, which will cause one eye to receive a competing signal. In such cases, amblyopia is all but assured if correction is not accomplished early in life. Ptosis, an inability to raise the upper eyelid, will have the same effect, especially if unilateral. Ptosis is typically caused by eye muscle anomalies or Duane anomaly and should also be corrected to avoid visual impairment.

The Ears

The ears are of particular importance to specialists in the communicative sciences because of their obvious connection to hearing and speech and language development. Although this seems so obvious as to be almost absurd to mention, clinicians should ask themselves if they actually ever pay much attention to ear structure, size, position, or orientation. Each of these factors may have a direct impact on hearing and they often represent clinical features of well known syndromes which reflect anomalies of cranial structure.

Ear Structure

Anomalies of ear structure include microtias, malformations of individual ear components (such as the helix or lobule), abnormal morphogenesis, and the degree of adherence of the ear to the temporal bone. Microtia is typically described in terms of the degree of abnormality of the external ear on a scale from Grade I through Grade III. In Grade I microtia, the ear is small, but the external canal is patent, (although it may be smaller than normal) and all of the normal ear structures are present (Figure 5–34). In

Grade II microtia, the external ear is malformed, and the external canal is usually present but is usually stenotic (ending in a blind pit or alley) or severely narrowed. The middle ear space is small and the ossicles are malformed or fused. Some components of the external ear may be abnormal, such as the lobule or helical rims (Figure 5–34). In Grade III microtia, the external ear is severely malformed or completely absent, the external canal is absent, and the middle ear space is either absent or nearly absent with severely malformed or absent ossicles (Figure 5–34). The degree of hearing loss is well correlated to the degree of microtia. Almost all microtias have some degree of conductive hearing loss, with Grade III microtias presenting with maximal conductive impairment. In some cases, Grade III microtias may also be accompanied by sensorineural hearing loss, although this is not common.

Malformations of individual ear components are typically found in the helix or lobule. Tragal or anthelical anomalies, or isolated anomalies of the external canal, are not as common. Helical rim anomalies include thickening or overfolding of the helical rims, as seen in velo-cardio-facial syndrome (Figure 5–35) or thinning of the helical rims as is often seen in Treacher Collins syndrome or Nager syndrome (Figure 5–35). Lobule anomalies may be subtle, such as creases in the lobules seen in Beckwith-Wiedemann syndrome (Figure 5–36) and absent or adherent lobules as seen in velo-cardio-facial syndrome (see Figure 5–35).

Abnormal morphogenesis is exemplified by Grade II and Grade III microtias, but in cases where this type of severe malformation is not present, errors in morphogenesis can be inferred from the presence of ear tags or preauricular pits. Tags and pits are associated with a number of syndromes, including OAVS, BOR syndrome, and Townes syndrome, among others.

Normally, the auricles sit close to the temporal bone without being adherent to it or being separated to the point that the ears

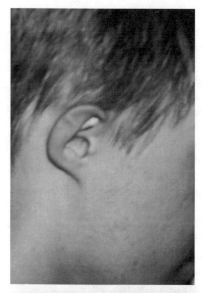

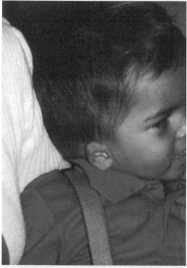

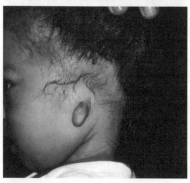

Figure 5–34. Grades of microtia, showing a Grade I microtia (top), Grade II (middle) and Grade III (bottom).

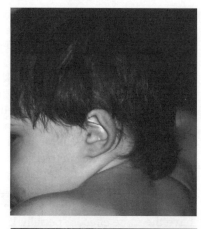

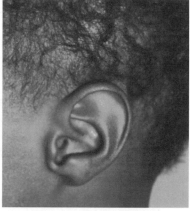

Figure 5–35. Helical rim anomalies, including overfolded helices in velo-cardio-facial syndrome (top) and thin helical rims in Nager syndrome (bottom). Also note the adherent lobules in the velo-cardio-facial syndrome ear at left.

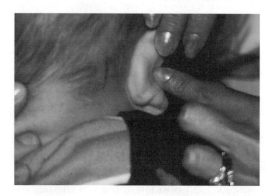

Figure 5–36. Creases in the lobule of a patient with Beckwith-Wiedemann syndrome.

stick out. Adherent ears may be found in a number of syndromes, including achondroplasia, but a more common anomaly is an ear that is protuberant or cup-shaped. Protuberant ears are common in syndromes where hypotonia is a common feature because the muscles inserted into the base of the auricle which overlie the temporal bone act to keep the auricles close to the cranium. If these muscles are weak or hypotonic, protuberant ears often result. Protuberant ears may be seen in Down syndrome, velo-cardio-facial syndrome, Langer-Giedion syndrome, fetal alcohol syndrome, and Weaver syndrome.

Ear Size

Microtia, already discussed above, is a somewhat more common finding associated with multiple anomaly syndromes than large ears. Very often, small ears or microtia not only assist in the diagnostic process, but also suggest conductive hearing loss as a part of the phenotypic spectrum. Large ears, on the other hand, do not connote hearing loss or malformation of the middle ear. Large ears are more typically associated with syndromes that have some degree of cognitive impairment, which is not necessarily the case with small ears (although it may be for certain syndromes). Large ears may be found in Beckwith-Wiedemann syndrome, Weaver syndrome, Sotos syndrome, Langer-Giedion syndrome, and Kabuki make-up syndrome, all of which are commonly associated with some degree of cognitive impairment. Anthropometric measurements of the ear become important for establishing their size because "eyeballing" the size of the ear may result in mistaken interpretations of the true size relative to the cranium and face. When the face is small, the ears tend to look large, even when by measurment they are small. In the case of protruding ears, it is necessary to flatten the ear before measurement so its true linear size can be determined. In general, ear size is not necessarily reflective of an underlying middle ear anomaly and

hearing loss unless the syndrome is known to have middle ear malformations as a clinical feature, or if cleft palate is a common feature in the syndrome and chronic middle ear effusion is a secondary consequence.

Ear Position

The ears should normally be positioned at a level comparable to that of the eyes. Specifically, if an imaginary line is drawn connecting the palpebral fissures of the eye and that line is extended back to-ward the ear (assuming that the eyes are not upslanting or downslanting), the line should intersect at least one third of the ear. Of course, if the ear is small, especially in its upper portion, it may distort this type of judgment. If the ear falls below the imaginary line, it is considered to be low set. Clinically, there is no circumstance that could lead to "high set" ears. Low set ears typically have been considered to be associated with cognitive impairment, but this is certainly not true for all syndromes. For example, the ears are often low set in Stickler syndrome and Crouzon syndrome. In both of these cases, the low position of the ears is related to the kyphosis and acute angulation of the posterior basicranium. Cognitive impairment is not typical of either of these syndromes.

The ears may also be posteriorly displaced. In syndromes where the cranial base angle is obtuse, the posterior basicranium is rotated away from the face, thus causing the ears to be more posteriorly displaced, as in Robinow syndrome and velo-cardio-facial syndrome.

Although many syndromes have abnormalities of ear position and accompanying hearing loss, the location of the ears is not responsible for the hearing impairment. Usually, the reason for the ear position abnormality and the hearing loss are the same, such as abnormalities in the structure of the skull base (which contains the temporal bone and the hearing mechanism) that are related to a primary skeletal dysplasia, which affects the middle ear and the resulting location of the outer ear. For example, in Treacher Collins syndrome, nearly all individuals have some degree of conductive hearing loss secondary to middle ear space and ossicular anomalies. These anomalies occur within the context of an abnormal skull base that is severely kyphotic, acutely angled, and deficient in the normal air spaces that exist in the cranium (including the middle ear, the ethmoid and sphenoid sinuses, and nasal chamber). Conductive hearing loss and skull base anomalies are frequently associated, and because the external ear sits over the temporal bone, which is a part of the skull base, the position of the ear will also be affected by an abnormal angulation of the basicranium.

Ear Orientation

Ear orientation is similarly affected by the rotation of the skull base and/or the position of the temporal bone. Normally, the ear is oriented in a vertical position on the side of the head, but in some syndromes, the ear is posteriorly rotated. Anterior rotation is not observed because the skull base cannot be so abnormally angulated as to cause this type of anomaly. Posterior angulation of the ear is typical in syndromes where the posterior basicranium is rotated posteriorly (i.e., acutely angled and kyphotic). As in anomalies of ear position, the angle of the ear per se does not affect hearing acuity, but if the angle of the ear is related to a syndrome in which hearing loss is caused by abnormalities in the formation of the basicranium (as in the section above), then an accompanying hearing loss should be anticipated and searched out.

The Teeth

Anomalies of the dentition are common in the general population and may be more frequent than nearly any other type of abnormality in humans. Therefore, when studying a particular syndrome, it is important to be sure that anomalies of the dentition occur with a higher frequency than expected in the general population. For example, certain teeth are frequently congenitally absent in humans (other than the third molar or "wisdom teeth"), such as the maxillary and mandibular lateral incisors. One or more premolars (bicuspids) are congenitally absent in approximately 3% of the general population.

Dental anomalies include abnormalities of number, size, structure, eruption pattern, and spacing and may occur in the primary dentition, the secondary (permanent) dentition, or both. Dental anomalies are commonly associated with multiple anomaly syndromes, especially those with craniofacial features, ectodermal dysplasia, or metabolic anomalies that could interfere with formation of the various dental components.

Abnormalities of Number

Teeth may be too few in number (called **anodontia** if all of the teeth are absent) or too many teeth may be present **(supernumerary teeth)**. As a practical issue, anomalies occurring in the primary dentition are usually of minimal concern because the primary teeth (sometimes called the deciduous or baby teeth) begin to exfoliate at around 6 years of age and anomalies in the primary denittion do not necessarily predict anomalies in the secondary teeth.

Congenital tooth absence is more common than the presence of supernumerary teeth. Congenital tooth absence can be expected in syndromes that involve ectodermal dysplasia because major components of the teeth are derived from the ectoderm in the developing embryo. Therefore, congenital tooth absence is a common manifestation in EEC syndrome, Rapp-Hodgkin syndrome, and Hay-Wells syndrome (Figure 5–37). Congenitally missing teeth may also be found in syndromes that do not have ectodermal dysplasia, including velo-car-

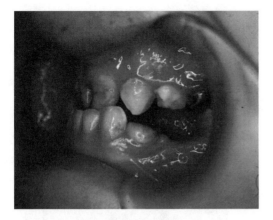

Figure 5–37. Hypodontia in EEC syndrome. Note the absence of the maxillary lateral incisors, as well as the deficient enamel.

dio-facial syndrome, Ellis-van Crevald syndrome (a syndrome of short stature and skeletal dysplasia), and Coffin-Lowry syndrome. Because congenitally missing teeth are so common in the general population, the clinician should not necessarily be concerned if a patient is missing one or two teeth, especially if they are commonly absent teeth, such as second premolars or lateral incisors. Missing teeth may be familial features and inherited as a separate trait. If the parents do not show any other anomalies, but do have missing teeth, it is possible that they have transmitted this trait to their child separately. Therefore, if the clinician notices that teeth are absent, the following should be determined:

1. Be certain that the teeth are congenitally absent and have not been extracted.
2. Be certain that the teeth are congenitally absent and are not impacted (and therefore unable to erupt).
3. Ask the parents if they are missing any teeth.

The congenital absence of teeth can be confirmed with dental radiographs, specifically a panoramic radiograph which will be able to identifiy the teeth that are present,

both erupted and unerupted. Parents may be unaware if they are missing any teeth. Therefore, clinicians should be familar with normal dental anatomy so they can determine which teeth are present.

A particular concern would be the congenital absence of a central incisor or, more precisely, the presence of only a single central incisor. As mentioned earlier in this chapter, a single central incisor is a part of the spectrum of holoprosencephalic disorders and strongly suggests an underlying brain malformation.

The clinical finding of missing teeth has a major implication for the growth and development of the jaws. Growth of the maxilla and mandible are largely dependent on the presence of teeth in the alveolar bone of the upper and lower jaws. Both the horizontal and vertical growth of the jaws is affected by the presence and degree of eruption of the teeth, which can affect facial appearance, jaw function, and occlusion. Growth of alveolar bone in both jaws is highly dependent on the presence of the teeth and the dental roots. As teeth move through the jaws, they migrate vertically until the crown of the tooth erupts through the alveolar bone and gingiva. As the root continues to move, new alveolar bone is formed around the root. The further the tooth erupts, the more alveolar bone forms around the tooth. The fewer teeth there are in the jaw, the less horizontal growth typically occurs. The more vertical eruption that occurs, the greater the vertical growth of the jaws. Similarly, the smaller the roots of the teeth, the less vertical growth there will be in the jaws. If teeth are congenitally absent, little alveolar bone forms and the height of the lower face becomes very short because of the lack of vertical development of the maxilla and mandible.

Excessive eruption of the teeth can cause increased facial height (often referred to as "long face" or vertical maxillary excess). Vertical maxillary excess (Figure 5–38) is common in indivduals with hypotonia, neuromuscular disease and primary myo-

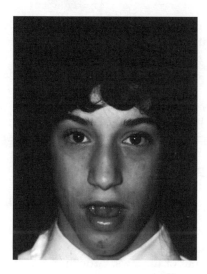

Figure 5–38. Vertical maxillary excess in an adolescent female with hypotonia resulting in increased lower face height.

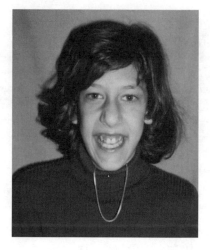

Figure 5–39. Excessive gingiva showing during smiling in an individual with vertical maxillary excess.

pathies (such as muscular dystrophies), cerebral palsy, and other forms of central nervous system disorders resulting in central hypotonia. People who are hypotonic nearly always have a chronic open-mouth posture. Because the mouth is in a chronically open position, the teeth continue to erupt vertically, therefore continuing to form new alveolar bone around the roots and increasing the alveolar height of both the maxilla and mandible. The reason for the continued eruption of the teeth is that the "signal" for teeth to discontinue their vertical migration is when they contact the corresponding teeth in the opposing jaw. In other words, unless the teeth are in the maxilla are in occlusion with the teeth of the mandible, they continue to erupt, thus forming new bone around them and causing the jaws to continue to grow vertically, resulting in a long lower third of the face. Because the alveolar bone is abnormally long in the vertical dimension in these disorders, during smiling, an excess of gingiva shows (Figure 5–39). If the majority of the vertical maxillary excess is posterior (at the molars), an anterior open-bite will develop because the teeth will occlude on the molars first (Figure 5–40). This will cause

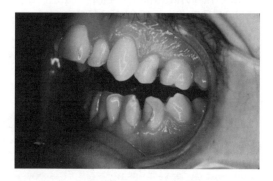

Figure 5–40. Anterior skeletal open-bite in an individual with vertical maxillary excess.

the mandible to be positioned in a more open position and therefore limit oral opening. Temporomandibular joint problems often occur in adult life. The presence of the open-bite essentially always results in a "tongue thrust" because of the open space between the teeth. Although it is tempting to believe that the tongue thrust causes the open-bite, this is not the case. Such open-bites are skeletal, not dental, in nature. The tongue thrust does not cause the open-bite. The contrary is true: the open-bite results in the tongue thrust.

Conversely, if some or most of the teeth are congenitally absent, there will be a reduction in vertical maxillary and mandibular growth because of a lack of alveolar bone height. In syndromes where the teeth are abnormally small or deficient in enamel so that they become severely decayed and may be lost or extracted, it is also probable that vertical facial height is reduced. Therefore, in syndromes of ectodermal dysplasia, such as Rapp Hodgkin syndrome or EEC syndrome, there may be deficient alveolar bone and reduced facial height.

Therefore, shortening or lengthening of the face is typically a secondary finding (in essence, a sequence) in most multiple anomaly syndromes. In syndromes with vertical maxillary excess, hypotonia should be suspected as one of the clinical features. In syndromes with reduced facial height, hypodontia, anodontia, or tooth abnormalities should be suspected. These findings have direct treatment implications. In syndromes with hypotonia and open-mouth posture, orthodontic management should be initiated to prevent the excessive eruption of the teeth (a procedure known as **intrusion**) and resultant open-bite. When the open-bite is already present, management of the tongue thrust by speech therapy or "myofunctional" techniques will not correct the tongue thrust, nor will they assist in closing the open-bite.

Abnormalities of Size

Abnormalities in the size of teeth may also have secondary effects on function and appearance, although of a somewhat different nature than anomalies of tooth number. Teeth that are too small will result in spacing problems if the jaws are of normal size. Teeth that are too large will result in crowding problems if the jaws are of normal size. However, excessive tooth size, especially if expressed in the roots of the teeth, may drive additional jaw growth and make the mouth appear larger than normal. Tooth size is quite variable in humans, both between racial subgroups and

between individuals within a racial subgroup. But normative studies and controlled studies have shown small teeth in a wide variety of syndromes, including velo-cardio-facial syndrome, EEC syndrome, Rapp-Hodgkin syndrome, frontometaphyseal dysplasia, and Ellis-van Creveld syndrome. Obviously, in syndromes of ectodermal dysplasia where enamel formation may be deficient, the teeth will be smaller. In velo-cardio-facial syndrome, hypocalcemia is a common finding, and this, too, may contribute to thinner enamel and smaller teeth. Large teeth are less common than small teeth. The best known syndrome with large teeth is the XYY chromosomal aneuploidy. Individuals with this syndrome have few dysmorphic findings, but large teeth are a consistent finding.

Abnormalities of Tooth Structure

Many types of structural tooth anomalies are caused by the basic mechanisms of gene action. Anomalies of enamel formation, root formation, and tooth shape occur in a large number of syndromes. Enamel formation has already been discussed in the context of tooth size. Defects in the enamel may also result in pitted teeth, as in tuberous sclerosis and tricho-dento-osseous syndrome. Root formation anomalies include taurodontism, short roots (as in Ehler-Danlos syndrome), pyramidal roots, globular roots, and resorbed roots. Various anomalies of tooth shape occur in syndromes, include peg-shaped teeth (common in Down syndrome), shovel-shaped teeth, and globular teeth. Opalescent teeth are found in osteogenesis imperfecta. Abnormalities in the tooth pulp may also be found in Ehlers-Danlos syndrome, including stones in the pulp chamber of the teeth.

Abnormalities of Eruption Pattern

A number of multiple anomaly syndromes have abnormal eruption patterns, including early eruption of primary or secondary teeth, late eruption, and failure of eruption (including impaction of teeth). One form of early eruption, which may be accompanied by supernumerary teeth, is the presence of natal teeth in the newborn child. Natal teeth are often found in children with cleft lip and palate (both syndromic and nonsyndromic), Ellis-van Creveld syndrome, Hallermann-Streiff syndrome, and holoprosencephaly. Natal teeth typically are lost early and may be structurally abnormal and/or supernumerary. Primary teeth may also be lost early, as often occurs in Down syndrome. Delayed eruption or failure of eruption of teeth is most noticeable and clinically significant in the secondary dentition. One of the best known syndromes with delayed or failed dental eruption is cleidocranial dysplasia syndrome, an autosomal dominant genetic condition with late fusion of the cranial sutures, small teeth, delayed or failed eruption, and absent clavicles (Figure 5–41). Very often, if teeth do not erupt, it is because the tooth buds are aligned in an abnormal position or because there is no room for the teeth in the dental arch secondary to overretained primary teeth or severe crowding.

Anomalies of Spacing

As mentioned previously, dental spacing disorders can occur secondary to abnormalities of tooth size. If tooth size is normal, abnormalities of jaw size or morphology will result in spacing disorders (Figure 5–42). For example, the maxilla tends to be wide and broad and the mouth large in Williams syndrome. The mandible tends to be smaller than the maxilla. The maxilla shows spacing problems because of its broad form. Spacing problems are further exacerbated by small teeth and short roots in Williams syndrome.

In cases where the jaws are small and the teeth are of normal size, crowding is a common finding. For example, in Stickler syndrome, both the maxilla and mandible are hypoplastic (Figure 5–43). Both jaws tend to have crowding problems requiring orthodontic management.

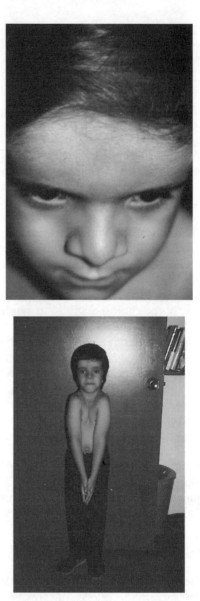

Figure 5–41. A 6-year-old male with cleidocranial dysplasia, including delayed closure of the cranial sutures resulting in an abnormal head shape (top), and absent clavicles allowing his shoulders to come together (bottom).

The Hair

The amount, color, and texture of hair in humans is extremely variable from person to person. So is the position of the anterior and posterior hairline. Although there is

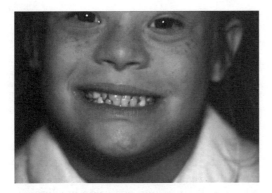

Figure 5–42. Spacing abnormality of the maxilla in a patient with Down syndrome.

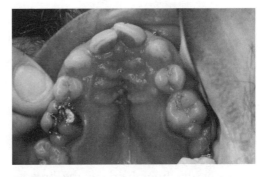

Figure 5–43. Crowding of the maxilla in a patient with Stickler syndrome.

some uniformity of hair color and texture in some racial subgroups, the number of possible combinations of hair color and texture is extremely large, and it is therefore important for clinicians to be careful about jumping to conclusions about hair anomalies. Hair texture and morphology anomalies are best detected by microscopic examination and will therefore not be discussed in detail in the context of this chapter, which is focusing on anomalies that can be easily observed on even casual inspection. However, coarse hair has been described in de Lange syndrome, several of the lysosomal storage diseases, and Menkes syndrome.

Anomalies of hair color (as long as the hair is not dyed) and amount can be seen from a short distance. Anomalies of the anterior and posterior hairline are also easily assessed by visual inspection. Hair color may be abnormal for the entire scalp, or only portions of the head hair may be abnormally colored. Patients with EEC syndrome (ectrodactyly, ectodermal dysplasia, and clefting) tend to have very light colored hair, usually very blond or platinum blond (almost white). The same is true for several other syndromes involving ectodermal dysplasia. Syndromes other than those associated with ectodermal dysplasia may also have abnormal patches of

hair color, such as the white forelock so familiar in Waardenburg syndrome. There are a number of syndromes that have sensorineural hearing loss associated with patches of depigmented hair.

Anomalies of the amount of scalp hair are best assessed by examining the scalp very closely to see how many hair follicles there are per square centimeter. However, obvious anomalies of hair abundance can be observed without such finite detail. Sparse hair is easier to assesss than abundant hair. Sparse scalp hair is seen in many syndromes of ectodermal dysplasia, including EEC syndrome, Rapp-Hodgkin syndrome, Hay-Wells syndrome, and hypohydrotic ectodermal dysplasia. Sparse hair is also associated with syndromes of premature aging or aged appearance, including proegeria, granddad syndrome, Cockayne syndrome, and Werner syndrome. A number of other syndromes, such as tricho-rhino-phalangeal syndrome, oculodento-digital syndrome, and homocystinuria, also have alopecia or sparse hair as a clinical feature. Abundant scalp hair is common in velo-cardio-facial syndrome, Coffin-Siris syndrome, de Lange syndrome, and Pena-Shokeir syndrome. Hair which appears to be thick on the scalp may be indicative of a small head circumference. In other words, the head is smaller than normal, but the number of hair follicles is normal, therefore causing the scalp hair to appear dense.

Abnormalities of the Hairline

The position of the anterior hairline is directly related to the appearance of the forehead, and therefore the entire facial region. Frequently, the position of the anterior hairline is a reflection of the height of the forehead and the anterior projection of the frontal bone, which is largely driven by the internal force of brain growth. The more posterior the front hairline, the broader and higher the forehead. The shorter the forehead, the lower the anterior hairline. The height of the frontal bone is driven by the development of the frontal lobes while the anterior projection is increased if the frontal horns of the ventricles are enlarged secondary to hydrocephalus. Macrencephaly (discussed earlier in this chapter) will also result in a broad and expansive forehead and posteriorly displaced hairline. Therefore, syndromes with macrencephaly or hydrocephalus are likely to have a posteriorly displaced anterior hairline. A posteriorly displaced anterior hairline may also be found in a number of syndromes in which there is a structural malformation of the cranium as in cleidocranial dysplasia (see Figure 5–41), but clinicians should be suspicious of an underlying brain anomaly if there are abnormalities in the position of the anterior hairline.

A low anterior hairline is common in syndromes in which the development of the frontal lobes is deficient, as in holoprosencephaly, fetal alcohol syndrome, and fetal hydantoin syndrome. Therefore, a low anterior hairline should alert the clinician to the possibility of cognitive dysfunction, or the diagnosis of a syndrome known to be associated with a deficiency of anterior brain development.

The posterior hairline is not correlated to brain development, but rather to the length and structure of the neck and the status of the underlying vertebrae. The anomaly of the posterior hairline may be abnormally low if the neck is very short, the cervical vertebrae are fused, or if there is webbing of the neck. If the neck is short, it is almost always because there is an underlying cervical vertebra anomaly, such as the Klippel-Feil anomaly (fusion of two or more cervical vertebra, hemivertebrae, and other vertebral anomalies associated with short neck and/or webbed neck), torticollis, or abnormally formed or shaped vertebrae. Vertebral anomalies are also common in oculo-auriculo-vertebral spectrum, including fusions and hemivertebrae which may result in a low posterior hairline. A low posterior hairline is also seen in syndromes that have webbing of the neck as a finding, including Turner syndrome and Noonan syndrome. The webbing of the neck in Turner syndrome is caused by congenital lymphedema of the neck, which gradually subsides leaving webbing and a low posterior hairline. Therefore, although a low set hairline itself is abnormal, the implications of the low set hairline are more important for the process of diagnosis and treatment planning.

The Hands

A patient's hands are easily visible to the clinician and even minor anomalies of the hands may be of importance in the diagnostic process. Features of the hands of importance to assess include the number of digits, the size of the hands, the length of the digits relative to the palms, the structure of the digits, the flexion creases of the digits and hands, the fingernails, and the texture of the skin.

Number of Digits

Anomalies of the number of digits may occur on one hand, or both. There may be too many or too few digits, although **polydactyly** (too many digits) is probably more common than **hypodactyly** (too few digits). Polydactyly may occur as an isolated genetic trait, but it is also a feature of Townes syndrome, the oral-facial-digital syndromes (there are eight different types),

Smith-Lemli-Opitz syndrome, Rubinstein-Taybi syndrome, Carpenter syndrome, Ellis-van Creveld syndrome, Greig syndrome, lacrimo-auriculo-dento-digital syndrome, acrocallosal syndrome, and more than 50 other disorders. Among the syndromes that feature polydactyly are a number of multiple anomaly disorders that are usually incompatible with life, such as trisomy 13 and Meckel-Gruber syndrome.

Polydactyly is categorized according to the position of the extra digit or digits. If the digit is on the thumb side of the web space between the thumb and index finger, the polydactyly is **preaxial** (Figure 5–44). If the polydactyly is on the index finger side of the web space, the polydactyly is **postaxial** (Figure 5–44). The type of polydactyly is important to differentiate because it is often

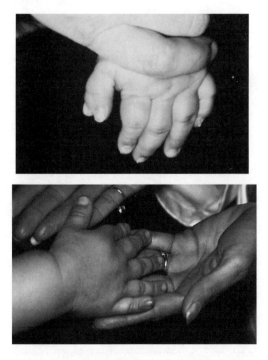

Figure 5–44. Forms of polydactyly, including preaxial polydactyly (top) where the extra digit is on the thumb side of the web space between the thumb and index finger, and postaxial polydactyly (bottom) where the extra digits are on the index finger side of the web space.

specific to the syndrome. For example, in lacrimo-auriculo-dento-digital syndrome (often referred to by the acronym LADD syndrome), the polydactyly is preaxial with anomalies of the thumb including duplication. In oral-facial-digital syndrome, Type V, the polydactyly is always postaxial, whereas in other forms of oral-facial digital syndrome, the polydactyly is often preaxial and postaxial.

Polydactyly does not always involve the formation of a complete digit. Sometimes there is a small nub or bud located in a preaxial position near the thumb or postaxially near the small finger. Polydactyly is often asymmetric with one hand being normal, or perhaps one hand being more severely involved than the other. There are, however, many syndromes with bilateral effects.

Hypodactyly may involve the complete or partial absence of one or more digits (Figure 5–45). Hypodactyly is also often asymmetric although bilateral effects are common. Syndromes where the clinician is likely to encounter complete absence of one or more digits include EEC syndrome, hypoglossia-hypodactyly syndrome, Nager syndrome (absent thumbs), and Miller syndrome. Hypoglossia-hypodactyly syndrome is of particular interest to speech pathologists because the tongue is either absent or severely hypoplastic. However, patients have been seen who have acoustically acceptable or normal speech production (Witzel, personal communication, 1996). Partial agenesis of the digits can occur in many syndromes, including de Lange syndrome, Nager sydrome, Aase syndrome, Fanconi pancytopenia syndrome, VATER association, Rothmund-Thomson syndrome, Laband syndrome, and Coffin-Siris syndrome. Absence of the thumb is a particularly serious problem because of its effect on manual dexterity. Therefore, children with absent or malformed thumbs should be referred to a qualified hand surgeon. A procedure known as policization is designed to move a postaxial digit into apposition with the rest of the digits so it can function as a thumb.

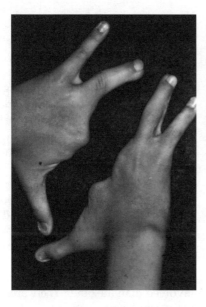

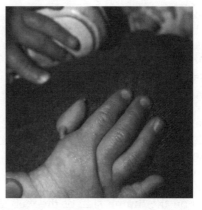

Figure 5–45. Forms of hypodactyly including absence of postaxial digits in EEC syndrome (left) and partial absence of the thumbs in Rothmund-Thomson syndrome (right).

The Size of the Hands

Small hands are a far more common clinical finding in multiple anomaly syndromes than large hands. Small hands may be found because of structural deficiency of the peripheral skeleton, poor vascularization of the distal structure (small hands are usually accompanied by small feet), anomalies specific to individual bones in the peripheral skeleton such as the metacarpals (the bones constituting the palms), or the distal phalanges (the bones of the finger tips). The width of the hand may also be narrow and the fingers may be slender. There are anthropometric normals for the size of the hands and the length of the middle finger (Figure 5–46). Palmar length is measured from the flexion crease that separates the palm from the wrist to the flexion crease that separates the base of the middle finger from the top of the palm. Middle finger length is measured from the flexion crease at the base of the middle finger to the middle finger tip. In velo-cardio-facial syndrome, the hands and fingers are

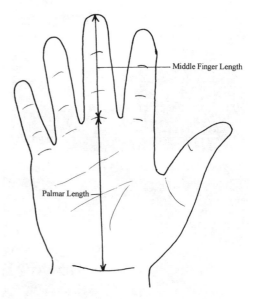

Figure 5–46. Drawing of the points for taking hand measurements. Palmar length is taken from the flexion crease between the wrist and base of the middle finger; middle finger length from the flexion crease at the base of the middle finger to the finger tip. Anthropometric norms are available for these measurements, as are norms for the proportion of length between the middle finger and palmar lengths.

small by measurement and the palms and fingers are slender with tapered digits (Figure 5–47). Although the large majority of patients with velo-cardio-facial syndrome are not of very short stature (most fall within the low normal range of height), the hands tend to be abnormally small. If the hands are small in association with a syndrome of short stature, such as achondroplasia or diastrophic dysplasia, this cannot be considered to be abnormal because the skeletal dysplasia and hypoplasia exists throughout the body. Small hands are a clinical feature of many syndromes, including de Lange syndrome, Prader-Willi syndrome, and Mohr syndrome.

Large hands (by measurement) can be found in the syndromes of overgrowth, such as Sotos syndrome and Weaver syndrome, but may also be found in syndromes with connective tissue dysplasia, such as Marfan syndrome and Ehlers-Danlos syndrome. A number of syndromes of hamartomatous growths may have anomalies associated with the limbs that cause large and malformed hands, as in Klippel-Trénaunay-Weber syndrome, Proteus syndrome, and Maffucci syndrome.

The Length of the Digits Relative to the Palms

Norms have also been established for the proportionality between the length of the palm and the middle finger. Anomalies of this proportion have diagnostic labels that should be recognized by clinicians so that such abnormalities can be described to other professionals. **Brachydactyly** is the term applied to digits that are short in relation to the palmar length (Figure 5–48). The prefix **brachy-** means short. Brachydactyly is common in Down syndrome, achondroplasia and other chondroplasias resulting in short stature, the lysosomal storage diseases, and Aarskog syndrome, to name a few.

Arachnodactyly refers to fingers which are long in relation to the palms (the prefix **arachno-** meaning "spidery"). Arachnodactyly (Figure 5–49) is less common than brachydactyly, but occurs in syndromes related to connective tissue dysplasias or anomalies. Arachnodactyly may be found in Marfan syndrome (related to a mutation in a fibrillin gene), Shprintzen-Goldberg syndrome (related to a similar type of mutation), and Stickler syndrome (caused by

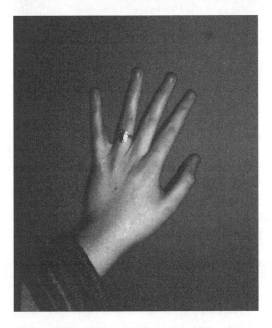

Figure 5–47. The hand of a patient with velo-cardio-facial syndrome demonstrating small, narrow hands with tapered, slender digits.

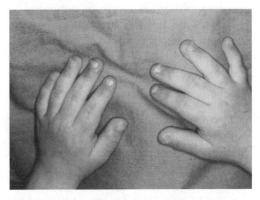

Figure 5–48. Brachydactyly in a patient with Down syndrome. The fingers are short in relation to the length of the palm.

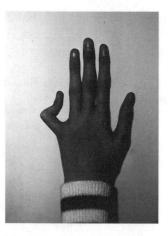

Figure 5–49. Arachnodactyly in a patient with Shprintzen-Goldberg syndrome. The fingers are long in relation to the palm.

a mutation in a collagen II gene). Arachnodactyly is often accompanied by joint contractures or hyperextensibility of the joints because of the basic connective tissue disorders that cause the anomaly. Because the number of syndromes with arachnodactyly is relatively small, the finding is an important diagnostic aid.

The Structure of the Digits

There are a number of malformations of the fingers which, although generally minor in nature, represent errors in morphogenesis that may be of diagnostic significance. These include abnormalities in the linearity of the fingers, the mobility of the joints, the proportionality of the digital segments, the number of phalanges in the digit, and the appearance of the spaces between the digits. The fingers are normally straight without deviation from a line drawn connecting the center of the base of the digit to the center of the finger tip (Figure 5–50). When the tip of the finger deviates inward, this minor anomaly is known as **clinodactyly** and is associated with a large number of syndromes that have limb anomalies as a

feature. Although clinodactyly is not pathognomonic for any diagnosis, its presence in a child with developmental delay, language disorders, or hearing impairment should lead the clinician to seek out a possible underlying syndromic diagnosis.

If the fingers deviate outward, this is known as an ulnar deviation and is a much less common finding than clinodactyly. Ulnar deviations usually connote a more severe connective tissue abnormality, which results in contractures. Freeman-Sheldon syndrome is an autosomal dominant genetic disorder with craniofacial and limb anomalies, including cleft palate, micrognathia, Robin sequence, joint contractures, and ulnar deviation of the hands and fingers (Figure 5–51).

Each finger of the hand is divided into either two or three segments, each separated by a joint and flexion crease. Two fingers, the thumbs, have only two segments; the other eight fingers have three. Each segment corresponds to an underlying bone. The bones of the fingers are known as **phalanges** with the bones closest to the palm known as the proximal phalanges, the bones in the finger tips known as the distal phalanges. In the fingers other than the thumb, the bones separating the proximal from the distal phalanges are known as the middle phalanges. The length of each segment of the finger reflects the underlying length of the phalanges. Each segment of the finger is usually of nearly equal length, with some minor variability, for all of the fingers. In many syndromes, however, there is a disproportion between the length of the segments with the proximal, middle, or distal phalanx being abnormally short. For example, in fetal hydantoin syndrome and otopalatodigital syndrome, the distal phalanges typically are abnormally short.

Absence of one or more phalanges or the presence of extra phalanges may also be diagnostic of multiple anomaly syndromes. Individuals with Laband syndrome, which typically includes cognitive impairment

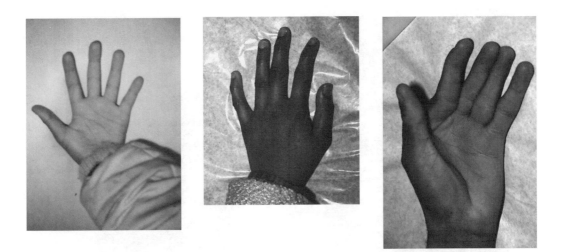

Figure 5–50. Photograph of a hand showing the normal linear structure of the fingers (left) compared to hand showing clinodactyly with the fingers bending toward the thumb in a patient with Larsen syndrome (center) and a hand showing ulnar deviation with the fingers bending away from the thumb toward the ulna in a patient with Freeman-Sheldon syndrome (right).

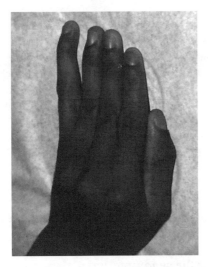

Figure 5–51. Ulnar deviation of the hands in Freeman-Sheldon syndrome.

associated with coarse facial appearance, have absence of the distal phalanges on all of the fingers. A number of syndromes have extra phalanges in the thumbs. Triphalangeal thumbs are found in Townes syndrome and several other syndromes with sensorineural hearing loss, including LADD syndrome.

The spaces between the digits refer to the separation between the fingers that allows normal manual dexterity and manipulation by each finger separately. In some syndromes, these spaces may be partially or completely obliterated. In general terms, this is known as **syndactyly**. Actually, syndactyly has more than one form and a particular form may be more common to one syndrome, than another. If the fingers are fused only by skin or soft tissue, this is known as a **soft tissue syndactyly** or **cutaneous syndactyly**. This is a fairly common anomaly in humans, particularly between the second and third toes. Syndactyly is less common on the fingers, but is not rare in multiple anomaly syndromes. Soft tissue syndactyly may be found in EEC syndrome between the ring and small finger, in Miller syndrome, Fraser syndrome, and triploidy among over 50 other multiple anomaly syndromes. The other form of syndactyly is **osseous syndactyly**, which occurs when one or more phalanges on the adjacent fingers are fused together. Osseous syndactyly is most common in Apert syndrome (Figure 5–52), which often demon-

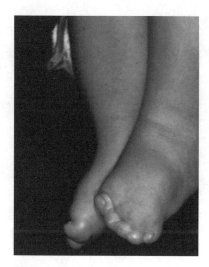

Figure 5–52. Osseous syndactyly in Apert syndrome.

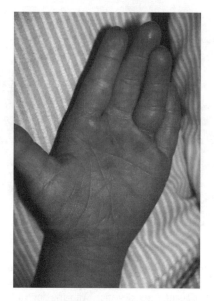

Figure 5–53. A transverse palmar crease, often called a simian crease, in a patient with Down syndrome.

strates fusion of multiple digits. Osseous syndactyly is found in relatively few syndromes and is therefore a strong diagnostic clue.

The Flexion Creases of the Digits and Hands

The creases of the palms and fingers of the hand reflect the underlying anatomy and physiology of the bones and muscles. For example, when two phalanges are fused (**symphalangism**) so that the joint between them cannot bend, the flexion crease is often absent. Therefore, if inspection of the palmar surface of the hands shows anomalies of the flexion creases on the digits, the clinician should suspect an underlying structural anomaly of the finger and refer the patient for proper work-up. Palmar creases may also be informative. For example, a transverse palmar crease (often referred to as a simian crease) is a common finding in a number of syndromes, but has become most closely associated with Down syndrome (Figure 5–53). However, Down syndrome is such an obvious diagnosis to most clinicians that the transverse palmar crease is of little diagnostic importance.

However, in less familiar syndromes, such as Aarskog syndrome, Cohen syndrome, Smith-Lemli-Opitz syndrome, triploidy, 5p- and 18q- deletion syndromes, the detection of a transverse palmar crease in association with other anomalies should raise an index of suspicion for a particular diagnosis.

Fetal alcohol syndrome has a distinctive palmar crease, which may provide a diagnostic clue, even if the mother denies the use of alcohol during pregnancy (Figure 5–54). The fetal alcohol palmar crease is a single crease that runs across the palm and exits between the index and middle fingers. Although this crease is not pathognomonic for the syndrome and it also occurs in a small percentage of the general population, in a child with other features consistent with fetal alcohol syndrome, its presence may be of diagnostic significance.

Although unusual flexion crease patterns on the palm may be diagnostic clues for specific syndromes, it should be understood that there is enormous variability in palmar crease patterns and no pattern is diagnostic in the absence of other anom-

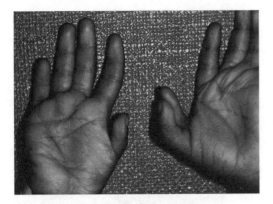

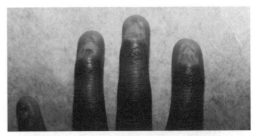

Figure 5–55. Absence of the fingernails in Rapp-Hodgkin syndrome which is also accompanied by sparse scalp hair, dental enamel hypoplasia, and cleft palate.

Figure 5–54. A palmar crease intersecting the interdigital space between the second and third fingers, often referred to as the fetal alcohol crease. This crease is commonly found in fetal alcohol syndrome.

alies. In other words, an individual with a fetal alcohol crease, but no other anomalies is not very likely to have fetal alcohol syndrome. However, in an individual with microcephaly, cleft palate, small eyes, a ventriculoseptal defect, and developmental delay (findings consistent with a number of syndromes), the presence of the fetal alcohol crease may help the clinician to narrow the diagnostic search considerably.

The Fingernails

Anomalies of the fingernails are minor malformations that have little functional significance. Absence of the finger- or toenails often implies an underlying deficiency of the distal phalanges. A number of syndromes are characterized by small or absent nails for this reason, including fetal hydantoin syndrome, fetal alcohol syndrome, popliteal pterygium syndrome, and Turner syndrome. Another cause of nail deficiency is ectodermal dysplasia in which absence or hypoplasia of the nails is often accompanied by sparse scalp hair, eyelashes, and dental enamel, as in EEC syndrome, Rapp-Hodgkin syndrome (Figure 5–55), and Hay- Wells syndrome.

Fingernail length and shape are also of diagnostic importance. The fingernail usu-

ally occupies approximately one half of the distance from the distal finger joint to the finger tip (Figure 5–56). In some syndromes, the fingernails are short, occupying far less than half the distal phalangeal length. In velo-cardio-facial syndrome, the nails are short (Figure 5–57) and are located on tapered finger tips. Other anomalies of the nails in multiple anomaly syndromes include hyperconvex nails (multiple pterygium syndrome), deep set nails (Weaver syndrome), and nails with linear splits (craniofrontonasal dysplasia syndrome).

The Texture of the Skin

The texture of the skin on the hands is particularly easy to examine and prone to anomalies if connective tissue dysplasias, autoimmune disease, hamartomatous growths, or other fibrous tissue disorders are present. For example, in velo-cardio-facial syndrome, there is an adolescent onset of rheumatoid disease, which is often expressed in red or purplish scaly skin, especially on the palms of the hands, although it is present on the feet, as well. Hamartomas and ectodermal dysplasias have already been discussed elsewhere in this chapter.

The Skin

The skin, a portion of which is easily visible to the examier, may express several

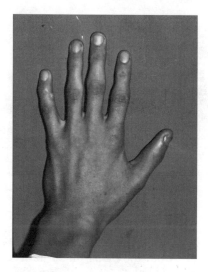

Figure 5–56. Normal fingernail length. Note that the nail occupies approximately one half the length of the distal joint of the finger.

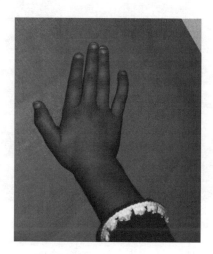

Figure 5–57. Short fingernails in velo-cardio-facial syndrome.

obvious anomalies. There may be loose and redundant skin, as in Setleis syndrome; areas of abnormal pigmentation or depigmentation, as in Gorlin syndrome and LEOPARD syndrome; the presence of abnormal growths, as in neurofibromatosis; thick and scaly skin, as in Hurler-Scheie syndrome; and the presence of vascular lesions, as in Sturge-Weber syndrome, ataxia-telangiectasia syndrome, and Maffucci syndrome. Even common skin problems, such as eczema and acne, may be syndromic features. Eczema is a common manifestation in Dubowitz syndrome and acne vulgaris is common in Apert syndrome. If the clinician is aware of the underlying type of skin anomaly and what it may be related to (i.e., connective tissue dysplasia or hypervascularization), the appearance of the skin may serve as an appropriate clue to initiate or continue the diagnostic search.

Overall Height and Weight (Somatic Size)

Normal stature covers a wide range and may further be variable in relation to racial type, racial subgroups, and even nutrition-

al influences (such as the absence of certain nutrients essential to normal bone growth). However, using the proper growth curves for comparison, it is possible to determine if a child or adult is of normal stature by a simple height measurement. Normal is defined as falling within two standard deviations of the mean in either direction. Thus, approximately 96% of the general population falls within the normal growth curve, while 2% are abnormally short and 2% are abnormally tall. There are many syndromes of short stature, some involving severe skeletal dysplasias, as in achondroplasia, diastrophic dysplasia, Russel-Silver syndrome, and other syndromes of both proportionate and disproportionate short stature (what used to be called "dwarfing"). However, many other syndromes with short stature are not related to skeletal dysplasias, such as Prader-Willi syndrome, Turner syndrome, Down syndrome, de Lange syndrome, Rubinstein-Taybi syndrome, and several hundred others. Chromosomal syndromes and teratogenic syndromes typically have short stature as a feature. In many syndromes of short stature, there are often severe major malformations which extend to many regions of the body.

Large stature is a less common syndromic association, occurring in only a handful of syndromes that have overgrowth as a feature, including Sotos syndrome, Weaver syndrome, and Beckwith-Wiedemann syndrome (which has early overgrowth that eventually subsides). Overgrowth syndromes are often accompanied by some type of endocrine abnormality and are also usually associated with some degree of cognitive deficiency and behavioral abnormality, such as psychiatric disorders.

Excessive weight gain is another form of overgrowth. Perhaps the best studied syndrome in the respect is Prader-Willi syndrome. Children with this disorder have insatiable appetites that often must be controlled with drastic procedures, such as locking the refrigerator or keeping food out of reach. There are a number of other syndromes with severe obesity, including Laurence-Moon-Biedl syndrome and Cohen syndrome. In some other syndromes, such as Down syndrome, obesity may be of later onset and secondary to other features of the syndrome, such as inactivity, obstructive sleep apnea, and poor behavioral management.

SUMMARY

This rather extensive chapter was not meant to provide a complete list of syndromes or diseases that have specific findings. Rather, it was meant to provide the fuel for the logical approach to diagnosis while leaving the clinician with the notion that a gestalt approach of putting pieces together is an essential part of the process. More specific information on individual syndromes will follow in Appendix I. But the message is clear; the clinician must be sensitive to differences in an individual's structure and function so they can ask intelligent questions and provide an informed pathway for the triage of those patients.

REFERENCES

Ades, L. C., Morris, L. L., Power, R. G., Wilson, M., Haan, E. A., Bateman, J. F., Milewicz, D.M., & Sillence, D. O. (1995). Distinct skeletal abnormalities in four girls with Shprintzen-Goldberg syndrome. *American Journal of Medical Genetics, 57*, 565–572.

Arvystas, M., & Shprintzen, R. J. (1984). Craniofacial morphology in the velo-cardio-facial syndrome. *Journal of Craniofacial Genetics and Developmental Biology, 4*, 39–45.

Cohen, M. M., Jr. (1982). *The child with multiple birth defects.* New York: Raven Press.

Cohen, M. M., Jr. (1987). The Elephant Man did not have neurofibromatosis. *Proceedings of the Greenwood Genetics Center, 6*, 187–192.

Farkas, L. G. (1981). *Anthropometry of the head and face in medicine.* New York: Elsevier.

Farkas, L. G., & Munro, I. R. (1987). *Anthropometric facial proportions in medicine.* Springfield, IL: Charles C. Thomas.

Farkas, L. G., & Posnick, J. C. (1992). Growth and development of regional units in the head and face based on anthropometric measurements. *Cleft Palate-Craniofacial Journal, 29*, 301–302.

Farkas, L. G., Posnick, J. C., & Hreczko, T. M. (1992a). Anthropometric growth study of the ear. *Cleft Palate-Craniofacial Journal, 29*, 324–329.

Farkas, L. G., Posnick, J. C., & Hreczko, T. M. (1992b). Anthropometric growth study of the head. *Cleft Palate-Craniofacial Journal, 29*, 303–308.

Farkas, L. G., Posnick, J. C., & Hreczko, T. M. (1992c). Growth patterns of the face: a morphometric study. *Cleft Palate-Craniofacial Journal, 29*, 308–315.

Farkas, L. G., Posnick, J. C., Hreczko, T. M., & Pron, G. E. (1992a). Growth patterns of the nasolabial region: A morphometric study. *Cleft Palate-Craniofacial Journal, 29*, 318–324.

Farkas, L. G., Posnick, J. C., Hreczko, T. M., & Pron, G. E. (1992b). Growth patterns in the orbital region: A morphometric study. *Cleft Palate-Craniofacial Journal, 29*, 315–318.

Franceschetti, A., & Klein, D. (1949). Mandibulo-facial dysostosis: New hereditary syndrome. *Acta Ophthalmologica, 27*, 143–224.

Fraser, F. C. (1970). The genetics of cleft lip and cleft palate. *American Journal of Human Genetics, 22*, 336–352.

Goldberg, R., Marion, R., Borderon, M., Wiznia, A., & Shprintzen, R. J. (1985). Phenotypic overlap between velo-cardio-facial syndrome and the DiGeorge sequence. [Abstract]. *American Journal of Human Genetics, 37,* 54.

Goldenhar, M. (1952). Associations malformatives de l'oeil et de l'oreille, en particulier le syndrome dermöide epibulbaire-appendices auriculaire-fistula auris congenita et ses relations avec la dysostose mandibulo-faciale. *Journal Génétic Humane, 1,* 243–282.

Golding-Kushner, K. J. (1995). Treatment of articulation and resonance disorders associated with cleft palate and VPI. In R. J. Shprintzen & J. Bardach (Eds.), *Cleft palate speech management: A multidisciplinary approach* (pp. 327–351) St. Louis: Mosby.

Golding-Kushner, K. J., Weller, G., & Shprintzen, R. J. (1985). Velo-cardio-facial syndrome: Language and psychological profiles. *Journal of Craniofacial Genetics and Developmental Biology, 5,* 259–266.

Gorlin, R. J., Cohen, M. M., Jr., & Levin, L. S. (1990). *Syndromes of the head and neck* (3rd ed.). New York: Oxford University Press.

Jones, K. L. (1992). *Smith's recognizable patterns of human malformation* (5th ed.). Philadelphia: W. B. Saunders.

Jones, M. C. (1988). Etiology of facial clefts: prospective evaluation of 428 patients. *Cleft Palate Journal, 25,* 16–20.

LeBlanc, E. M., & Cisneros, G. J. (1995). The dynamics of speech and orthodontic management in cleft lip and palate. In R. J. Shprintzen & J. Bardach (Eds.), *Cleft palate speech management: A multidisciplinary approach* (pp. 305–326). St. Louis: Mosby.

Levin, L. S., & Jorgenson, R. J. (1972). Familial otodental dysplasia: A "new" syndrome. *American Journal of Human Genetics, 24,* 61.

MacKenzie-Stepner, K., Witzel, M. A., Stringer, D. A., Lindsay, W. K., Munro, I. R., & Hughes, H. (1987). Abnormal carotid arteries in the velocardiofacial syndrome: A report of three cases. *Plastic and Reconstructive Surgery, 80,* 347–351.

Mansour, A., Wang, F., Goldberg, R., & Shprintzen, R. J. (1987). Ocular findings in the velo-cardio-facial syndrome. *Journal of Pediatric Ophthalmology, 24,* 263–266.

Mitnick, R. J., Bello, J. A., Golding-Kushner, K. J., Argamaso, R. V., & Shprintzen, R. J. (1996). The use of magnetic resonance angiography prior to pharyngeal flap surgery in patients with velocardiofacial syndrome. *Plastic and Reconstrive Surgery, 97,* 908–919.

Papolos, D. F., Faedda, G. L., Veit, S., Goldberg, R., Morrow, B., Kucherlapati, R., & Shprintzen, R. J. (1996). Bipolar spectrum disorders in patients diagnosed with velo-cardio-facial syndrome: Does a hemizygous deletion of chromosome 22q11 result in bipolar affective disorder? *American Journal of Psychiatry, 153,* 1541–1547.

Rollnick, B. R., & Pruzansky, S. (1981). Genetic services at a center for craniofacial anomalies. *Cleft Palate Journal, 18,* 304–313.

Saal, H. M., Bulas, D. I., Allen, J. F., Vezina, L. G., Walton, D., & Rosenbaum, K. N. (1995). Patient with craniosynostosis and marfanoid phenotype (Shprintzen-Goldberg syndrome) and cloverleaf skull. *American Journal of Medical Genetics, 57,* 573–578.

Shprintzen, R. J. (1982). Palatal and pharyngeal anomalies in craniofacial syndromes. *Birth Defects Original Article Series, 18*(1), 53–78.

Shprintzen R. J. (1995). A new perspective on clefting. In R. J. Shprintzen & J. Bardach (Eds.), *Cleft palate speech management: A multidisciplinary approach* (pp. 1–15). St. Louis: Mosby.

Shprintzen, R. J., & Goldberg R. (1982). A recurrent pattern syndrome of craniosynostosis associated with arachnodactyly and abdominal hernias. *Journal of Craniofacial Genetics and Developmental Biology, 2,* 65–74.

Shprintzen, R. J., Goldberg, R., Golding-Kushner, K. J., & Marion, R. (1992). Late-onset psychosis in the velo-cardio-facial syndrome. *American Journal of Medical Genetics, 42,* 141–142.

Shprintzen, R. J., Goldberg, R. B., Lewin, M. L., Sidoti, E. J., Berkman, M. D., Argamaso, R. V., & Young, D. (1978). A new syndrome involving cleft palate, cardiac anomalies, typical facies, and learning disabilities: Velo-cardio-facial syndrome. *Cleft Palate Journal, 15,* 56–62.

Shprintzen, R. J., Goldberg, R., Young, D., & Wolford, L. (1981). The velo-cardio-facial syndrome: A clinical and genetic analysis. *Pediatrics, 67,* 167–172.

Shprintzen, R. J., Siegel-Sadewitz, V. L., Amato, J., & Goldberg, R. B. (1985). Anomalies associated with cleft lip, cleft palate, or both. *American Journal of Medical Genetics, 20,* 585–595.

Sood, S., Eldadah, Z. A., Krause, W. L., McIntosh, I., & Dietz, H. C. (1996). Mutation in fibrillin-1 and the marfanoid-craniosynostosis (Shprintzen-Goldberg) syndrome. *Nature Genetics 12*, 209–211.

Tessier, P. (1976). Anatomical classifications of facial, cranio-facial, and latero-facial clefts. *Journal of Maxillofacial Surgery, 4*, 69–92.

Williams, M. A., Shprintzen, R. J., & Goldberg, R. B. (1985). Male-to-male transmission of the velo-cardio-facial syndrome: A case report and review of 60 cases. *Journal of Craniofacial Genetics and Developmental Biology, 5*, 175–180.

Williams, M. A., Shprintzen, R. J., & Rakoff, S. J. (1987). Adenoid hypoplasia in the velo-cardio-facial syndrome. *Journal of Craniofacial Genetics and Developmental Biology, 7*, 23–26.

Witzel, M. A. (1995). Communicative impairment associated with clefting. In R. J. Shprintzen, & J. Bardach (Eds.), *Cleft palate speech management: A multidisciplinary approach* (pp. 137–166). St. Louis: Mosby.

Young, D., Shprintzen, R. J., & Goldberg, R. (1980). Cardiac malformations in the velo-cardio-facial syndrome. *American Journal of Cardiology, 46*, 643–648.

CHAPTER

6

SYNDROMIC IMPLICATIONS FOR TREATMENT

The previous chapters in this text, have discussed the importance of syndromic diagnosis because of the potential effects on treatment planning. The three factors accompanying the diagnosis (the phenotypic spectrum, the natural history, and the prognosis) have been demonstrated to be of importance to clinicians of all types (medical, dental, and behavioral) because of the predictive power they have in understanding the disorder and allowing anticipation of suspected problems. In this chapter, examples of types of multiple anomaly syndromes will be discussed in relation to the manner in which the diagnosis and accompanying natural history and prognosis affect treatment recommendations and outcomes. An example of each of the following types of syndromes will be discussed: syndromes with static structural anomalies, syndromes with progressive structural anomalies, syndromes with a static neurological disorder, syndromes with a progressive neurological disorder, syndromes with static hearing loss (both sensorineural and conductive), syndromes with progressive

hearing loss (both sensorineural and conductive), syndromes with early behavioral disorders, and syndromes with late onset behavioral disorders.

SYNDROMES WITH STATIC STRUCTURAL ANOMALIES

Static structural anomalies are present at birth and do not get worse or develop into another anomaly or set of anomalies in a sequential manner. Ventriculoseptal defect (VSD), a hole between the chambers of the heart, is a common form of congenital heart anomaly, which occurs in a large number of syndromes, including velo-cardio-facial syndrome, Down syndrome, and Kabuki make-up syndrome, to name a few. VSD is a static anomaly in that it does not get larger with time. In fact, in many cases of isolated VSD (when not associated with other heart anomalies), the hole may spontaneously close. Static skeletal anomalies include spinal fusions, spina bifida, short limbs associated with achondroplasia and other syndromes of short stature, or fusion of two or more cervical vertebrae as in the Klippel-Feil anomaly. Static organ anomalies may include a single missing kidney, anophthalmia (unilateral or bilateral), omphalocele (herniation of the gut through the abdominal wall), and Hirschsprung aganglionic megacolon (absence of innervation to a segment of the large intestine). Although these possible anomalies have little in common in terms of embryology or effect on the child, they are similar in that many can be successfully treated and the others may not cause severe restrictions on life. Anomalies that can be treated successfully do not typically cause major residual problems, although minor modifications in lifestyle or medical management may be necessary. For example, patients who have had structural heart anomalies repaired often require prophylactic antibiotics (known as SBE prophylaxis to prevent bacterial endocarditis) if there is risk of the oral or nasal mucosa being scratched and contaminated, such as during a dental procedure or nasal endoscopy.

Even short limbs can now be lengthened with a procedure known as distraction in which a cut is made in a bone and traction is applied to it to lengthen the bone slowly. As pressure is exerted to lengthen the bone slowly, new bone forms in the areas of the cuts so that the bone is lengthened permanently. Distraction has been applied to the arms, legs, and even the mandible. Other anomalies that cannot be treated, or for which patients refuse treatment, often do not impair life sufficiently to require surgery. For example, people of short stature can adapt to their size in many ways and still lead successful lives, blind people can live independently, and individuals with Klippel-Feil and other spinal anomalies learn to adapt their movements to their limited neck movements.

Therefore, treatment decisions regarding static structural anomalies must be put within the context of the ubiquitous "risk-to-benefit" ratio health care professionals are always considering. Clinicians must weigh all of the factors that accrue to risk and realistically assess the benefit to the patient. For example, in the case of the VSD, although

cardiac surgery presents a risk to the patient, so does leaving the problem untreated if the VSD is large and not spontaneously closing. If not repaired, the patient may have a reduced quality of life and quantity of life. Therefore, the benefits outweigh the risk. The same decisions relate to communicative disorders and their treatments. Although the risks are rarely life-threatening, they may impinge on the quality of life, and in some cases, the benefits may not be clearly known. It is not mandatory to fix an anomaly simply because it can be fixed.

In the way of examples for communicative impairment, microtia and cleft palate present as two static structural anomalies that are relatively common in humans. Specifically, let us look first at a grade II microtia. Grade II microtia (see Figure 5–34) may occur as an isolated anomaly or a part of a spectrum of anomalies, as in oculo-auriculo-vertebral spectrum (OAVS) or Treacher Collins syndrome. When unilateral with a normal hearing ear on the opposite side, a microtia results in some degree of hearing impairment with respect to laterality, sound localization, and impaired shadowing effect, but the large majority of people function normally with one normal hearing ear. Surgery can be done to reconstruct an external canal and middle ear, although the expertise is not widespread. If surgery goes well, hearing in the low normal or mildly impaired range may be achieved. Because grade II microtia essentially always involves absence of some ossicles, or very abnormal ossicles with fixation of the footplate of the stapes, it becomes necessary to fenestrate the inner ear or free the fixation. Complications therefore include the possibility of infection or destruction of the inner ear mechanism and the possibility of substituting a total deafness for a maximal conductive hearing loss. Although this complication is unusual, it must be considered in determining if this risk supersedes the benefit of having better binaural hearing. If a syndromic entity is added to the mix, the decision becomes more complicated. For example, in OAVS, the anatomy of the middle ear and temporal bone is very abnormal, and the facial nerve often courses through the middle ear space and may be found passing through the footplate of the stapes. This abnormal position of cranial nerve VII adds additional risk to middle ear reconstruction, which increases the risk portion of the ratio. The decision to go ahead with surgery therefore needs to be a combination of well-informed professionals and properly counseled parents. The audiologist needs to be able to articulate the possible gains in hearing and the advantage such gains will have for the patient over the prospect of a long-term unilateral maximal conductive hearing loss. In my experience, patients with OAVS have typically opted to avoid surgery because of the potential risks and the relatively small advantage provided by the increase in hearing in the microtic ear. The use of amplification, even if in selective environments (such as school), becomes an alternative in treatment planning, which might not otherwise be considered as strongly if surgery were not so complicated.

The risk-to-benefit ratio may also be influenced by the cognitive status of the patient, which may alter the benefit of reconstructive surgery. In cases where the prognosis indicates that the patient will have very severe intellectual impairment, the value of reconstructive surgery becomes dubious. However, in cases where there is a mild or borderline impairment, the question becomes more important with regard to either reconstructive surgery or amplification. Recent research suggests that even mild conductive hearing losses may contribute to an educational disadvantage (Gravel, Wallace, & Ruben, 1995). Although extensive data do not exist with regard to unilateral hearing losses, a clinical judgment may be influenced by the possibility that any hearing impairment could have an influence on learning and language development.

Cleft palate, without cleft lip, presents as a static structural anomaly with obvious implications for resonance disorder during speech. In most centers in the U.S., the palate is repaired at approximately 1 year of age. The sole reason for palate repair is to provide the structure necessary for the normal development of speech. Although results vary from surgeon to surgeon and may be influenced by both the timing and technique of surgery, most centers report that 80 to 85% of their patients develop normal speech after primary palate repair (palatoplasty). Because normal speech cannot be achieved unless the palate is repaired, the very small risk involved in the surgery in normal healthy patients is very small compared to the benefit of normal speech in 80% of more of the cases. Even in the cases that do not develop normal speech on the first operation, secondary surgery almost always resolves the problem. Risk may be altered by coexisting heart anomalies or other health-related issues, but such conditions can usually be resolved or minimized eventually. However, in cases where there is a very poor prognosis for the development of speech because of severe intellectual impairment, the benefit of palate repair is negated. Cleft palate does not interfere with feeding, as exemplified by the fact that palatoplasty is not accomplished until 1 year of age and children feed perfectly well until that time with minimal modifications (Sidoti & Shprintzen, 1994). Therefore, in nearly all cases, the only reason to repair the palate is to allow normal speech development. If speech is unlikely to develop, palate repair should not be considered, or, at the very least, it should be deferred until there is an indication that language development will occur. In cases where there is a poor prognosis for speech and language development, the risks far outweigh the benefit.

SYNDROMES WITH PROGRESSIVE STRUCTURAL ANOMALIES

Progressive structural anomalies show change over time, either gradual or sudden, so that treatment planning needs to account for the natural history of the anomaly. In some cases, the progression of the anomaly is only relative to the continued normal growth and development of surrounding structures. For example, in OAVS, which has already been described in this chapter, the mandible is smaller than normal, primarily unilaterally. The asymmetry is caused by a hypoplasia of one or more parts of the mandible, including the body (corpus), the ascending ramus, the coronoid process, or the condyle. The condyle and even the ramus may be completely absent, if not very deficient. Even though the deficient side of the mandible grows, it grows more slowly than the normal side and therefore, over time, the smaller side of the face becomes progressively smaller in comparison to the larger side.

In other cases of progressive structural anomalies, the anomaly's natural history is truly changeable with time. An example would be the von Recklinghausen form of neurofibromatosis (NF type I). The earliest manifestation of the skin lesions is the café-au-lait spots, which are often concentrated in the axillary area (near the arm pits). With increasing age, more café-au-lait lesions form all over the body and eventually may develop into raised lumps (neurofibromas), which are benign tumors. These tumors often grow larger and may eventually require surgical removal. In this case, the structural anomaly is truly progressive. Other examples of such progressive anomalies include cystic hygromas, some hemangiomas, hemihypertrophy, Klippel-Trénauney-Weber syndrome, and Maffucci syndrome.

There are two different types of craniometaphyseal dysplasia based on the mode of inheritance: an autosomal dominant and autosomal recessive form. Although each type is essentially the same clinically, the autosomal recessive form has a more consistent and severe expression (Gorlin, Cohen, & Levin, 1990). The most severe expressions of the autosomal dominant variety of craniometaphyseal dysplasia are similar in expression to the autosomal recessive form, but in general the majority of the autosomal dominant cases are less severely involved. Craniometaphyseal dysplasia involves a progressive overgrowth of the craniofacial skeleton, especially in the nasal region with severe sclerosis of the interorbital space, nasal lumen, and the entire nasal bone complex. With age, there is significant progressive sclerosis of the temporal bone and petrous pyramid with compression of one or more cranial nerves. Optic atrophy may occur because of compression of the optic foramena and the optic nerves.

Craniometaphyseal dysplasia has a number of progressive changes that impact directly on communicative impairment. The natural history of the syndrome involves a progressive change in speech resonance and hearing acuity. Speech may become increasingly hyponasal with the progression of the bony overgrowth in the nasal capsule. With compression of the cranial nerves, facial paresis may develop and could possibly impair articulation and oral resonance. Hearing loss, both conductive and sensorineural, also becomes progressive after a relatively late onset (usually in the second decade of life) and can become severe. The hearing loss may be accompanied by progressive balance disorders and vertigo. Therefore, the management of patients with craniometaphyseal dysplasia should take into account the anticipated worsening of middle ear, inner ear, auditory nerve, and vestibular abnormalities, as well as progressive nasal airway obstruction. Contrary to what might be expected for other craniofacial syndromes, in craniometaphyseal dysplasia, audiometric assessments should be done more frequently with age. For example, in the large majority of craniofacial syndromes, middle ear disease (chronic serous otitis with middle ear effusion) is more common in infancy and early childhood and often resolves by the age of 8 years or shortly thereafter. Therefore, it is typical in children with other syndromes, such as craniofrontonasal syndrome or Robinow syndrome, to recommend more intensive audiometric assessments early in life rather than in adult years. Because of the natural history of craniometaphyseal dysplasia syndrome, the opposite would be recommended.

SYNDROMES WITH A STATIC NEUROLOGICAL DISORDER

Static neurologic disorders are common in a large number of chromosomal, genetic, and teratogenic syndromes. Any malformation of the central nervous system, even more specifically the brain, will result in a static encephalopathy causing functional deficits that almost always include a communicative disorder. Static encephalopathies may be the result of any number of possible central nervous system (CNS) malformations, such as failure of development of the frontal region in holoprosencephaly, cerebellar dysgenesis in velo-cardio-facial syndrome, agenesis of the corpus collosum in craniofrontonasal syndrome, encephalocele in Roberts syndrome, primary microcephaly in Seckel syndrome, cortical atrophy in Pena-Shokeir I syndrome, or white matter hypoplasia in COFS syndrome (cerebro-oculo-facio-skeletal syndrome, or Pena-Shokeir II). In general, static neurologic anomalies are evident early in life, with developmental delays, delayed motor milestones, and possible cognitive deficits. Speech and language impairments are common. Obviously, the type of impairment is dependent on the specific portion of the CNS that has been damaged, maldeveloped, or underdeveloped. Once the nature of the disorder and its extent is determined, it is usually possible to devise an appropriate treatment plan with a predictable outcome because the disorder will not become worse over time. However, in some cases, the extent of the disorder will be so severe as to prevent significant habilitation with treatment, as is the case with alobar or partially lobar holoprosencephaly.

Mild developmental delay and cognitive impairment are common clinical findings in Beckwith-Wiedemann syndrome. Neonates and infants with Beckwith-Wiedemann syndrome are often "floppy babies" (hypotonic). Language milestones are often mildly delayed and speech is impaired by a combination of low muscle tone, a large tongue, and class III malocclusion related to mandibular prognathism. As is often true in other syndromes with overgrowth, children with Beckwith-Wiedemann syndrome often have macrencephaly, which is often indicative of a static generalized brain dysplasia. However, because the problem is static and present at birth, it is possible to determine the extent of the deficit early in life and also determine the child's potential. Therefore, every effort should be made to enroll such children in early therapy programs, including speech and language therapy and early stimulation, physical therapy for hypotonia, and occupational therapy. As is often true in static neurologic disorders, the child's responsiveness to therapy is often a strong predictor of the eventual prognosis.

SYNDROMES WITH A PROGRESSIVE NEUROLOGICAL DISORDER

Progressive neurological disorders in multiple anomaly syndromes are of three types:

1. Syndromes with a late or progressive onset of a degenerative process involving the cells and tissues of the brain.
2. Syndromes with progressive cranial anomalies that have a secondary effect on the developing brain.
3. Syndromes with neoplastic activity that directly or indirectly affects the central nervous system.

In general, syndromes with progressive courses are not easily treated and the progression of the intellectual or performance deficits is irrevocable. However, there are some exceptions in all three categories of progressive neurological disorders, which are treatable or even preventable.

Syndromes with a Late or Progressive Onset of a Degenerative Process Involving the Cells and Tissues of the Brain

Although not a common occurrence, a handful of multiple anomaly syndromes have degenerative neurologic dysfunction. Many of the lysosomal storage diseases, most of which are autosomal recessive genetic disorders, have degeneration of the central nervous system because of accumulation of metabolic waste products in the intracellular matrix of the brain. Thus, deterioration of cognitive and motor skills is a common complication of syndromes such as Tay-Sachs disease, Hunter syndrome, and Hurler syndrome.

Syndromes with premature senility also result in degeneration of the central nervous system, often because of demyelinization. There are a number of syndromes with premature senility as a clinical feature, including Cockayne syndrome, Werner syndrome, Down syndrome (Alzheimer's disease), and Xeroderma pigmentosum. Other syndromes with neurologic degeneration include Refsum syndrome, a syndrome of deafness which is an autosomal recessive genetic disorder, ataxia-telangiectasia, and homo cystinuria.

In the syndromes cited above, the biological mechanisms are different, but all are essentially untreatable at the present time because the progressive disorders represent a set of genetic instructions that is encoded into the entire daily activities of the body's cells. While it is possible that someday these abnormal processes may be stopped with gene therapy, at the present time, these syndromes all have an irreversible course with poor prognoses. Therefore, treatment plans should take into consideration the ultimate poor outcomes for the types of progressive disorders that will ultimately be immune to treatment.

For example, in Cockayne syndrome, children often appear normal at birth, but by the age of 2 years or after, the presentation of the syndrome becomes obvious and there is progressive neurological degeneration. With time, patients develop ataxia and athetosis, progressive mental retardation, central hearing disorder, and, on occasion, blindness. There is progressive calcification of the cerebral cortex and cerebellum. Demyelinization also occurs in the subcortical white matter with advancing age. Because of the progressive anatomical changes in the central nervous system, attempts at remediation of the cognitive and hearing impairments meet with failure.

Syndromes with Progressive Cranial Anomalies That Have a Secondary Effect on the Developing Brain

In the cases cited in the previous section, the degenerative process is in the central nervous system itself. There are multiple anomaly syndromes, however, where the central nervous system is intact and normal, but the surrounding cranial structures progressively impinge on the central and/or peripheral nervous systems, eventually resulting in progressive deterioration of function. In some cases, the progression of the disorder is reversible or correctable, as in many of the syndromes of craniosynostosis, such as Crouzon syndrome, Saethre-Chotzen syndrome, Jackson-Weiss syndrome, and milder forms of Pfeiffer syndrome. In these syndromes of craniosynostosis, the premature fusion of the calvarial sutures can cause compression of the brain and increased intracranial pressure. If the compression is severe enough and an aqueductal stenosis develops, hydrocephalus may occur, resulting in even more serious brain deformity. Therefore, early cranial reconstruction can relieve the intracranial pressure and prevent the potential for progressive brain damage. However, in some syndromes of craniosynostosis, such as Carpenter syndrome, Apert syndrome, Pfeiffer type III, and Shprintzen-Goldberg syndrome, many or all cases have intrinsic brain anomalies as well as craniosynostosis. Therefore, even though the craniosynostosis may be corrected with cranial reconstruction in these syndromes, affected individuals still have cognitive impairments of varying degree. However, the craniosynostosis should be corrected even if there is evidence of cognitive impairment because any deformation of the brain will result in additional cognitive impairment superimposed on the preexisting anomaly.

When progressive cranial anomalies involve the skull base, the problem is more serious because the foramena at the base of the skull permit the entry of vital nerves, blood vessels, and the spinal structures into the intracranial space. A number of syndromes have progressive anomalies of bone deposition and/or bone growth that affect the entire craniofacial complex, including the skull base. Some of these disorders, such as van Buchem disease and sclerosteosis, are rare and generally isolated to specific populations, such as South Africans of Dutch descent (Afrikaners) in sclerosteosis and European Dutch in van Buchem disease. In frontometaphyseal dysplasia, there is a generalized skeletal distortion of the skull base, the ribs, the spine, and the facial bones causing a prominent brow, chin, and "pugilistic" facies. Progressive mixed hearing loss occurs in nearly all cases, as well as hyponasality and airway obstruction in many cases.

Perhaps the best known, although one of the rarest syndromes of progressive bone growth, is craniodiaphyseal dysplasia. The reason the syndrome is so well recognized (though not by name) is its representation in the movie *Mask*. Craniodiaphyseal dysplasia is an autosomal recessively inherited genetic disorder that causes progressive

and severe thickening of the bones of the skull and face. There is severe bony invasion of the nasal region, the skull base, and temporal bones. Eventually, the choanae become closed with excessive bone, causing obstructive apnea. There is a progressive mixed hearing loss as bone continues to invade the temporal bone and middle ear space. The optic foramena also becomes compromised by bony growth, causing visual impairment or blindness. The constant bony overgrowth of the calvarium, facial bones, and skull base eventually causes compression of the brain, increased intracranial pressure, headaches, and even progressive cognitive deterioration. Most patients have a dramatically shortened life span. Because the bony changes are progressive and continuous, treatment other than palliative management of life-threatening conditions almost always results in failure. Therefore, although the types of decision that must be made are unpleasant and frustrating to clinicians who wish to help, the prognosis for successful management is essentially nil.

Syndromes with Neoplastic Activity that Directly or Indirectly Affect the Central Nervous System

Neoplasias may be either benign or malignant growths, which represent tissues that are by themselves abnormal or normal tissues that are located in an abnormal place. Neurofibromatosis, one of the most common genetic diseases in human, involves progressive neoplastic activity. A number of of syndromes with neoplastic activity have been described elsewhere in this text, including Down syndrome, Proteus syndrome, Beckwith-Wiedemann syndrome, Maffucci syndrome, tuberous sclerosis, Gorlin syndrome, Cowden syndrome, Klippel-Trénauney-Weber syndrome, and hemihyperplasia. By their very nature, neoplasias (because they are growths) are progressive, whether benign or malignant, and therefore usually require treatment.

Neoplasias can interfere with communication in many ways, depending on the location and growth velocity of the space-occupying mass. For example, auditory nerve tumors will have a direct effect on the neural component of hearing, whereas growths known as oral teratomas, which disrupt palatal fusion, may cause cleft palate and speech resonance. Diffuse or isolated brain lesions can cause language and cognitive impairment. Other neoplasias may disrupt metabolic or endocrine processes that can indirectly affect communication. For example, pituitary tumors would have no direct impact on speech or voice, but if pituitary dysfunction causes a disturbance in normal growth (including growth of the vocal tract), the voice is likely to be high pitched and the resonance of voice and speech will likely be thin.

Multiple mucosal neuroma syndrome is an autosomal dominant disorder, although the majority of cases appear to be new mutations. Individuals with this syndrome develop multiple neoplasias of the mucous membrane in the mouth, eyes, nose, larynx, and pharynx. As a result, if the neoplasias are present in infancy, there is often failure-to-thrive with airway obstruction. It is therefore important to recognize this disorder in the differential diagnosis so that neoplasias can be removed to resolve these early disorders of the upper and lower airway. Neoplasias often develop on the tongue, the buccal mucosa, and the lips can become very puffy and distended. All of these growths may contribute to disorders of speech production because of physical obstruction or hindrance of the articulators. In this case, even though the process is progressive and tumors may recur, neoplasias that interfere with speech, feeding, or breathing should be removed to improve the quality of life for the patient. In some cases, if the growth is in the larynx, these procedures may be life-saving.

SYNDROMES WITH STATIC HEARING LOSS (BOTH SENSORINEURAL AND CONDUCTIVE)

Genetic contributions to hearing loss include malformations of the external ear and middle ear, anomalies of the inner ear, and anomalies of the auditory nerve. In general, static hearing loss is related to structural anomalies of the middle ear or inner ear, of which there are many examples. Hundreds of syndromes have hearing loss as a common or occasional feature. For an excellent compendium of syndromes of hearing loss, the reader is referred to the recent text by Gorlin et al. (1995), *Hereditary Hearing Loss and Its Syndromes*.

In many syndromes, hearing loss is related to chronic middle ear disease and effusion, which will cause a fluctuating mild loss. This secondary effect may be related to cleft palate, which is known to cause abnormalities of Eustachian tube function or other craniofacial anomalies, which may contribute to failure for the middle ear to ventilate normally or to harbor microbe-rich middle ear fluid. For example, in syndromes of craniosynostosis, the cranial base, which surrounds the Eustachian tube, is abnormally angled and the progressive synostosis of the synchondroses results in a lack of expansion of the middle ear space and the maxillary sinuses. Individuals with craniosynostosis usually are not able to breathe through their noses and are chronic mouth breathers, thus not allowing normal air passage around the Eustachian orifice in the nasopharynx. The nasal cavity tends to be partially or completely shut by choanal stenosis and it often fills easily with mucus. Therefore, there tends to be a generalized lack of ventilation of the airspaces of the craniofacial complex, including the middle ear.

Bilateral malformations of the conducting mechanism of the ear may be found in Treacher Collins syndrome, Townes syndrome, Nager syndrome, BOR syndrome (often mixed hearing loss), Miller syndrome, Wildervanck syndrome (often mixed hearing loss), otopalatodigital syndrome, and Apert syndrome, although the mechanisms in each syndrome are somewhat different. For example, microtia and malformation of the ossicles with fixation of the footplate of the stapes are common findings in Treacher Collins syndrome and Nager syndrome. Similar unilateral anomalies are found in oculo-auriculo-vertebral dysplasia, although on occasion, this disorder may also have bilateral anomalies. In Apert syndrome, the middle ear space may be slightly reduced in size, but the major contributor to conductive hearing loss is fixation of the footplate related to the synostosis, which also occurs in the cranium and other joints in the body. Malformations of the ossicles are not a clinical feature of Apert syndrome.

Static sensorineural hearing loss is also a feature of hundreds of syndromes. Congenital sensorineural hearing loss may vary from mild to total and may present as a primary feature of syndrome with only a few anomalies or as one of many major anomalies in complex disorders involving many of the body's systems. For example, perhaps the most common cause of deafness in the United States is Usher syndrome, an autosomal recessive disorder that has only two major findings: sensorineural hearing loss and retinitis pigmentosa. It is likely that the majority of children who are both deaf and blind have Usher syndrome. Although the retinitis pigmentosa is progressive and may eventually result in blindness, the hearing loss is not progressive and is usually profound.

Many syndromes of deafness are accompanied by pigmentary anomalies of the skin and/or hair (the integument). All of these disorders present with static sensorineural hearing loss. If a clinician notes pigmentary anomalies, audiometric assessment is clearly indicated. Examples of syndromes with integumentary anomalies and deafness are Waardenburg syndrome, LEOPARD syndrome, Refsum syndrome, autosomal recessive piebald trait with deafness, autosomal dominant piebald trait with ataxia and deafness, vitiligo with achalasia and deafness, and another 20 or more syndromes.

The treatment of patients with sensorineural hearing loss might seem very straightforward to audiologists. If the patient is a candidate for amplification, an appropriate hearing aid should be selected for the type of hearing loss. If not, an alternative form of communication should be taught. However, Usher syndrome presents an excellent example of how the diagnosis, or even the anticipation of a diagnosis, can affect patient care. It is estimated that 10% of patients with congenital profound hearing loss have Usher syndrome (Gerber, 1990). Because a very high percentage of congenitally deaf children have Usher syndrome, but the retinitis pigmentosa is not evident at birth (and cannot be detected in its early stages without complete fundoscopic examination of the eyes) and no other distinctive anomalies are associated with the syndrome, children with Usher syndrome may simply be considered to be deaf. Because the onset of retinitis pigmentosa may not occur until the second decade of life and then progresses, it becomes important to diagnose the syndrome as early as possible in order to prepare the patient for the impairment of both major sensory inputs (vision and hearing). Because vision may be severely impaired, the use of speech reading as a primary means of receiving language input may be compromised in the long run, and patient should be prepared to learn other forms of communication skills.

SYNDROMES WITH PROGRESSIVE HEARING LOSS (BOTH SENSORINEURAL AND CONDUCTIVE)

Progressive hearing loss may be indicative of a progressive cranial malformation, as discussed above in craniodiaphyseal dysplasia and van Buchem disease. It may also be a sign of a developing neoplasia of the auditory nerve, as in neurofibromatosis type II. In cranial anomalies that secondarily cause hearing loss, the hearing loss may be conductive, sensorineural, or mixed. Of course, in the case of acoustic neuromas, the problem is strictly neural. Progressive sensory hearing loss is an unusual finding.

Because the risks of treatment may be high, or treatment may be essentially impossible in many disorders with progressive hearing loss, consideration should be given to improving the patient's quality of life without risking the patient's quantity of life. The recurrence of the progressive problem and/or the inevitability of its progression must be assessed in relation to the risk-to-benefit ratio discussed earlier.

Refsum syndrome, an autosomal recessive disorder, has progressive hearing loss, which often begins as an asymmetric mild loss in the second or third decade of life and progresses to a severe hearing loss by the fourth decade of life. There is a more severe effect in the high frequencies. Refsum syndrome also has retinitis pigmentosa, degenerative neurological findings (including ataxia, sensory abnormalities, anosmia, parasthesia, and possible eventual paralysis), and ichthyosis. Unlike Usher syndrome where the hearing loss is the initial finding, the retinitis pigmentosa usually precedes the onset of hearing loss in Refsum syndrome. Diagnosis becomes very important because the course of the syndrome is related to phytanic acid accumulation, which can be controlled to some extent by diet. The progression of the syndrome can be dramatically altered by changing the diet.

SYNDROMES WITH EARLY BEHAVIORAL DISORDERS

In the context of this section, a behavioral disorder will refer to psychological, temperament, and psychiatric disorders, even though it is recognized that speech, language, and learning disorders are behavioral problems. A substantial number of multiple anomaly syndromes have, as a result of brain malformation or biochemical imbalance, behaviors that are maladaptive. Although it is more common to think of *temperament* as an adult concept, infants and young children do have temperaments, which have been described in the literature as "irritable," "laconic," "affable," "immature," or "congenial." These characteristics become associated with syndromes when observations of many children with the same disorder show a remarkable consistency in temperament. Thus, the "affectionate" nature of children with Down syndrome, the "cocktail party manner" in children with Williams syndrome, and the violent temper tantrums in children with de Lange syndrome are well-recognized patterns of behavior common to, but not necessarily specific to, these multiple anomaly disorders.

An example of a syndrome in which overall behavior may affect treatment planning is Williams syndrome. Discussed earlier in Chapter 5 with reference to physical findings and the causation of the syndrome, which has been linked to the deletion of the elastin gene on the long arm of chromosome 7 (7q11.23 to be precise), Williams syndrome has attracted a lot of attention from clinicians of many backgrounds because of the unusual behavior patterns displayed by affected children. Williams syndrome has a broad phenotype that includes cardiac anomalies (including VSD, supravalvular aortic stenosis, supravalvular pulmonic stenosis), hypercalcemia, dental enamel hypoplasia, microdontia, kidney anomalies, esotropia, developmental delay, and mild to moderate mental retardation in the large majority of cases. Their early childhood behavior is friendly and "chatty," with a very loquacious pattern of speech which is quite sophisticated in the structure of its grammar and language use for a child with a cognitive impairment. However, much of what is said makes little sense. There is often impulsive behavior which can be very maladaptive. However, because their early language usage seems disproportionate to their actual performance, it would be easy to overestimate the level of intelligence, and therefore the level of need for a particular child. Therefore, if Williams syndrome is suspected as a diagnosis, extensive neuropsychological testing should be done to determine the true nature of the cognitive disturbance so that proper services can be provided.

SYNDROMES WITH LATE ONSET BEHAVIORAL DISORDERS

The relation of behavioral disorders and psychiatric illness to genetic syndromes is just beginning to draw attention from both the psychiatric and genetic community. Only a handful of disorders that have a predisposition to late-onset behavioral disorders or psychiatric illness as a feature have been identified. In most instances, the association of late-onset behavioral disorders is coupled with a history of cognitive impairment, learning disabilities, or mental retardation. Both Down syndrome and the so-called Fragile X syndrome (X-linked mental retardation or Martin-Bell syndrome) have been associated with late-onset psychosis. It is also well known that males with an XYY chromosome complement exhibit impulsive and aggressive behavior that often becomes expressed as criminal behavior in adult life.

It is tempting to believe that the observation of behavioral problems in individuals with multiple anomaly syndromes is caused by social isolation, poor treatment by parents and siblings, poor self-image, or constant teasing. However, when the same pattern of behavior is consistently observed in many individuals with a particular syndrome, it is very unlikely that the disturbance is related to experience, rather than biology. In fact, clinicians should be sensi-

tive to the notion that any and all abnormalities, physical or behavioral, that occur in a child with multiple anomalies simply represent another feature of the multiple anomaly syndrome.

Another problem with psychological, temperament, or psychiatric disorders is that many of them cannot be diagnosed until adulthood. Childhood schizophrenia or bipolar affective disorder is not understood very well, and the early behavioral precursors, or prodromal findings, have not been fully delineated. Therefore, it is possible that findings like hyperactivity or attention deficit disorder are actually early diagnostic signs of a more serious psychiatric problem, which will develop later as the diagnostic standards become applicable (Papolos et al., 1996).

Velo-cardio-facial syndrome (VCFS) was delineated in 1978, but it was not until 1992 that psychiatric disorders were recognized as a feature of the syndrome. In part, this is because the majority of patients with this common syndrome who were seen early in the process of the description of the syndrome were young children or infants. The psychiatric findings did not become obvious until they reached their teen or adult years. However, several cases who had serious and significant psychiatric illness were seen by this author as early as 1975. At that time, it was presumed that their psychological problems were related to their educational difficulties, ostracization by their peers, and failure to integrate into society. It was not realized, at that early phase of syndrome delineation, that their failure to integrate into society was a symptom, not an outcome. It is now known that the majority of patients with VCFS have some form of bipolar affective disorder (Papolos et al., 1996). Nearly 70% of cases assessed by Papolos et al. were found to manifest disorders ranging from dysthymia to psychotic manic depressive illness. The finding of eventual psychiatric illness presents a difficult counseling dilemma and special consideration of the advisability of invasive procedures that would normally positively affect the quality of life. Early in life, many infants with VCFS are irritable and have a temperament that makes it difficult to have a normal parent-baby bonding. Babies with VCFS may have serious heart anomalies that require surgery and hospitalization, feeding problems are common, and health is impaired by frequent upper and lower respiratory illness. Their irritability may be expected, but the fact that it probably represents an early manifestation of their poor social interaction adds an enormous amount of stress in dealing with their problems. Because of this chronic irritability, attempts at feeding babies with VCFS become very problematic and are often abandoned in favor of gastrostomy or long-term gavage feeding. In the overwhelming majority of cases, feeding can be accomplished with effort and only minor modification. Therefore, clinicians need to accept the behavioral problems presented by the children and forge ahead in spite of them. In childhood, patients with VCFS have many phobias and are generally fearful of doctors and even minimally invasive procedures. Because hypernasality is a very common finding in VCFS, children require nasopharyngoscopy and multi-view videofluoroscopy prior to consideration for pharyngeal flap surgery. It is the rare child with VCFS who will cooperate fully with this procedure, and many clinicians will avoid doing the examination until the child is older, hoping that additional maturity will help. Unfortunately, the phobias do not resolve with age and may get worse. Therefore, it has been my practice to inform the parents that the child will be likely to struggle, scream, and resist the procedure, but that by restraining the child (I usually have the parent hold the patient) the examination can be successfully accomplished. In fact, it has been my experience that, once the endoscope is inserted and the child realizes that the thing they fear most has already been accomplished, in many cases their affect goes flat and they become cooperative. This approach is not recommended with other patients, but certainly works well in VCFS because of the understanding of the psychological manifestations.

SUMMARY

In summary, the cases and circumstances presented in this chapter are only representative of the many hundreds of syndromes, which have a variety of clinical features that can signal the experienced clinician to alter approaches to management. Because there are so many multiple anomaly syndromes, it should be realized that the approach to patient diagnosis and treatment is nearly as individual as the syndrome. It is therefore vital that speech-language pathologists and audiologists not only be sensitive to the possibility of a syndromic diagnosis, but also be as knowledgeable as possible of the phenotypes expressed in the more common syndromes so that proper care can be applied.

REFERENCES

Gerber, S. E. (1990). *Prevention: The etiology of communicative disorders in children.* Englewood Cliffs, NJ: Prentice-Hall.

Gorlin, R. J., Cohen, M. M., Jr., & Levin, L. S. (1990). *Syndromes of the head and neck* (3rd ed.). New York: Oxford University Press.

Gorlin, R. J., Toriello, H. V., & Cohen, M. M., Jr. (1995). *Hereditary hearing loss and its syndromes.* New York: Oxford University Press.

Gravel, J. S., Wallace, I. F., & Ruben, R. J. (1995). Early otitis media and later educational risk. *Acta Otolaryngologica, 115,* 279–281.

Papolos, D. F., Faedda, G. L., Veit, S., Goldberg, R., Morrow, B., Kucherlapati, R., & Shprintzen, R. J. (1996). Bipolar spectrum disorders in patients diagnosed with velo-cardio-facial syndrome: Does a hemizygous deletion of chromosome 22q11 result in bipolar affective disorder? *American Journal of Psychiatry, 153,* 1541–1547.

Sidoti, E. J., & Shprintzen, R. J. (1994). Pediatric care and feeding of the newborn with a cleft.

In R. J. Shprintzen & J. Bardach (Eds.), *Cleft palate speech management: A multidisciplinary approach* (pp. 63–74). St. Louis: Mosby.

Shprintzen, R. J., Goldberg, R., Golding-Kushner, K. J., & Marion, R. (1992). Late-onset psychosis in the velo-cardio-facial syndrome. *American Journal of Medical Genetics, 42,* 141–142.

Shprintzen, R. J., Goldberg, R. B., Lewin, M. L., Sidoti, E. J., Berkman, M. D., Argamaso, R. V., & Young, D. (1978). A new syndrome involving cleft palate, cardiac anomalies, typical facies, and learning disabilities: Velo-cardio-facial syndrome. *Cleft Palate Journal, 15,* 56–62.

CHAPTER

7

UNDERSTANDING LABORATORY TECHNIQUES

From the clinician's point of view, the process of diagnosis relies on judgment, knowledge of the spectrum of anomalies associated with the multitude of syndromes that have been delineated to date, and the ability to know the proper referral sources to assess and treat patients with multiple anomaly disorders. The clinician's role is enhanced by an aptitude for problem solving, and many geneticists regard the process of clinical diagnosis to be as much an art as a science. However, as the human genome project has progressed, the application of laboratory tests has become more commonplace. The growth of the use of laboratory tests has given the clinician new scientific tools which help to remove some of the uncertainty that occurs because of the overlap of phenotypes of many syndromes. The variability of expression of genetic disorders is also a source of possible diagnostic error. Laboratory tests, if accurate, may not have to rely on the perception of the clinician to identify the disorder.

A number of different types of diagnostic tests may be called upon either to aid the clinician or to definitively confirm the diagnosis. In general, there are two broad types of laboratory procedures: indirect and direct. Indirect tests do not directly identify the genetic or chromosomal error, but measure some byproduct of that error. There are many such indirect tests, which may be specific to a particular enzyme or metabolic agent or may be very routine laboratory procedures, such as a blood count or urinalysis. Even radiographs (X-ray assessments) can be utilized as indirect tests, especially when skeletal dysplasias are suspected. Direct tests assess the genome itself, whether at the chromosomal, genetic, or molecular levels.

INDIRECT TESTS

To recommend or utilize indirect tests, the clinician must know if there are specific physiological or biochemical features of syndromes that could be detected by such an analysis. There are many hundreds of such disorders, some of which can be diagnosed definitively by indirect tests, and others which can be included in the differential diagnosis without being identified specifically. Indirect tests are used frequently because they tend to be much less expensive than complicated direct analyses, and far more laboratories are available to perform them than molecular genetics labs. The use of indirect tests often evolves for disorders as the biochemical defects become better understood and laboratory procedures become more sophisticated. A good model for demonstrating the use of indirect tests are the lysosomal storage disorders. The lysosomal storage diseases, also often called the mucopolysaccharidoses, are a group of over a dozen separate genetic disorders that are caused by the deficiency of the group of enzymes that break down the complex carbohydrates known as the glycosaminoglycans (formerly known as mucopolysaccharides), dermatan sulfate, heparan sulfate, and keratan sulfate. With the exception of Hunter syndrome, the other lysosomal storage diseases all have autosomal recessive inheritance (Hurler syndrome, Scheie syndrome, Sanfilippo syndrome types A through D, Morquio syndrome types A and B, Maroteaux-Lamy syndrome types A and B, and Sly syndrome). Hunter syndrome (types A and B) is X-linked recessive.

In the earliest days of identification of the lysosomal storage diseases, if it was suspected that the child was affected, a simple indirect test known as a "spot test" was done to look for excessive amounts of glycosaminoglycans. These simple urine tests were usually sensitive to the detection of a lysosomal storage disorder, but were not necessarily specific to the individual disease. However, simple urine screenings could be done to determine if a child was likely to have a storage disease. If positive, this finding would then allow additional testing later on. It is now possible to assess the specific enzymatic deficiencies from blood. For example, it is known that Hurler syndrome has a deficiency of α L-Iduronidase. Because the enzymatic assays are done by extracting leukocytes (white blood cells) from the blood samples, it is possible to perform these tests prenatally from amniotic fluid or chorionic villus sampling. Because the genes for several of the lysosomal storage disorders have been mapped in humans, it will soon be possible to perform direct testing.

Another example of an indirect test in humans is a simple CBC (blood count). This common lab test can be used to assess the number of red and white blood cells, thus enabling the diagnosis of anemia (too few red blood cells and reduced hemoglobin) or leukocytosis (too many white blood cells). Anemia, leukocytosis, or thrombocytopenia (a low platelet count) may be features, singly or collectively, in a number of syndromes. Leukocytosis may be found in Down syndrome and radial aplasia-thrombocytopenia syndrome. Anemia is common in Fanconi pancytopenia syndrome, Peutz-Jeghers syndrome, Fabry syndrome, fetal rubella syndrome, and dyskeratosis congenita, to name a few. Thrombocytopenia is common in velo-cardio-facial syndrome, Fanconi pancytopenia, and radial aplasia-thrombocytopenia syndrome. Although anemia, leukocytosis, and thrombocytopenia are all common findings in the general population, when they occur in association with other anomalies, it must be suspected that they are a part of the phenotypic spectrum of that syndrome.

Radiographs

Radiography, or the use of X-rays and other imaging procedures for diagnostic purposes, is also a useful type of indirect test. Radiography may be useful in detecting skeletal dysplasias, cranial anomalies, brain malformations, the integrity of the internal organs, and even the structure and number of teeth. However, because there are few, if any, anomalies that are radiographically pathognomonic for a specific syndrome, X-ray examinations must be interpreted with caution, recognizing that more than one syndrome may express the same anomaly. For example, craniosynostosis is easily detectable using either two-dimensional planar radiographs (i.e., a standard skull film) or CT studies (computed tomography that is often reformatted by computer software into three-dimensional images). However, craniosynostosis is a finding in many syndromes, including Apert syndrome, Crouzon syndrome, Saethre-Chotzen syndrome, Pfeiffer syndrome, Jackson-Weiss syndrome, Carpenter syndrome, Antley-Bixler syndrome, Escobar syndrome, and Shprintzen-Goldberg syndrome. Craniosynostosis may also occur secondary to a primary microcephaly (a small head size caused by a lack of brain growth as discussed in Chapter 5). When the brain does not drive the skull to expand, the cranial sutures may fuse prematurely. In such cases, even though the synostosis is a secondary finding, it may provide diagnostic clues because there is a large cadre of syndromes that have primary microcephaly as a common finding, such as Seckel syndrome, de Lange syndrome, Rubinstein-Taybi syndrome, Dubowitz syndrome, and fetal alcohol syndrome. Magnetic resonance imaging can detect soft tissue anomalies, particularly of the central nervous system, such as the characteristic cysts near the ventricles in velo-cardio-facial syndrome, absence of the corpus callosum in craniofrontonasal syndrome, and communication between the ventricles in holoprosencephaly.

Dental radiographs may be valuable for identifying tooth structure anomalies, tooth number anomalies, jaw shape anomalies, or jaw size anomalies. Syndromes may be identified by a pattern of congenitally missing teeth, accessory teeth, the presence of micrognathia, maxillary deficiency, or mandibular prognathism. For example, a large lower jaw (macrognathia) is possibly an indicator of Beckwith-Wiedemann syndrome, or a small lower jaw with antegonial notching may be indicative of Stickler syndrome. However, because antegonial notching and a small lower jaw are found in a number of other syndromes (such as Treacher Collins syndrome, Nager syndrome, and Ehlers-Danlos syndrome).

The number of possible indirect laboratory tests is practically limitless because, with many thousands of multiple anomaly syndromes already delineated, there are so many physiologic and biochemical functions which might be impaired that lab procedures can be applied to quantify them according to what is known about the syndrome. By establishing the full range of the phenotypic spectrum of a syndrome, it is possible to come up with indirect laboratory procedures which will be sensitive to a diagnosis, although indirect tests are rarely specific. The goal for indirect tests should be to develop data from laboratory tests with the highest possible sensitivity, the highest possible specificity, the lowest number of false positives, and the lowest number of false negatives.

DIRECT TESTS

Direct assessments of the genome are now possible in a variety of ways, depending on the identification of specific etiologies of known disorders. Direct assessments may provide a detailed visual picture of the human chromosomes (as discussed earlier in Chapters 2, 3, and 5) with varying degrees of resolution. In the earliest days of chromosome analysis, it was not possible to distinguish all of the chromosomes from each other because groups of chromosomes are of similar size and difficult to identify individually without the advanced staining procedures available today. It is now possible to find even very tiny deletions and rearrangements of chromosomes which have come to light in only the last 5 years. However, many genetic abnormalities are too small to be detected by looking at the structure of the chromosomes and require molecular analysis of DNA to detect an error. Such errors may be deletions, point mutations (changes in a single base pair in a single gene DNA sequence), or even additions of DNA sequences to existing longer chains within a gene. If the specific genetic error is known, or if the DNA sequence of the normal gene that has been mutated is known, it is possible to utilize a number of direct tests to determine if the genome of a specific individual is normal for that region of DNA. The most common direct tests used include:

- Karyotypes (standard and high resolution)
- Southern blot
- Northern blot
- Western blot
- Fluorescent in situ hybridization (FISH), and
- Polymerase chain reaction (PCR).

Karyotypes

Chromosome analysis is a relatively new procedure when one considers that many diagnostic tests, such as diagnostic X-rays, have been available for nearly a century. The first karyotypes were performed in the late part of the 1950s, but the procedure at that time was quite crude and better forms of chromosome visualization did not become popular until the 1960s. Today, karyotypes may be performed with any tissue containing cells that can be grown in culture so that during the cell division's metaphase, the chromosomes become visible, may be photographed or imaged by computer, and stained so that small segments can be distinguished (banding, as described in Chapter 5). Standard karyotypes image the chromosomes in their normal size and state except for the banding induced by the staining techniques (such as Giemsa staining). Standard karyotypes are adequate for detecting larger chromosome rearrangements where at least an entire band is affected, such as trisomies, polyploidies, monosomies, deletions of large segments of chromosome, translocations, ring chromosomes, large inversions, iso-

chromes, and dicentric chromosomes (see Chapter 2). A newer technology for karyotypes is the high resolution karyotype, which stretches the chromosomes beyond their normal size so that even smaller rearrangements and deletions can be detected. In many cases, small rearrangements that are not visible on standard karyotyping, such as the 22q11 deletions in velo-cardio-facial syndrome and the 15q11 deletions in Prader-Willi syndrome, have been detected by high resolution karyotype. In general, karyotypes should be requested if the patient does not have a recognizable single gene disorder, but has small stature, significant developmental delay, mental retardation, more than one major anomaly, more than three minor anomalies, or severe craniofacial, limb, or heart anomalies.

The process of performing a karyotype is typically started by obtaining approximately 10 cc of peripheral blood (usually from the arm, although in small infants, it may be necessary to find larger veins elsewhere, such as in the leg, wrist, neck, or scalp). The lymphocytes (white blood cells) are extracted, grown in culture, and stained so that the nuclei and chromosomes become visible during mitosis. During metaphase, the banded chromosomes are clearly visible and can be photographed. The precise number of bands and structure are known for each chromosome so that any individual's chromosomes can be matched to well mapped standards. It is typical to analyze multiple cells for a number of reasons. First, not all cells in an individual are necessarily normal. Somatic mutations and aneuploidies can occur in only some cells if the mutation occurred after morphogenesis. Second, the cells potentially could be damaged in the process of preparation. Third, patients may have a mosaic aneuploidy. In other words, only a percentage of the individual's cells may be abnormal. For example, a phenotypic female may have 10% or 25% of her cells with a missing X chromosome. Individuals with 100% of their cells missing an X chromosome have Turner syndrome and typically have webbed necks, absent ovaries and uterus, poorly defined secondary sexual characteristics, and a variety of malformations including relative small stature, occasional cognitive impairments, heart anomalies, hyperconvex finger nails, and cleft palate. If only 10% or 25% of the person's cells are affected, the phenotype is less severe. There may be a uterus, some evidence of secondary sexual characteristics, relatively normal stature, and less pronounced webbing. Therefore, karyotypes typically involve the counting of minimally 10 cells, but more routinely 20 or more cells.

NEW TECHNOLOGIES FOR MEDICAL GENETICS

Even though karyotypic is a relatively new technology for medicine, more recent advances in molecular biology have opened the floodgates for the understanding of the mechanisms that cause genetic diseases. Broadly known as **recombinant DNA technology**, the use of these new procedures has become commonplace in the study of human illness and has even spread to the legal system in helping to identify people by genomic finger printing. Recombinant DNA technology utilizes the process of making an essentially limitless supply of DNA from a biological sample so that the DNA samples can be studied and their sequences decoded in a way relevant to studying human disease. Many people are familiar with the word **cloning**, although few actually understand what it is beyond the fanciful applications of the term to science fiction and popular movies like *Jurassic Park*.

Cloning

In simple terms, cloning is the process by which a sequence of DNA can be copied many times over so that a substantial amount of that DNA sequence can be obtained. The DNA sequence may be very short, or rather long, but cloning does not imply the creation of an entire organism by copying an entire organism's genome. In actual use, cloning becomes an important tool for obtaining sufficient quantities of DNA for study so that abnormalities in the sequence can be assessed to determine if they cause a disease.

Molecular Genetics and Applications to Human Disorders

Because DNA sequences constitute the genes and chromosomes, cloning provides a mechanism by which an individual's genetic make-up can be studied outside of the human body by manufacturing the DNA in culture. The term *recombinant DNA technology* was coined to connote the ability to take human DNA and combine it with nonhuman DNA, such as bacterial or yeast DNA, so that a large supply of the human DNA sequences can be harvested from the more rapidly growing host (such as *E. coli* bacteria or baker's yeast). The ultimate goal of these molecular techniques is to map the location of human genes on the chromosomes, identify the gene's DNA sequence, understand what that sequence does (meaning what protein is created in the process of gene expression), and determine the pathway by which that expression takes place (i.e., how does the gene's action produce a specific developmental process).

By identifying abnormal genes, it becomes possible to pinpoint the chromosomal location of the genes by the techniques to be described below, and to then see how the anomalies found in the abnormal individuals result from the abnormal DNA sequences. Thus, although clinically relevant, the process of identifying disease-causing genetic errors, scientists have an in vivo experiment which helps to decode the human genome.

HOW CHROMOSOMAL DNA IS STUDIED

Approximately 25 years ago, molecular biologists identified **restriction endonucleases** or **restriction enzymes.** This discovery was an important first step in the process of DNA analysis. Restriction endonucleases, derived from common bacteria, separate double-stranded genomic DNA into segments by recognizing a specific short DNA sequence (usually 4 or 6 base pairs). Such sequences of base pairs usually occur repeatedly within a person's genomic DNA. Therefore, a single restriction endonuclease can divide a person's genomic DNA into a million segments of varying size, more or less, depending on where the recognized sequence occurs in the genome. For example, a restriction endonuclease may recognize the six-base, double stranded pair sequence

G-A-A-T-T-C

C-T-T-A-A-G

The alert reader will note that the sequence shown above represents a palindrome (in other words, the sequence from one strand reads the same way front-to-back that the complimentary strand reads back to front). This recognition sequence is specific to the endonuclease *Eco*RI (derived from E. *coli*). Every time this sequence appears in the genome, the DNA is cut between the G (guanine) and A (adenine) base in each strand of the double stranded molecule. This creates two ends of the strands which look like this:

(LONG DNA STRAND)-G-	A-A-T-T-C-(LONG DNA STRAND)
(LONG DNA STRAND)-C-T-T-A-A	-G-(LONG DNA STRAND)

(break)

The unequal length of the ends of each of the strands in the double strand helix creates what is known as "sticky ends" because the uneven structure is the same for all of the cut strands and it is possible for

any of the strands of DNA to fit onto any of the other strands. This ability for strands that were not originally contiguous to combine with each other is known as **recombinance** and the resulting combinations are known as **recombinant DNA**. The process of gluing together the sticky ends of cut strands of DNA to form a recombinant DNA molecule is assisted by another enzyme known as a **DNA ligase**.

Not all endonucleases cut DNA sequences the same way. Some cleave DNA strands without the overlap and *sticky ends* left by *Eco*RI, leaving equal length strands at the end. These can also recombine with the assistance of a ligase. Also, each endonuclease creates a unique number and length of individual strands based on the short DNA sequence recognized and the locations where the same sequence occurs again. The longer the recognition chain of the endonuclease, the fewer times this sequence will appear within the genome and the fewer the number of cleavage sites. In other words, by simple probability alone, it is more likely that a four-base pair sequence will be found than a six-base pair sequence (relating this to an everyday human activity, it is easier to win a four-number lottery than a six-number lottery). Therefore, *Eco*RI with its six-base pair recognition will divide genomic DNA into fewer segments than the endonuclease *Sau*3A, which has a four base pair recognition sequence:

G-A-T-C

C-T-A-G

Growing More DNA for Study

Once human DNA has been cut up into bits, which are easier to study than very long segments (such as whole chromosomes), it becomes even easier to study the DNA if there are larger quantities of it for the various tests that must be applied. This is where recombinant DNA technology plays an important a role for molecular biologists and geneticists. One way in which additional human DNA can be obtained by cloning is to create **vectors**. A vector is a segment of DNA that will spontaneously replicate itself when placed in an appropriate host environment, such as a bacteria or yeast cells. The process works in the following way. Once human DNA has been cut into many segments by restriction enzymes, the short segments can become a part of a recombinant DNA molecule by having a ligase attach it to a DNA segment from a bacterial host, such as *E. coli*. Thus, a new DNA molecule, part human DNA and part *E. coli* DNA is formed, and because bacteria grow rapidly in culture, the recombinant DNA molecule, along with its human DNA segment, can be grown in abundance. A number of different types of vectors may be used in this process. Probably those most familiar to the reader will be those known as **plasmids**, **cosmids**, **bacteriophages**, and **yeast artificial chromosomes** because these terms frequently appear in the language of the molecular geneticist.

Plasmids

A plasmid is a fairly small circular double-stranded DNA molecule that has, within its DNA, sequence sites that can be cut by restriction endonucleases so that a human DNA segment can be inserted into the plasmid for cloning in bacteria or yeast. Plasmids occur naturally in bacteria and yeast cells, but the plasmid DNA is not a part of the cell's chromosomal DNA. In other words, the plasmid is contained within the bacterium or yeast cell, but is not attached to or a functioning part of the cell's chromosome. However, just like the cell's chromosome, plasmids replicate during normal mitotic cell division so that the two new cells formed from the single dividing cell each has the same copy of the plasmid. Plasmids do contain genes that may perform a function within the cell. For example, one gene,

which may be located on a plasmid within a bacterium, such as *E. coli*, renders the cell immune to antibiotics, such as ampicillin. Thus, bacterial cells that contain the drug-resistant plasmid gene will survive antibiotic therapy, while other *E. coli* bacteria will be killed. With the drug-resistant strain established and continuing to divide, large colonies of the drug-resistant bacteria will take hold to the exclusion of the *E. coli* that are not drug-resistant. This establishment of drug resistance is a potential menace for humans, it becomes a useful laboratory aid for growing plasmids with recombinant DNA in vivo. The typical plasmid is only 5 kilobases (kb), or 5,000 base pairs long (some slightly smaller, some as large as 100 kb). Because of the small size of cosmids, using them as a vector for DNA replication is suitable only for relatively small segments of human DNA.

By using restriction endonucleases, it is therefore possible to create a plasmid that contains a human DNA segment the molecular scientists would like to study. How then can the scientist be assured that the recombinant plasmid is contained within a particular *E. coli* cell? This process is assisted by the ability to have *E. coli* cells absorb plasmids combined with the ampicillin resistance afforded by some plasmids containing the gene that provides that resistance. Although plasmids cannot simply gain access to a bacterium by bumping up against its cell membrane, it is possible to chemically treat the bacterial cells so that they admit the plasmid. This process is known as *transformation*. Therefore, scientists can construct a plasmid that is known to have the antibiotic-resistant gene which is recombinant with the human DNA segment they wish to study. They will then mix the recombinant ampicillin-resistant plasmids with a large colony of *E. coli* cells and chemically treat them so that a few of the cells will transform and accept the plasmids. The entire colony is then placed on a medium that contains ampicillin. The ampicillin will kill the *E. coli* cells that did not admit the plasmid, thus establishing a colony of the antibiotic-resistant cells which also contain the human DNA segment. The drug-resistant cells will divide and reproduce rapidly (as *E. coli* do) so that a large amount of the recombinant DNA can be obtained. The largest recombinant DNA segment that can be inserted into a plasmid is approximately 20 kb in length, although most are smaller.

Bacteriophages

A phage is a virus, and a bacteriophage is a virus that infects bacteria. A specific bacteriophage known as **bacteriophage lambda**, or λ-phage, is an excellent vector for cloning large amounts of DNA which are larger than those segments which can be cloned in a plasmid vector. Bacteriophage lambda has a single double-stranded DNA molecule which governs its life cycle. This molecule is approximately 45,000 base pairs in length with much of the DNA in it being unnecessary for the continued life of the virus. These segments of unnecessary DNA can be replaced by using restriction enzymes to cut the bacteriophage DNA and recombine it with segments of human DNA. Because the bacteriophage DNA molecule is larger than that of a plasmid, the human DNA segment that can be recombinant with the virus is far larger (in the range of 25,000 base pairs, or 25 kb). With the recombinant DNA sequence in place, the bacteriophage serves as a vector by infecting an *E. coli* bacterium. Once a bacterium is infected, the bacteriophage reproduces rapidly, eventually destroying the *E. coli* cell, but leaving in its place hundreds of thousands of bacteriophages with the cloned human DNA sequence in very high concentration which can then be isolated for study.

Cosmids

Cosmids are essentially large plasmids, which will accommodate a recombinant segment of human DNA of 45,000 base pairs (45 kb). The production of longer human DNA inserts involves a combination of plasmid and λ-phage vectors. The term **cosmid** is derived from sites on the λ-phage DNA molecule known as *COS sites*. COS sites are specific base pair sequences which are separated by nearly 50 kb of DNA. Cosmids are produced by taking a typical plasmid of 5 kb length and by using recombinant techniques, inserting COS sites from λ-phages into the plasmid. This insertion then allows multiple fragments of DNA totaling up to 45 kb to be inserted into the new cosmid vector. The cosmid is then "packaged" into a λ-phage (i.e., inserted into a λ-phage which has this recombinant DNA molecule replacing its normal viral genome and the virus infects an *E. coli* cell, thus producing large amounts of the longer human DNA segments.

Yeast Artificial Chromosomes (YACs)

YACs provide the largest vector for cloning human DNA. YACs have the same structure as typical nuclear chromosomes, with arms, centromeres, and telomeres (see Figure 2–7 in Chapter 2). Yeast artificial chromosomes will accommodate a recombinant segment of human DNA of a megabase (1 million base pairs) in size. This is a large enough segment to contain many genes, so that a YAC will allow the cloning of a huge amount of DNA covering a fairly large region of the human genome.

WHAT TO DO WITH ALL OF THAT DNA

Using the techniques which have come with recombinant DNA technology allows molecular geneticists to clone large amounts of human DNA for study. The next logical question should be what the molecular scientist is going to do with the DNA. How can these cloned copies of small, medium, or large DNA segments be useful in diagnosing genetic illnesses or decoding the human genome?

A first step bringing some order to the large amount of human DNA which has been cloned is to create a sort of database of DNA sequences. For genetic studies, genomic DNA is stored for future study in repositories known as libraries. Libraries are often chromosome-specific, meaning that a researcher in one place may have all available clones for chromosome 12, and another researcher might have all available clones for chromosome 8. Researchers or clinicians interested in studying genetic material from a particular chromosomal source can contact these libraries and obtain DNA that contains all of the genes from the region of interest. By having large libraries of genetic material from each chromosome, it has become possible to develop methods to check a person's DNA to determine if it contains any abnormalities (mutations or deletions, for example) by comparing it to a region from these libraries which is known to be normal. This process is assisted by developing segments of DNA known as **probes**, which can be diagnostically informative when utilized in a process known as hybridization.

Hybridization

As mentioned above, the various procedures for cloning DNA using recombinant technology create large quantities of double-stranded DNA. Double-stranded DNA, what most people think about when they think of the DNA molecule (the "double helix" described by Watson and Crick and discussed in Chapter 2), can be separated into single strands by a process known as **denaturation**. Using heat or chemical solutions, double-stranded DNA can be separated into single strands. Because of the specific base pair sequence, these single strands can only be **renatured** with strands of DNA that have the complementary base pair sequence (remember, as discussed in Chapter 2, that adenine can only pair with thymine and guanine with cytosine). When a single stranded DNA sequence is renatured with a complimentary DNA sequence that is not from the original DNA source (meaning the same organism), but rather from another living source or from synthetic DNA (i.e., constructed in a laboratory), the matching of the

two DNA segments is known as **hybridization**. Hybridization presents an ideal opportunity to use segments of DNA to detect abnormalities in single-stranded copies of human genomic DNA.

Probes

Probes are cloned or synthetic DNA segments that are used to hybridize to a specific region in the human genome to determine if it is normal. Probes may be used to detect deletions of chromosomal material or mutations of specific genes in which the normal sequence of base pairs has been altered. Probes may also be used to detect abnormal transcriptions in RNA so that the identification of a genetic abnormality does not come from genomic DNA, but from the transcription of the genetic code into the mRNA derived from the nuclear DNA. A probe is typically a DNA molecule or a gene produced by recombinant DNA procedures which is used diagnostically to determine if a disease-causing genetic abnormality is present. Probes may be small (several hundred base pairs) or closer to the size of a gene (thousands of base pairs), depending on the specific defect being sought. There are a number of techniques for using probes diagnostically, including:

- Southern blotting,
- Northern blotting,
- Fluorescent in situ hybridization (FISH), and
- Polymerase chain reaction (PCR).

Southern Blots

This procedure was first described in 1975 by Southern and has been consistently used for identifying genetic disorders. All procedures used for assessing a person's genome must begin with the individual's genomic DNA contained within the chromosomes. The simplest tissue source for extracting DNA is blood, usually obtained by puncturing a vein in the arm (hence the term *periph-*

eral blood). The actual source of genomic DNA from a blood sample is the white blood cells (lymphocytes), because red blood cells do not have nuclei and therefore do not have chromosomes or genomic DNA. Red blood cells shed their nuclei during the process of cellular differentiation. Other sources of genomic DNA include skin tissue obtained from biopsies (using fibro-blasts as a cellular source), organ tissues obtained by biopsy (such as liver tissue), or in the case of prenatal diagnosis, amniotic fluid or chorionic villi samples. Perhaps the most benign source of DNA is a buccal smear or scraping. A buccal sample involves using an intraoral swab or brush to scrape the inside of the cheek. The cells of the buccal mucous membrane shed very easily and adhere to the swab. Although karyotypes cannot be performed with buccal cells, they do provide a source of DNA.

Once a tissue source has been obtained and DNA extracted, restriction enzymes are used to cut the genomic DNA into a million or more fragments. The DNA fragments are placed on an agarose gel medium, which is then subjected to a low level of electric current, a process known as **electrophoresis**. The electric current causes the DNA segments to move across the gel. Because of their lower weight, the smaller segments of DNA move more rapidly, and therefore farther along the gel than the larger segments. The different sizes of the cut segments of DNA cause the entire sample to be arrayed in a more or less orderly fashion across the gel tray. The DNA is denatured into single strands, which will subsequently allow hybridization with probes. The single-stranded DNA is then transferred to filter paper by blotting the gel (Southern *blotting*). The filter paper is then combined with a quantity of probe DNA to identify the presence or absence of an area of interest in the genomic DNA. The probe is labeled with a radioactive marker that does not interfere with the DNA sequence. Because the probe is specific to a particular sequence in the human DNA genetic code, it will hybridize only with that specific sequence and only if it is present. If that code is absent because it is mutated (so that the base pair sequence is no longer specific to the probe) or deleted (so that the code is absent), the probe will not hybridize with the person's DNA. The filter is then washed to remove all of the probe DNA that has not hybridized with the person's genomic DNA so that the only probe material left on the filter paper is that which has hybridized. If the radioactive probe has hybridized with the genomic DNA, then the DNA sample will expose a piece of X-ray film, leaving a signal that is detected as a dark band (Figure 7–1). If the probe is not taken up, the DNA sample will not expose the film.

Northern Blots

Northern blotting is a procedure similar to Southern blotting, except, instead of detecting DNA sequences in an individual's genomic DNA, Northern blots are applied to RNA to determine if a gene contained within a person's genome is transcribing a gene product (see Chapter 2). The technique for Northern blotting is nearly the same as in Southern blotting, except that the RNA must be obtained from a specific tissue and cell type. RNA cannot be cut by restriction enzymes, as can DNA, but individual RNA transcripts differ from each other in length because they represent a linear code of base pairs which are translations of genes. Since genes are not all the same size (in fact, they are all of different sizes), the RNA transcripts are all of different lengths. Therefore, RNA transcripts can be placed on an agarose gel tray and will respond to electrophoresis just like fragments of DNA that have been cut by endonucleases. Radioactively labeled probes are then used in the same way as in Southern blotting to obtain a signal that can be detected on X-ray film.

Fluorescent in situ Hybridization (FISH)

Fluorescent in situ hybridization (known by its acronym **FISH**) is a technique in which

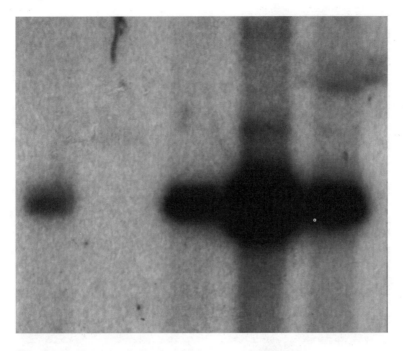

Figure 7–1. Example of a Southern blot.

probes are used to hybridize to chromosomal DNA. During FISH, a karyotype analysis is performed and during the metaphase of the cell division, the chromosomes are denatured so that the genomic DNA is single stranded. The chromosomes are then exposed to probes tagged with fluorescent rather than radioactive chemicals. The probes will hybridize to the chromosomal DNA only if the specific region under investigation is present and, if present, has the exact complementary sequence to the probe (just as in Southern blotting). Therefore, the fluorescent marker will appear under a fluorescent microscope (a microscope using a specific type of light which fluoresces the visual objective) only if the genetic region being studied is exactly complimentary to the probe's DNA sequence. If the region is deleted, or mutated, the fluorescent marker will not appear. Two fluorescent probes are use for each chromosome: one is the probe for the specific genetic region, the other is a probe specific for that chromosome's centromere or telomere. Therefore, if the chromosome is

normal, two fluorescent marks will appear; one at the centromere or telomere and one in the region of interest. If the region of interest is mutated or deleted, only a single fluorescent mark will appear at the centromere or telomere (Figure 7–2). The procedure is known as in situ hybridization because the genomic DNA is not cut by restriction enzymes, but is still on the chromosomes and there is no electrophoresis on an agarose gel, but the chromosome preparation is viewed directly on a slide.

Polymerase Chain Reaction (PCR)

The polymerase chain reaction (PCR) is a molecular genetics procedure well-recognized by the general public because of its frequent application in the legal community and because of its forensic value. PCR is a procedure that is relatively inexpensive, can be performed fairly quickly, and is able to take even an extremely small amount of DNA, as small as a single cell, to analyze an area of interest in the genome. PCR has been

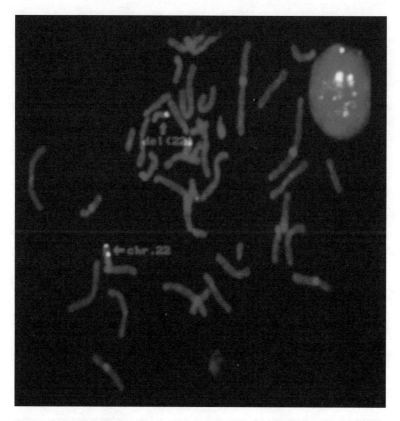

Figure 7–2. FISH (fluorescent in situ hybridization) of chromosome 22 in a patient with velo- cardio-facial syndrome. One copy of chromosome 22 has two fluoroescent markers; the other has only one, indicating a deletion.

applied to biological samples that are old or obtained from normal tissue loss from an individual, such as a lost hair or blood stains at a crime scene. In patient assessment, cheek scrapings provide a noninvasive and easily obtained source of cells for DNA analysis.

PCR does not require cloning to grow additional DNA. Basically, the "chain reaction" refers to the ability to continuously synthesize a specific short segment of DNA so that millions of copies of the segment can be obtained within hours. Rather than cutting the entire sample of a person's genomic DNA with restriction enzymes, PCR utilizes a specific and known target segment of DNA (a region of special interest to the geneticist), which is exponentially replicated.

THE CONFUSION CAUSED BY A CONSTANTLY CHANGING GENOME

The procedures described in the last section depend on the ability to know of specific DNA sequences or regions of interest within the genome in order to target them with probes that will hybridize to the segment under study. However, life is rarely perfectly simple, and even DNA analysis has a few curve balls to throw at the molecular geneticist. One major detour from perfect simplicity is something called a **polymorphism**. Polymorphisms are variations within a gene that result in differing gene effects when the gene is expressed. In other words, for a specific trait, multiple alleles (see Chapter 2) are known to exist at a particular gene locus. For example, the differences in blood groups (types) represent a polymorphism in the gene that mediates red blood cell antigen formation. Most people are familiar with the clinical importance of recognizing what a person's blood group is in order to allow him or her to receive transfusions. The inability of individuals to receive a transfusion from a person whose blood group is different from theirs because they have antigens that will reject the donor's blood group (except for type O blood in which the red blood cells do not contain any antigen) is caused by a variation in the allele located at the q34 band of chromosome 9. The variations that occur among individuals with different blood groups appear with significant frequency in the general population and are not therefore considered to be abnormal in the sense that a mutation causes a specific congenital anomaly. Therefore, the phenomenon of having two or more variations of a single gene at the same chromosomal location (locus) is known as a polymorphism. As more and more of the genome becomes decoded, larger numbers of polymorphisms are being found for specific genes. Polymorphisms help to illustrate that the human genome is complicated, fluid, and evolving. In fact, everyone's genome undergoes change. Even though we inherit 50% of our chromosomal DNA from our mothers and 50% from our fathers, our genomes are not exactly the sum of those two parts. That is because all cells, both somatic (the cells of the body not involved in reproduction) and germline (cells involved in the production of eggs and sperm) are constantly undergoing changes in the DNA sequence. These changes may involve the loss of some DNA sequences, the addition of some DNA sequences, or a substitution in the base pair sequence. Some of these changes, if they occur in one of the approximately 100,000 chromosomal genes in a germline cell, could result in mutations that cause anomalies in offspring. If the

changes occur in the DNA between the genes which does not have any coding function, the only thing that is changed is the length of the segment of random DNA which separates the genes. Thus, changes in our DNA sequences can occur with no effect on the developing person. Changes in the DNA coding sequences that occur in somatic cells are much more difficult to detect because their effects are not necessarily developmental. Mutations in somatic cells may cause cancers by altering the cell's growth rate. However, somatic mutations may also result in anomalies if the mutation occurs early in life, or even during embryogenesis. The earlier the somatic mutation occurs, the more likely the effects will be seen in many different parts of the resulting child. Somatic mutations resulting in congenital anomalies are difficult to detect and may often only be surmised if the nuclear genomic DNA shows no evidence of mutation. Therefore, it is appropriate to focus first on the chromosomal DNA in our search for changes in DNA structure.

Restriction Fragment Length Polymorphisms (RFLP)

Polymorphisms and the normal changes in the sequences that make up the chromosomal DNA can be detected by Southern blotting if the changes occur at a site normally cut by restriction enzymes. As explained earlier in the chapter, restriction enzymes (endonucleases) cut the genomic DNA at locations where a specific sequence is recognized. The constant changes that can occur in the genome may alter the sites where the endonucleases would normally cleave the DNA. A change could occur in one or more of the recognition sites. An alteration of even a single base pair at a normal endonuclease cleavage site would eliminate the sequence from recognition so that there would be fewer DNA segments and some of the segments would be longer than normal. Conversely, a change elsewhere in the DNA sequence could create a cleavage site where none existed before. Another mechanism for changing the length of the DNA segments after cutting by a restriction endonuclease is the addition or deletion of DNA between cleavage sites. Thus, mutations that insert or delete DNA from a region of interest will result in longer or shorter DNA segments. Therefore, in a region of the genome that is of specific interest and for which probes are available, Southern blotting can be used to determine if there are variations in the length of the cut DNA fragments. With a large number of restriction endonucleases available for cutting DNA at a variety of sites (determined by the specific sequence recognized by the enzyme), scientists can study the base pair sequence in the region of a given probe to determine if there are variations in length that might represent polymorphisms. These changes at the restriction sites are known as **Restriction Fragment Length Polymorphisms (RFLP)**. Studying polymorphisms can supply a great deal of understanding in regard to the complexities of understanding human traits that do not necessarily follow obvious patterns of inheritance and expression, as in dominant or recessive mutant genes.

An example is provided by a recent finding associated with velo-cardio-facial syndrome (VCFS). It has been established that there is a very high prevalence of bipolar affective disorder in patients with VCFS (Papolos et al., 1996). Approximately 70% of individuals with VCFS develop some type of affective disorder. A subset of patients with VCFS who have psychiatric illness develop the rapid cycling form of bipolar affective disorder (defined by the number of mood swings experienced over a set period of time). It is known that VCFS is related to a deletion of DNA from the 22q11 region of the genome. Within the deleted region is a gene known as COMT (catechol-O-methyltransferase, as discussed initially in Chapter 2). The COMT gene in-

activates catecholamines, substances that aid in regulating the amount of dopamines found in the brain. Decreased COMT activity has been linked to elevated dopamine levels in the brain (COMT deactivates dopamines) and elevated dopamine levels are known to accompany a variety of psychiatric disorders, including bipolar affective disorder. It has been found that there is a polymorphism of the COMT gene (Lachman et al., 1996) with two alleles: one that causes the secretion of high levels of catecholamines and one that results in a low level of catecholamines. The polymorphism in the COMT gene results in a three- to fourfold lower level of catecholamine activity in people who have the low-secreting allele. It was shown that this COMT polymorphism is associated with the development of bipolar spectrum disorders, and, in particular, the rapid cycling variant (Lachman et al., 1996). Every COMT allele found in the rapid cycling subgroup of VCFS patients was the low secreting COMT allele on the nondeleted chromosome. Because individuals with VCFS are deleted for 22q11.2 on one chromosome and are therefore deleted for one copy of the COMT gene, with the only present copy being the low-secreting COMT allele, these VCFS patients have a much lower level of COMT enzymatic activity, thereby significantly diminishing the capacity for catecholamine inactivation at brain synaptic terminals. This suggests that, in some patients with VCFS, an increase in catecholamine neurotransmission, caused by low COMT activity, can induce an unstable rapid cycling form of bipolar affective disorder. These findings may provide a valuable model for studying the evolution of early-onset bipolar disorder and may also provide clues to the biochemical pathways that may be involved in this common form of psychiatric illness. Thus, the presence of a normally occurring polymorphism (about 25% of the general population has the low-secreting form of the COMT allele) may explain unusual patterns of human behavior when found in association with a known genetic deletion.

SUMMARY

In summary, although the tests and procedures described above may seem a bit out of reach for speech-language pathologists and audiologists who are not laboratory scientists, the reality is that all clinicians who deal with patients who have genetic diseases should have at least a nodding acquaintance with the types of procedures that are being applied to discover the root of human physical and behavioral disease. Findings from tests such as karyotypes, FISH, and PCR-RFLP may be reported in medical records that accompany patients into clinical settings. Just as we would hope that geneticists

would understand some basics in reference to communicative impairment, so should we understand the basics of genetic science.

REFERENCES

Lachman, H. M., Morrow, B., Shprintzen, R. J., Veit, S., Parsia, S. S., Faedda, G., Goldberg, R., Kucherlapati, R., & Papolos, D. F. (1996). Association of codon 108/158 catechol-o-methyl transferase gene polymorphism with the psychiatric manifestations of VCFS. *American Journal of Medical Genetics, 67,* 468–472.

Papolos, D. F., Faedda, G. L., Veit, S., Goldberg, R., Morrow, B., Kucherlapati, R., & Shprintzen, R. J. (1996). Bipolar spectrum disorders in patients diagnosed with velo-cardio-facial syndrome: Does a hemizygous deletion of chromosome 22q11 result in bipolar affective disorder? *American Journal of Psychiatry, 153,* 1541–1547.

APPENDIX

1

SYNDROMES WITH SPEECH, LANGUAGE, HEARING, AND COGNITIVE IMPAIRMENTS

This table catalogues many syndromes that manifest speech, language, hearing, and cognitive impairment. This is a long, yet still limited list for several reasons. Very rare syndromes, such as those described in only one or several families, have generally not been included. Syndromes that may occasionally have communicative impairment, but where the link between the speech-language-hearing disorder and the syndrome is not well-established, have also been excluded. Syndromes are listed according to the broad categories of speech, resonance, voice, language, and hearing disorders. In some instances, the author or other investigators have had limited experience in assessing certain aspects of communication, and therefore the word *unknown* will appear. *N.A.* refers to *not applicable*, such as for resonance disorders in children who do not develop speech. Genetic, teratogenic, and mechanically induced syndromes are listed first, followed by a separate listing for chromosomal syndromes. For more extensive descriptions of the syndromes listed in this table, the reader is referred to three excellent texts which are referenced elsewhere in this text: *Syndromes of the Head and Neck* by Gorlin, Cohen, and Levin; *Hereditary Hearing Loss and Its Syndromes* by Gorlin, Toriello, and Cohen; and *Smith's Recognizeable Patterns of Human Malformation* by Jones.

Major Features	Speech Production	Resonance
Aarskog syndrome Hypertelorism, hypodontia, brachydactyly, inguinal hernias shawled scrotum, short stature, occasional cognitive impairment	Articulation disorders related to placement errors from jaw and dental anomalies; possible compensatory errors secondary to clefting and VPI; occasional delay secondary to mild cognitive impairment	Cleft palate has been reported; therefore may cause hypernasality
Aase-Smith syndrome I Joint contractures, hydrocephalus, cleft palate	Neurogenic delay or articulation impairment secondary to brain anomalies; possible compensatory errors secondary to clefting and VPI	Cleft palate common, often resulting in hypernasality
Aase-Smith syndrome II (Blackfan-Diamond syndrome) Hypoplastic anemia, triphalangeal thumbs, small stature, cognitive impairment, webbed neck, cleft lip	Neurogenic/cognitive delay; articulation impairment; possible compensatory errors secondary to clefting and VPI; possible obligatory errors secondary to cleft alveolus	Cleft lip ± cleft palate, may cause VPI and hypernasality
Abruzzo-Erickson syndrome Cleft palate, short stature, hypospadias, sensorineural hearing loss, ocular coloboma (iris, retina, optic nerve)	Possible compensatory articulation errors secondary to clefting	Cleft palate common, may cause VPI and hypernasality
Acanthosis nigracans Discolored hyperkeratotic skin, hypertrophic lingual papillae, malignancies, thickening of lips	Impaired articulation secondary to lesions (papillomas) of oral mucosa, including the tongue, lips, and palate	Normal
Achondroplasia Disproportionate short stature, short anterior cranial base, open-bite, maxillary hypoplasia, occasional hydrocephalus, obstructive apnea	Articulation disorder related to anterior skeletal open-bite	Hyponasality; muffled oral resonance
Acrocallosal syndrome Polydactyly, cognitive impairment, macrocephaly, agenesis of corpus callosum, small stature, prominent forehead, hernias (inguinal, umbilical)	Severely delayed or absent	Unknown
Acrodysostosis Cognitive impairment, cataracts, enamel hypoplasia, rounded face, delayed dental eruption, soft tissue calcifications	Delayed secondary to mild cognitive impairment	Hyponasality secondary to nasal obstruction
Acroosteolysis (see Hajdu-Cheney syndrome)		
AEC syndrome (see Hay-Wells syndrome)		
Aicardi syndrome Microphthalmia, agenesis of corpus callosum, brain anomalies, occasional cleft lip ± cleft palate	Very limited or absent	Cleft lip ± cleft palate an occasional finding, may result in hypernasality

Voice	Language	Hearing	Primary Etiology
Unknown	Occasional mild impairment	Not documented	X-linked recessive, mutation in FGD1 gene at Xp11.2
Unknown	Impairment secondary to brain anomalies	Conductive loss secondary to to chronic otits media related to cleft	Autosomal dominant
Unknown	Impairment secondary to brain/cognitive anomalies	Conductive loss secondary to chronic otitis media related to cleft	Autosomal recessive
Unknown	Unknown	Mixed loss, progressive sensorineural loss possible	X-linked recessive
Unknown	Normal	Conductive and/or sensorineural loss possible	Heterogenous, may be autosomal dominant
High pitched, thin	Usually normal	Conductive loss secondary to middle ear disease	Autosomal dominant, mutation in FGFR3 gene at 4p16.3
Unknown	Severely impaired	Unknown	Possibly autosomal recessive, possibly caused by 12p trisomy
Unknown	Mildly impaired secondary to cognitive impairment	Conductive loss secondary to middle ear disease	Autosomal dominant
Unknown	Severe impairment	Unknown	X-linked recessive, mutation at Xp22.31

Major Features	Speech Production	Resonance
Alagille syndrome Small stature, broad forehead, heart anomalies, vertebral anomalies, hepatic anomalies, occasional cognitive impairment, small genitals	May be delayed secondary to mild cognitive impairment	Unknown
Albers-Schönberg syndrome Dense but fragile bones, macrocephaly, cranial nerve palsies, distorted teeth, hypocalcemia, hydrocephalus, mixed or sensorineural hearing loss, eventually lethal.	May be delayed or impaired secondary to facial paresis, or cognitive impairment (about 20% of cases)	Unknown
Albinism, late onset sensorineural hearing loss	Normal	Normal
Albright osteodystrophy (see Acrodysostosis)		
Alport syndrome Nephritis, sensorineural hearing loss myopia, stridor, apnea, dysphagia	Normal	Normal
Alström syndrome Obesity, mildly short stature, nystagmus, loss of vision, baldness (males), diabetes mellitus, renal anomalies, scoliosis, sensorineural hearing loss	Normal	Normal
Amelogenesis imperfecta Hypoplasia of the dental enamel	Articulation impairment secondary to tooth loss	Normal
Amnion rupture sequence Facial clefts, digit amputations, ringlike constrictions on limbs, possible cranial defects	Articulation impairment common in cases where amniotic bands deform or disrupt oral structures, possible compensatory articulation secondary to cleft palate; possible obligatory errors secondary to cleft alveolus	Cleft lip ± cleft palate may result in VPI and hypernasality; oral resonance may be distorted by disruption of oral structures
Anderson syndrome Maxillary hypoplasia, mandibular prognathism, scoliosis, thin calvarium	Articulation impairment secondary to malocclusion caused by abnormal jaw growth and position	Normal
Angelman syndrome Cognitive impairment, microcephaly, mandibular prognathism, large mouth optic atrophy, seizures, ataxia	Nearly all cases have no speech development	N.A. (no speech)
Aniridia-Wilms tumor syndrome Absent iris, mental retardation, microcephaly, cranial asymmetry, long thin face, Wilms tumor and other malignancies	Delayed or absent speech development secondary to cognitive impairment	Unknown

Voice	Language	Hearing	Primary Etiology
High pitch	May be delayed and/or impaired secondary to mild cognitive impairment	Normal	Autosomal dominant Deletions reported at 20p11.23 → 20p12.2
Unknown	May be delayed and/or impaired secondary to hearing loss or cognitive impairment	Neural, may result in total deafness secondary to auditory nerve compression	Autosomal recessive
Normal	Normal	Late onset sensorineural loss, progressive	X-linked recessive
Normal	Normal	Sensorineural loss, variable severity, progressive	Heterogenous, with mutations found in 3 different type IV collagen genes at Xq22 (X-linked dominant), and 2 autosomal recessive genes
Normal	Normal	Sensorineural loss with onset at approximately 5 yrs. of age, cochlear in origin, progressive	Autosomal recessive
Normal	Normal	Normal	X-linked form caused by mutation of amelogenin gene on Xq
Laryngeal anomalies not common	May be impaired if cranium and brain are involved	Usually normal; may be mild conductive impairment secondary to otitis media from cleft anomalies	Intrauterine mechanical disruption
Normal	Normal	Normal	Autosomal recessive
N.A.	No speech or language development	Normal	Deletion of 15q11 → 13 from maternal chromosome 15
Unknown	Impaired secondary to cognitive impairment	Normal	Deletion of 11p13, most cases sporadic

Major Features	Speech Production	Resonance
Antley-Bixler syndrome Craniosynostosis, malformed ears, arachnodactyly, synostosis of the radius and humerus, femoral bowing, digital anomalies, heart anomalies, imperforate anus, kidney anomalies	May be delayed secondary to cognitive impairment (hydrocephalus may occur); articulation impairment secondary to midface hypoplasia	Hyponasal (nasal obstruction common)
Apert syndrome Craniosynostosis, syndactyly, symphalangism, short upper arms, hydrocephalus, cognitive impairment, choanal stenosis/atresia, acne, upper airway obstruction, occasional cleft palate	Often delayed secondary to cognitive impairment, chronic upper airway obstruction, and severe occlusal anomalies; cleft palate may result in compensatory articulation	Hyponasality secondary to choanal stenosis or atresia; hypernasality secondary to cleft palate; mixed resonance common; abnormal oral resonance secondary to reduced pharyngeal dimensions
Arthrogryposis (see Distal arthrogryposis syndrome)		
Ascher syndrome Drooping eyelids, horizontal fold in upper lip with soft tissue redundancy, thyroid enlargement (benign)	Articulation impaired by redundant and loose tissue of the upper lip	Normal
Ataxia-telangiectasia Thin flaccid facies, athetosis, relative small stature, cerebellar ataxia, progressive cognitive deterioration, telangiectasias of ears and conjunctiva	Early development normal until onset of cerebellar ataxia with accompanying dysarthria	Initially normal, eventually may become hypernasal secondary to hypotonia and dysarthria
Baller-Gerold syndrome Craniosynostosis, hypoplasia of the radius, occasional missing thumbs, possible cognitive impairment, anal anomalies, occasional heart anomalies	Onset may be delayed secondary to cognitive impairment and/or motor delay	Unknown
Bamatter syndrome Lax skin, giving the face an aged appearance, hypotonia, inguinal hernia, hypoplastic alveolar bone	Onset may be delayed secondary to hypotonia; articulation may be impaired by lax facial skin and muscle and malocclusion from prognathism	Unknown
Bannayan-Riley-Ruvalcaba syndrome Large size at birth, macrocephaly, cognitive impairment, pigmented spots on penis, intestinal polyps	Often delayed and impaired secondary to cognitive impairment and neurologic disorders	Unknown
Bardet-Biedl syndrome Obesity, cognitive impairment, polydactyly, retinitis pigmentosa, hypogonadism, occasional heart anomalies, strabismus	Delayed speech onset and impaired articulation secondary to cognitive impairment and hypotonia; in cases with severe retardation, there may be very limited speech	Unknown
Basal cell nevus syndrome Basal cell carcinomas, macrocephaly, rib anomalies, scoliosis, strabismus, occasional cognitive impairment	May be delayed in a small percentage secondary to CNS anomalies and cognitive impairment (under 5%); compensatory articulation disorder may occur secondary to cleft lip/palate (under 5%)	Hypernasality may be found secondary to cleft palate in a small percentage

Voice	Language	Hearing	Primary Etiology
Unknown	May be impaired secondary to cognitive impairment	Conductive hearing loss may occur secondary to middle ear disease, reduced middle ear volume, or external canal stenosis	Autosomal recessive (presumed)
Hoarseness, breathiness may be caused by calcification of the larynx	Often delayed and/or impaired secondary to cognitive disorder, hydrocephalus, and/or brain anomalies	Conductive hearing loss common secondary to middle ear effusion, reduced middle ear volume, fixation of stapes footplate	Autosomal dominant mutation in FGFR2 gene (fibroblast growth factor receptor 2) on chromosome 10 (10q25 →10q26)
Normal	Normal	Normal	Autosomal dominant
Begins normal, then spasmodic dysphonia may develop	Initial development normal, then cognitive impairment develops close to 10 years of age	Normal	Autosomal recessive mutation in ATM gene located on chromosome 11 (11q22 → q23)
Unknown	May be delayed or impaired secondary to cognitive impairment	Unknown	Autosomal recessive
Unknown, but small stature may result in high pitch	Unknown	Unknown	Autosomal recessive
Unknown	Usually delayed and impaired secondary to cognitive impairment and neurologic disorders	Unknown	Autosomal dominant
Unknown	Delayed and impaired secondary to cognitive impairment	Unknown	Autosomal recessive mapped to multiple chromosome sites (3, 15, 16q, 11q)
Normal	May be delayed/impaired in cases with CNS anomalies and cognitive impairment	Normal	Autosomal dominant mapped to 9q

Major Features	Speech Production	Resonance
Beckwith-Wiedemann syndrome Large at birth, mandibular prognathism omphalocele or umbilical hernias, hypotonia, possible cognitive impairment, accelerated growth, macroglossia, creases in ear lobes, enlarged liver, spleen, and kidneys, inguinal hernias, occasional heart anomalies, occasional hypoglycemia	May be delayed secondary to cognitive impairment and hypotonia; articulation disorders secondary to large tongue and malocclusion (prognathism) common; possible compensatory articulation secondary to cleft palate	Hypernasality secondary to cleft palate is possible; hypotonia may also contribute to hypernasality; oral resonance may be impaired secondary to large tongue
Bencze syndrome Facial asymmetry, strabismus, amblyopia, submucous cleft palate	Compensatory articulation secondary to cleft palate is possible; minor articulation impairment may be found secondary to malocclusion (facial asymmetry)	Hypernasality secondary to cleft palate and VPI is possible
Berardinelli syndrome Absence of facial subcutaneous fat, enlarged liver and heart, cognitive impairment, hirsutism, hypertrophic tonsils and adenoids, penile or clitoral enlargement	Delayed speech onset is probable in nearly half of cases secondary to cognitive impairment	Abnormal oral resonance secondary to enlarged tonsils is common; muffled oral resonance, hyponasality secondary to enlarged adenoids
Berman syndrome Lysosomal storage disease, puffy face, strabismus, variable cognitive impairment	Delayed speech onset with progressive ataxic speech production; sensorineural hearing loss may also contribute to speech impairment if the onset is early	Hypernasality may develop secondary to progressive neuropathy
Binder syndrome Hypoplastic midface, absence of anterior nasal spine, flattened nose	Abnormalities of articulatory placement secondary to maxillary hypoplasia	Normal
Bixler syndrome Cleft lip and palate, hypertelorism, microtia, short stature, cognitive impairment, heart anomalies, kidney anomalies, short stature, anomalous ossicles	Delayed onset secondary to cognitive impairment; articulation impairment secondary to maxillary hypoplasia; possible compensatory articulation caused VPI secondary to cleft palate; possible obligatory errors secondary to cleft alveolus	Possible hypernasality secondary to cleft palate
Blepharonasofacial syndrome Telecanthus, broad nasal root, midfacial hypoplasia, hyperextensible joints, cognitive impairment	Usually delayed secondary to cognitive impairment; possible abnormal articulatory placement secondary to maxillary hypoplasia	Unknown
Blepharophimosis syndrome Short palpebral fissures, telecanthus, cup-shaped ears, hypogonadism, hypotonia, occasional cognitive impairment	May be delayed secondary to cognitive impairment	Normal
Bloch-Sulzberger syndrome Incontinentia pigmenti, alopecia, strabismus, eye anomalies, cognitive impairment, dental anomalies	May be delayed or impaired secondary to cognitive impairment; dental anomalies may interfere with articulation	Normal
Bloom syndrome Small stature, deficient subcutaneous fat, occasional cognitive deficiency, psychiatric illness, neoplasias	May be delayed or impaired in cases with cognitive impairment	Normal

Voice	Language	Hearing	Primary Etiology
Hoarseness	Language often delayed and/or impaired secondary to cognitive impairment (usually mild)	Conductive loss from chronic middle ear disease secondary to cleft palate	Autosomal dominant IGF2 gene at 11p15.5 with imprinting (inherited from maternal chromosome)
Unknown	Unknown	Conductive hearing loss from chronic middle ear disease secondary to cleft palate	Autosomal dominant
Unknown	Delayed/impaired in approximately 50% of cases secondary to cognitive impairment	Unknown	Autosomal recessive
Unknown	Impaired secondary to progressive cognitive and neurologic degeneration	Variable progressive sensorineural hearing loss ranging from moderate to severe	Autosomal recessive
Normal	Normal	Normal	Unknown
Unknown	Delayed and impaired secondary to cognitive impairment	Conductive loss caused by both microtia and middle ear disease secondary to cleft	Probable autosomal recessive
Unknown	Usually delayed secondary to cognitive impairment	Unknown	Autosomal dominant
Normal	May be impaired secondary to cognitive impairment	Normal	Autosomal dominant, mapped to 3q23
Normal	May be impaired secondary to cognitive impairment	Normal	X-linked dominant lethal in males
High pitch	May be impaired in cases with cognitive impairment	Normal	Autosomal recessive linked to 15q26.1

Major Features	Speech Production	Resonance
BOF syndrome **(branchio-oculo-facial syndrome)** Cleft lip-palate, lacrimal duct stenosis, eye anomalies, conductive hearing loss, malformed auricles, premature grey hair, preauricular pits, cervically displaced thymus gland, thin skin on neck	Possible compensatory articulation errors secondary to cleft and VPI; obligatory articulation errors secondary to cleft alveolus	Possible hypernasality secondary to clefting
BOR syndrome **(branchio-oto-renal syndrome)** Conductive hearing loss, sensorineural hearing loss, ossicular anomalies, cochlear anomalies, vestibular anomalies, branchial clefts, preauricular pits, malformed auricles, lacrimal duct stenosis, renal anomalies	Possible delay secondary to hearing loss	Abnormal resonance as seen in "deaf speech" may occur
Börjeson-Forssman-Lehman syndrome Short stature, obesity, cognitive impairment, hypotonia, hypogonadism, coarse facies, seizures, large "puffy" ears	Delayed or absent, depending on degree of cognitive impairment	Unknown
Borud syndrome Sensorineural hearing loss, myopathy, cardiomyopathy, encephalopathy, ataxia	Late onset deterioration secondary to progressive encephalopathy and myopathy	Unknown
Brachial plexus neuropathy Cleft palate, hypotelorism, facial asymmetry, upslanting deep-set eyes, parasthesia of arms and hands, small stature, reduced reflexes	Possible compensatory articulation secondary to cleft palate	Possible hypernasality secondary to cleft palate
C syndrome Trigonocephaly, microcephaly, hypotonia, micrognathia, macrostomia, polydactyly, short limbs, hip dysplasia, contractures, hemangiomas, heart malformations, cryptorchidism, redundant skin, early mortality	Usually no speech development because of severe cognitive impairment	N.A.
Caffey-Silverman syndrome Thickening of cortical bones, including mandible, ribs, and limbs, tissue of face, chest, and limbs, infantile fever and irritability	Unknown, but it is presumed that enlargement of the mandible may alter articulation and result in malocclusion which will affect articulatory placement	Unknown, presumed normal
Campomelic syndrome Growth deficiency (prenatal onset), brain malformation, delayed bone maturation, micrognathia, flat midface and nasal bridge, short palpebral fissures, shortening and malformation of the limbs, anomalous trachea and bronchi, anomalous male genitalia, neonatal death is common, few survive into childhood	Most patients do not survive long enough to develop speech, therefore, speech development parameters are unknown	Unknown
Camurati-Engelmann syndrome Progressive diaphyseal dysplasia, long	Normal	Normal

Voice	Language	Hearing	Primary Etiology
Unknown	Normal	Conductive loss, usually mild to moderate	Autosomal dominant
Normal	May be impaired secondary to hearing loss	Conductive, sensorineural, or mixed loss, may be progressive, ranges from mild to profound	Autosomal dominant
High pitch	Impaired or absent, depending on degree of cognitive impairment which ranges from moderate to severe	None known	X-linked recessive
Unknown	Early development normal	Progressive sensorineural hearing loss	Mitochondiral (exclusively maternal inheritance)
Hoarseness secondary to recurrent laryngeal nerve dysfunction	Normal	Normal	Autosomal dominant
N.A.	Usually no language development	Unknown	Autosomal recessive chromosome 3 aneuploidies have been implicated
Unknown, presumed normal	Unknown, presumed normal	Unknown	Autosomal dominant
Unknown, but anomalous lower airway must affect voice production	Most do not live long enough to develop language; those who have survived have been severely retarded	Nearly all surviving cases have had severe hearing loss, with both conductive and sensorineural components secondary to ossicular malformations and cochlear anomalies	Autosomal recessive mapped to SOX9 gene at 17q25
Unknown	Nomal	Sensorineural hearing loss (usually progressive), in less	Autosomal recessive

Major Features	Speech Production	Resonance
Camurati-Engelmann syndrome *(continued)* bowed limbs, delayed walking, bone pain, scoliosis, possible facial distortion from thickening of cortical bone, possible optic atrophy, possible hearing loss		
Cardio-facio-cutaneous syndrome (CFC) Large appearing forehead with bitemporal depressions, sparse scalp hair, depressed nasal root, short neck, ptosis, skin anomalies (hyperkeratosis or ichthyosis), small stature cognitive impairment, hypotonia, cardiac anomalies	Delayed speech onset secondary to cognitive impairment and hypotonia	Abnormal oral resonance related to short neck
Carpenter syndrome Craniosynostosis, polydactyly, syndactyly heart anomalies, small stature, cognitive impairment, occasional skeletal anomalies, occasional hernias, scoliosis	Delayed onset in most cases secondary to cognitive impairment; articulatory impairment secondary to constricted maxilla	Hyponasality secondary to small nasal capsule; abnormal oral resonance secondary to short neck
Cartilage-hair hypoplasia Small stature, short limbs, bowed legs, small hands, short vertebrae, lordosis, light fragile hair, hyperextensible hands	Normal	Normal
Cat eye syndrome Coloboma of iris, choroid, and retina, hypertelorism, occasional microphthalmia, cognitive impairment, anal anomalies, kidney anomalies, short stature, hernias, heart malformations, occasional cleft palate, occasional malformed external ears, malrotation of gut	Usually delayed onset secondary to cognitive impairment; possible compensatory articulation secondary to cleft palate	Possible hypernasality secondary to cleft palate
Catel-Manzke syndrome Cleft palate, micrognathia, clinodactyly, club foot, heart anomalies	Compensatory articulation may occur secondary to cleft palate, articulatory placement may be impaired by micrognathia	Hypernasality may occur secondary to VPI from cleft palate
Cerebro-costo-mandibular syndrome Severe micrognathia, small stature, small chest, rib anomalies, cognitive impairment, feeding problems, tracheal anomalies, elbow anomalies, vertebral anomalies	Articulation disorder secondary to small mouth and difficulty with normal placement; speech delay secondary to cognitive impairment; poor breath support	Abnormal oral resonance secondary to small oropharynx and short neck
Cerebro-oculo-facial-skeletal syndrome Hypoplastic cerebral white matter, microcephaly, hypotonia, severe small stature, prominent nasal root, large ears, small eyes, micrognathia, limb contractures, kidney anomalies, hirsutism, rocker bottom feet, early death	No speech development	N.A.
CHARGE association Ocular Coloboma, Heart anomalies, choanal Atresia, growth Retardation, Genital anomalies, Ear anomalies, cognitive impairment, unilateral facial paresis, occasional cleft palate, feeding disorders	Delayed speech onset secondary to cognitive impairment; articulation impairment secondary to paresis; possible compensatory articulation secondary to cleft palate	Hyponasality secondary to choanal atresia, possible cul-de-sac resonance if palate is cleft; possible hypernasality secondary to clefting

Voice	Language	Hearing	Primary Etiology
		than 10% of cases	
Thin voice	Delayed and impaired language secondary to cognitive impairment	Normal	Autsomal dominant possibly linked to 7q
Unknown	Delayed and impaired secondary to cognitive impairment	Probably normal in most cases	Autosomal recessive
High pitched	Normal	Normal	Autosomal recessive linked to chromosome 9p
Unknown	Usually delayed and impaired secondary to cognitive impairment	Possible conductive hearing loss secondary to malformed external ears and/or middle ear effusion secondary to cleft palate	Extra segment of chromosome 22 (entire short arm) inserted at the long arm near 22q11
Unknown	Normal	Conductive hearing loss secondary to middle ear effusion from cleft palate is likely	Unknown
Thin, hoarse	Delay and impairment secondary to cognitive disorder	Normal	Autosomal recessive
N.A.	No language development	Unknown	Autosomal recessive
Hoarseness	Delayed and impaired language secondary to cognitive impairment	Sensorineural and mixed hearing loss common, pure conductive least common, ranging from mild to profound, usually asymmetric with ossicular anomalies possible	Etiologically heterogenous

Major Features	Speech Production	Resonance
Christian syndrome Craniosynostosis, microcephaly, cleft palate, arthrogryposis, cognitive impairment, dysphagia, seizures, micrognathia, torticollis, hirsutism, early death from respiratory failure	Usually no speech development	N.A.
Cleidocranial dysplasia Absent or hypoplastic clavicles, delayed closure of cranial sutures, broad forehead, late dental eruption, finger anomalies, delayed mineralization of pubic symphysis, occasional osteosclerosis, hearing loss, and cleft palate	Possible compensatory articulation secondary to cleft palate and VPI	Possible hypernasal resonance secondary to cleft palate
Clouston syndrome Thickened skin on palms and soles of feet, excess pigmentation of skin in multiple locations (elbows, axillae, knuckles), sparse or absent hair (alopecia), dysplastic finger and toenails, strabismus, cataracts, cognitive impairment, short stature	Possible speech delay secondary to cognitive impairment	Normal
Cockayne syndrome Short stature, deficient subcutaneous fat, progressive cognitive impairment, progressive peripheral neuropathy, retinal pigment anomalies, photosensitivity of the skin, enlarged liver, cryptorchidism, central hearing impairment	Initial development in infancy and toddler years normal, then progressive deterioration of speech with dysarthric component	Initially normal, may become hypernasal with progressive dysarthria
Coffin-Lowry syndrome Short stature, cognitive impairment, coarse facies, hypodontia, dental spacing, short sternum, scoliosis, puffy hands, flat feet, microcephaly, hypotonia	Usually no speech development secondary to severe cognitive impairment	N.A.
Coffin-Siris syndrome Short stature, cognitive impairment, severe hypotonia, microcephaly, coarse facial appearance, small or absent 5th fingers, hyperextensible joints, sparse scalp hair, hirsutism on body	Often no speech or very limited speech development secondary to cognitive impairment	N.A.
COFS syndrome (see Cerebro-oculo-facial-skeletal syndrome)		
Cohen syndrome Obesity, short stature, delayed puberty, cognitive impairment, hypotonia, scoliosis, hyperextensible joints, narrow face, high nasal root, downslanting eyes, microcephaly	Delayed onset secondary to cognitive impairment/hypotonia, misarticulations secondary to open-bite and maxillary constriction	Normal
Cornelia de Lange syndrome (see de Lange syndrome)		
Cowden syndrome Multiple hamartomas, neuromas, polyps, goiter, breast lesions, papillomas on lips and tongue	May be impaired by lesions on lips, tongue, and gingiva	Normal
Craniodiaphyseal dysplasia Severe thickening of the bone of the	Often delayed with progressive deterioration of articulation	Hyponasal secondary to nasal obstruction from

Voice	Language	Hearing	Primary Etiology
Inspiratory stridor from laryngomalacia	Usally no language development	Unknown	Autosomal recessive
Possible hoarseness	Normal	Possible conductive or mixed hearing loss	Autosomal dominant linked to deletion at 6p21
Normal	Possible language delay and impairment secondary to cognitive impairment	Normal	Autosomal dominant linked to 13q
High pitch	Initial onset normal, followed by deterioration of all cognitive functioning, including language	Perceptual (central) hearing impairment	Autosomal recessive
Unknown	Usually no language development	Normal	X-linked recessive linked to Xp22
High pitch	Often limited or no language development secondary to cognitive impairment	Normal	Autosomal recessive
Unknown	Almost always delayed secondary to cognitive impairment	Normal	Autosomal recessive
Hoarseness and breathiness secondary to laryngeal polyps	Normal	Occasional sensorineural hearing loss	Autosomal dominant linked to 10q22
Normal	Usually delayed secondary to cognitive impairment with	Mixed hearing loss secondary to osseous growth	Autosomal recessive

Major Features	Speech Production	Resonance
Craniodiaphyseal dysplasia (*continued*) face and skull, hypertelorism, eventual optic atrophy (possible blindness), hearing loss, progressive cognitive deterioration, early death is common	secondary to bony overgrowth of jaws and palate	bony overgrowth
Craniofrontonasal dysplasia syndrome Hypertelorism, orbital dystopia, cleft lip ± cleft palate, longitudinal splitting of fingernails, agenesis of corpus callosum, strabismus, craniofacial asymmetry, sloping, shoulders, occasional cognitive impairment	Articulatory impairment secondary to malocclusion and/or cleft; possible compensatory articulation secondary to cleft; occasional delay secondary to cognitive impairment	Hypernasality may occur secondary to cleft; occasional hyponasality or mixed resonance secondary to small nasal capsule
Craniometaphyseal dysplasia Bony overgrowth of face and skull, hypertelorism, nystagmus, hearing loss	Progressive articulatory impairment secondary to abnormal bony growth of jaws and palate; possible lip incompetence caused by progressive facial paresis	Progressive hyponasality from bony overgrowth in nasal cavity
Cri-du-chat syndrome (see Chromosomal syndromes, 5p-)		
Crouzon syndrome Craniosynostosis (multiple sutures), maxillary hypoplasia, exorbitism, hearing loss, cognitive impairment (not common), cleft lip/palate (not common)	Usually normal onset and development; articulatory impairment secondary to Class III malocclusion and midface deficiency	Often hyponasal secondary to small nasal capsule
Cryptophthalmos syndrome (see Fraser syndrome)		
DeBarsy syndrome Small stature, cognitive impairment, wrinkled skin, hyperextensible joints, athetosis, hypotonia, large ears, microcephaly, corneal clouding	Severely delayed or absent, depending on severity of cognitive impairment; dysarthria	Unknown
de Lange syndrome Short stature, cognitive impairment, limb reduction (arms), digital anomalies, coarse facies, synophrys, microcephaly, irritability, seizures, hypertonia, lack of facial expression, cleft palate, low anterior hairline, long eye lashes, anomalous auricles, hirsute ears, short neck, somatic hirsutism, renal anomalies, multiple hernias, pyloric stenosis, intestinal anomalies, cardiac malformations, micrognathia, Robin sequence possible	Usually severely delayed or absent, neurogenically based articulation disorders	May be hypernasal secondary to VPI caused by cleft palate
DeMyer sequence (see Holoprosencephaly)		
Diastrophic dysplasia Short stature, short limbs, flexion abnormalities of multiple joints, scoliosis, "cauliflower ears," abnormal thumb placement, short tubular bones with broad metaphyses, occasional cleft palate and Robin sequence	Usually normal onset, although may have compensatory articulation secondary to VPI from cleft palate	May be hypernasal secondary to VPI caused by cleft palate
DiGeorge sequence (see Velo-cardio-facial syndrome)		

Voice	Language	Hearing	Primary Etiology
	progressive deterioration with increasing brain compression from bony overgrowth	in the tympanum and eventual compression of the auditory nerve	
Normal	Occasionally delayed secondary to possible cognitive impairment	Conductive hearing loss caused by middle ear effusion secondary to cleft	X-linked dominant
Normal	Progressive deterioration secondary to compression of CNS	Moderate to severe mixed hearing loss	There is both an autosomal dominant and autosomal recessive form
Normal	Usually normal	Conductive hearing loss common secondary to frequent middle ear effusion and reduced volume of middle ear	Autosomal dominant mutation in FGFR2 gene (fibroblast growth factor receptor 2), chromosome 10q23 → 26
Unknown	Severely impaired or absent depending on severity of cognitive impairment	Unknown, probably normal	Autosomal recessive
Low pitch, often hoarse; cry in infancy is low pitched	Severely delayed, impaired, or absent secondary to cognitive impairment	Conductive loss may occur secondary to middle ear effusion in cases with clefts; sensorineural hearing loss from mild to profound in approximately 50% of cases	3q25.1–26.2 trisomy
High pitch	Usually normal	Occasional conductive pathology caused by middle ear disease secondary to cleft palate	Autosomal recessive mutation in DTDST gene

Major Features	Speech Production	Resonance
Distal arthrogryposis syndrome Multiple contractures of limbs and digits, "clenched" hands, hip dislocation, ulnar deviation of fingers, occasional limitation of jaw opening, occasional cleft palate, Robin sequence may occur	Usually normal, but jaw limitation may result in late onset and articulatory impairment into childhood (contractures usually respond to therapeutic management); possible compensatory articulation if cleft is present	May be hypernasal if cleft is present; oral resonance may be impaired if jaw movement is limited
Down syndrome (see Chromosomal syndromes, Trisomy 21)		
Dubowitz syndrome Small stature, low birthweight, microcephaly, cognitive deficiency, short palpebral fissures, telecanthus, ptosis, micrognathia, eczema, sparse scalp hair, late dental eruption, occasional cleft palate, attention deficit hyperactivity disorder	Often delayed speech development secondary to cognitive impairment; possible compensatory articulation secondary to cleft palate and VPI	May be hypernasal if cleft is present
Dysautonomia Hypotonia, poor suck in infancy, absent reflexes, delayed motor milestones, ataxia, decreased pain sensation, indifference to pain, digestive problems, progressive scoliosis, macular erythema, decreased tearing leading to corneal ulceration, absent or decreased papillae on tongue, drooling, absent/hypoactive gag, sad facial expression, mild facial asymmetry, frequent early death from pulmonary compromise secondary to aspiration	Dysarthria	Hypernasality secondary to dysarthria and rhythm problems
Dyskeratosis congenita Hyperpigmented skin, excessive sweating on palms and soles, decreased sweating elsewhere, hyperkeratosis of skin, thin hair, thin build, cognitive impairment, sparse scalp hair, anemia, hypoplastic nails, small male genitals, dysphagia, hearing loss	Delayed secondary to cognitive impairment	Normal
Dysosteosclerosis Cranial anomalies, frontal bossing, patent anterior fontanel, short stature, frequent skeletal fractures, dental anomalies, late dental eruption, progressive thickening of the cranial bones leading to cranial nerve dysfunction, skeletal sclerosis	Normal onset of speech, later deterioration secondary to facial paresis, progressive neurologic dysfunction, and impinging skeletal sclerosis on the brainstem	Initially normal, followed by eventual hyponasality caused by cranial overgrowth
EEC syndrome (ectrodactyly-ectodermal dysplasia-clefting) Cleft palate ± cleft lip, ectrodactyly, absent or hypoplastic nails, syndactyly, sparse hair, decreased pigmentation of the hair and skin, absent punctae in lower eye lids, missing or abnormal teeth, enamel hypoplasia, photophobia, occasional cognitive impairment, occasional kidney anomalies	Frequent compensatory articulation secondary to clefting which is most often bilateral complete; occasional delay secondary to cognitive impairment; misarticulations secondary to missing or malformed teeth (hypohidrosis)	Frequent hypernasality secondary to VPI caused by clefting

Voice	Language	Hearing	Primary Etiology
Normal	Usually normal	Usually normal	Autosomal dominant
High pitch, hoarseness	Delayed and impaired in most cases secondary to cognitive impairment	Usually normal	Autosomal recessive
Monotone	Normal	Normal	Autosomal recessive linked to 9q31, found mostly in Ashkenazic Jews of Eastern European origin
Hoarseness	Delayed and impaired secondary to cognitive impairment	Conductive hearing loss secondary to middle ear malformation; sensorineural hearing loss	Etiologically heterogenous X-linked form linked to Xp28
Initially normal, subsequent hoarseness	Initially normal followed by deterioration as sclerosis progresses	Initially normal followed by progressive conductive and sensorineural hearing loss; otosclerosis is also common	Autosomal recessive
Hoarseness and breathiness are common caused by lack of normal secretions of vocal cords (hypohidrosis)	Delayed and/or impaired on occasion secondary to cognitive impairment	Conductive hearing loss common secondary to ossicular anomalies; possible chronic middle ear effusion secondary to clefting	Autosomal dominant

Major Features	Speech Production	Resonance
Edwards syndrome Short stature, obesity, nystagmus, blindness, cognitive impairment, acanthosis nigricans, diabetes mellitus, sensorineural hearing loss	Delayed onset secondary to cognitive impairment	Unknown, but probably affected by severe sensorineural hearing loss
Ellis-van Creveld syndrome Small stature, short limbs, polydactyly, short narrow chest, anodontia, short upper lip, labial frenula, heart anomalies, dysplastic nails	Misarticulations related to absent or abnormal teeth; abnormal bilabial production caused by short upper lip	Normal
Epstein syndrome Progressive renal failure, thrombocytopenia, sensorineural hearing loss	Speech production impaired by high-frequency sensorineural hearing loss in many cases	Resonance may be impaired by severe hearing loss
Escobar syndrome Small stature, downslanting drooping eyes, hypertelorism, micrognathia, cleft palate, lack of facial expression, webbing of neck, popliteal pterygium, pterygia at elbows, cryptorchidism in males, absent labia in females, fusion of vertebrae	Impaired articulation secondary to limited mouth opening and poor oral movements; possible compensatory articulations secondary to cleft palate and/or tongue backing from micrognathia	Hypernasality common; abnormal oral resonance secondary to limited oral opening and reduced oral size with tongue backing
Fabry syndrome Multiple dark nodules on skin clustering in several areas (umbilical area, genitals, knees), corneal opacity, hematuria, renal failure, severe burning pain in extremities, headaches, seizures, vascular abnormalities in brain, occasional cognitive deficiency, occasional coarse facies, heart disease, occasional hemiplegia, hypohidrosis	Possible speech delay related to cognitive impairment; occasional articulatory impairment caused by thickened lips	Abnormal oral and pharyngeal resonance caused by build-up of ceramide trihexoside in the upper and lower airway mucosa
Facioscapulohumeral muscular dystrophy Weakness of facial and shoulder muscles, upper arm weakness, progressive course spreading to other muscle groups, cognitive impairment in about a third of cases, retinal vascular anomalies, hearing loss	Articulation impairment possibly caused by progressive muscle weakness	Possible hypernasality caused by pharyngeal and palatal muscle weakness
Fanconi pancytopenia syndrome Short stature, microcephaly, cognitive impairment in a quarter of cases, small or absent thumbs bilaterally, hip dislocation, renal anomalies, small genitals in males, hematologic disorders (pancytopenia), nystagmus, strabismus, hearing loss	Possible delay if cognitive impairment is present	Normal
Fechtner syndrome Late onset renal dysfunction, large platelets, thrombocytopenia, cataracts, hearing loss	Normal development	Normal
Femoral hypoplasia unusual facies Absence or hypoplasia of the femurs, cleft palate, micrognathia, upslanting	Possible compensatory articulation pattern secondary to cleft palate and VPI	Possible hypernasality secondary to cleft palate and VPI

Voice	Language	Hearing	Primary Etiology
Unknown	Delayed onset secondary to cognitive impairment	Progressive sensorineural hearing loss	Autosomal recessive
Unknown	Occasional delay or disorder secondary to cognitive impairment in a small percentage of cases	Normal	Autosomal recessive
Normal	Normal	Progressive sensorineural hearing loss with onset in childhood (usually after age 5), usually resulting in moderate to severe loss	Autosomal dominant
Normal	Normal	Possible conductive impairment caused by middle ear effusion secondary to cleft palate	Autosomal recessive
Hoarse voice secondary to hypohidrosis and accumulation of ceramide trihexoside in the pharynx, larynx, and trachea	Usually normal, but may be delayed or impaired secondary to cognitive impairment	High-frequency sensorineural hearing loss common; diminished vestibular response	X-linked recessive mutation in alpha-galactosidase A gene mapped to Xp22
Hoarseness and breathiness possible	May be delayed or impaired secondary to cognitive impairment	Bilateral sensorineural hearing loss, highly variable, from mild to profound; cochlear pathology	Autosomal dominant deletion of 4q35 → qter
Unknown	May be delayed or impaired secondary to cognitive impairment	Conductive hearing loss in approximately 10% of cases caused by ossicular anomalies or external canal stenosis	Autosomal recessive mapped to 16q24
Normal	Normal	High-frequency sensorineural hearing loss, late onset (usually after age 20 years), variable severity	Autosomal dominant
Normal	Normal	Possible conductive hearing loss caused by chronic otitis media secondary to cleft palate	Unknown, autosomal dominant inheritance has been proposed,

Major Features	Speech Production	Resonance
Femoral hypoplasia unusual facies (*continued*) eyes, mildly dysmorphic ears, hypoplastic female genitalia, syndactyly		
Fetal alcohol syndrome Cognitive impairment, low birthweight, microcephaly, short palpebral fissures, heart anomalies, short nose, flat philtrum, cleft palate ± cleft lip, digital anomalies, joint abnormalities	Speech delay; articulatory impairment secondary to poor motor skills; compensatory articulation secondary to clefting; dyspraxia	Possible hypernasality secondary to cleft palate and VPI
Fetal hydantoin syndrome Cognitive impairment, growth deficiency, cleft palate ± cleft lip, short nose, flat philtrum, hyoplastic distal phalanges and nails of hands and feet, low anterior hairline, cardiac anomalies, genital anomalies	Speech delay secondary to mild cognitive impairment; compensatory articulation secondary to clefting	Possible hypernasality secondary to cleft palate and VPI
Fetal warfarin embryopathy Small nose, skeletal anomalies, hypoplastic nails, low birthweight, cognitive impairment	Speech delay secondary to cognitive impairment	Unknown
FG syndrome Cognitive impairment, macrocephaly, plagiocephaly, upsweeping anterior hairline, downslanting palpebral fissures, strabismus, micrognathia, cleft palate, imperforate anus, genital anomalies, umbilical hernia, hearing loss	Speech delay secondary to cognitive impairment; compensatory articulation secondary to cleft palate	Hypernasality secondary to cleft palate; abnormal oral resonance secondary to sensorineural hearing loss
Fibrodysplasia ossificans progressive Progressive ossification and calcification of connective tissues	Normal	Normal in early childhood, with possible nasal resonance abnormalities secondary to restriction of palatal aponeurosis from advancing calcification
Filiform adhesions-clefting syndrome Cleft lip-palate, skinlike adhesions connecting the upper and lower eye lids	Normal	Possible hypernasality secondary to clefting and VPI
Fountain syndrome Coarse facial appearance, swollen lips, cognitive impairment, hearing loss, skeletal thickening	Delayed and severely impaired secondary to cognitive impairment, profound sensorineural hearing loss, and, in some cases, grossly distorted lips	Abnormal resonance patterns secondary to profound sensorineural hearing loss
Fragile X (see X-linked mental retardation)		
Fraser syndrome Cryptophthalmos (eyes covered by a layer skin so that they appear absent), scalp hair growing forward onto the forehead, cup-shaped ears, notching of the nostrils, syndactyly, small and abnormal genitals in both males and females, laryngeal stenosis, cognitive impairment	Usually delayed, occasionally absent secondary to cognitive impairment	Normal
Freeman-Sheldon syndrome "Whistling face" appearance, keel-shaped	Impaired articulation secondary to limited oral opening; possible	Hypernasality possible secondary to cleft palate and

Voice	Language	Hearing	Primary Etiology
			maternal diabetes has been implicated
Hoarseness common	Delayed and impaired with global cognitive impairment a consistent finding	Chronic otitis media common with possible conductive hearing loss resulting	Maternal consumption of alcohol during pregnancy
Normal	Delayed and impairment secondary to cognitive impairment	Chronic otitis media common with possible conductive hearing loss resulting	Maternal use of hydantoin (an anticonvulsant) if blood levels exceed safe levels
Unknown	Delayed and impairment secondary to cognitive impairment	Unknown	Maternal use of warfarin, a blood thinner
Hoarseness common	Delayed and impairment secondary to cognititive impairment	Sensorineural hearing loss common; possible conductive component secondary to middle ear effusion	X-linked recessive
Hoarseness from restricted movement of vocal cords	Normal	Both conductive and sensorineural hearing loss, conductive more common secondary to advancing calcification of the ossicles and connective tissues, onset usually in early childhood	Autosomal dominant
Unknown	Normal	Possible conductive hearing loss caused by chronic middle ear disease secondary to clefting	Autosomal dominant
Unknown	Severely impaired or absent verbal language secondary to combination of cognitive impairment and hearing loss	Often profound sensorineural hearing loss for all frequencies except 250 and 500 Hz where there may be very low levels of hearing	Autosomal recessive
High pitched; hoarse	Impaired and delayed secondary to cognitive impairment	Normal	Autosomal recessive
Normal	Usually normal, but may be delayed or impaired if cognitive	Possible conductive hearing loss caused by chronic middle ear	Autosomal dominant mapped to 11p15.5

Major Features	Speech Production	Resonance
Freeman-Sheldon syndrome *(continued)* forehead, micrognathia, limited oral opening, ulnar deviation of fingers, multiple joint contractures, relatively short stature, cleft palate, Robin sequence, occasional cognitive impairment	compensatory articulation secondary to cleft palate and VPI	VPI; abnormal oral resonance secondary to limited oral opening
Friedreich ataxia Ataxia with onset at approximately 10 years of age, peripheral neuropathy, scoliosis, progressive contractures, optic atrophy, cardiac arrhythmias beginning in the third decade of life, hearing loss, nystagmus, occasional diabetes	Onset and early development are normal	Normal
Frontometaphyseal dysplasia Prominent supraorbital ridge, pointed chin, enlarged foramen magnum, generalized skeletal dysplasia, hearing loss	Normal	Hyponasality occasionally develops secondary to bony dysplasia and subsequent nasal obstruction
GAPO syndrome The acronym signifies *G*rowth retardation, *A*lopecia, *P*seudoanodontia, and *O*ptic atrophy, small stature	Articulation may be impaired secondary to unerupted primary and secondary denitition,	Normal
Golabi-Rosen syndrome Cognitive impairment, overgrowth, macrostomia, prominent nasal root, macrencephaly, macroglossia, postaxial polydactyly, broad fingers, small nails, heart anomalies, renal anomalies, hernias	Speech delay and impairment common and variable depending on the degree of cognitive deficiency; articulation impairment caused by large tongue	Normal
Goldberg-Shprintzen syndrome Hirschsprung aganglionic megacolon, cleft palate, lower lip pit or mound, short stature, cognitive impairment, long curled eyelashes	Impaired secondary to both cognitive impairment and cleft palate	Hypernasality secondary to cleft palate
Goldenhar syndrome (see Oculo-auriculo-vertebral spectrum)		
Goltz syndrome Skin anomalies, nail anomalies, dental enamel hypoplasia, oral papillomas on lips, syndactyly, small eyes, strabismus, cognitive impairment, small stature	Articulation may be impaired by dental anomalies and oral mucosal lesions; cognitive impairment may be present and may cause speech delay	Normal
Gorlin syndrome (see Basal cell nevus syndrome)		
Hajdu-Cheney syndrome Small stature, bone anomalies, lack of ossification of cranial sutures, thick eyebrows and lashes, prominent ear lobes, short mandibular ramus, abnormal positioning of the mandibular condyles, small chin, abnormal skull shape, possible compression of the cerebellum through the foramen magnum, premature tooth loss, resorption of alveolar bone, vertebral anomalies, short fingers and nails	Articulation placement problems caused by early tooth loss and resorption of alveolar bone	Normal

Voice	Language	Hearing	Primary Etiology
	Impairment is present	Disease secondary to clefting	
Normal	Normal	Mild to moderate sensorineural hearing loss	Autosomal recessive mapped to the long arm of chromosome 9
Hoarseness	Normal	Progressive mixed hearing loss	X-linked recessive
Normal	Normal	Normal	Autosomal recessive
Unknown	Delayed and impaired with variable severity depending on the degree of cognitive impairment	Normal	X-linked recessive
Normal	Delayed and impaired secondary to cognitive impairment	Conductive hearing loss caused by otitis media	Autosomal recessive
Unknown	May be impaired if cognitive impairment is present	Normal	X-linked dominant, probably lethal in most males, mapped to Xp22
High pitch, thin	Normal	Occasional conductive and/or sensorineural hearing loss	Autosomal dominant

Major Features	Speech Production	Resonance
Hallermann-Streiff syndrome Small face with very thin, pointed nose, severe micrognathia, obstructve apnea, frontal bossing, wide cranial sutures, microphthalmia, cataracts, nystagmus, hypo/anodontia, small stature, occasional cognitive impairment, sparse scalp hair, lashes, and eyebrows	Articulation impairment caused by severe micrognathia which makes normal tongue placement difficult	Occasional hyponasality secondary to small nasal capsule
Hay-Wells syndrome Attachment of upper and lower eyelids at the lateral margins, hypo/anodontia, absent or severely hypoplastic fingernails, sparse or absent scalp hair, midface deficiency, cleft palate, hypohidrotic ectodermal dysplasia	Articulation placement problems secondary to maxillar deficiency; possible compensatory articulation secondary to cleft palate and VPI	Hypernasality secondary to cleft palate is possible
Hecht syndrome Abnormal muscle development with limited oral opening, abnormal hand function, enlarged mandibular coronoid process	Limited oral opening may affect articulatory placement and rapidity of tongue movement	Oral resonance may be dampened or muffled by limited oral opening
Helwweg-Larsen syndrome Anhidrotic ectoderal dysplasia with near complete absence of sweating, hypodontia, hearing loss	Articulation may be impaired by dental anomalies	Normal
Hemifacial microsomia (see Oculo-auriculo-vertebral spectrum)		
Hemihypertrophy Asymmetry of face and body with one side excessively large, neoplasias including Wilm's tumor, skin pigmentary anomalies, hair anomalies, unilaterally enlarged teeth, genital anomalies, renal anomalies, occasional cognitive impairment	Articulation may be impaired by unilateral enlargement of the tongue; shift in occlusion caused by unilateral dental hypertrophy may cause malocclusion and lateral open-bite which may impair articulation	Normal
Hemimaxillofacial dysplasia Unilateral enlargement of the maxillary alveolus, small and missing teeth on affected side, excessive facial hair on affected side	Articulatory distortion secondary to missing/hypoplastic teeth and lateral open-bite	Normal
Herrmann syndrome Late onset (onset after age 30) light-induced myoclonic seizures, progressive neurologic degeneration, ataxia, dementia, diabetes, kidney disease, hearing loss	Normal onset, subsequent deterioration of articulatory skills	Normal
HMC syndrome *H*ypertelorism, *M*icrotia, *C*left lip-palate, heart anomalies, renal anomalies, small stature	Possible compensatory articulation secondary to cleft palate and VPI	Possible hypernasality secondary to cleft palate and VPI
Holoprosencephaly Brain anomalies ranging from incomplete septation of the brain, absence of olfactory bulbs and tracts, hypotelorism (cyclopia in most severe	Delay or complete absence of speech depending on severity of brain anomalies; compensatory articulation secondary to clefting	Possible hypernasality secondary to clefting; possible hyponasality secondary to obstruction of nasal cavity

Voice	Language	Hearing	Primary Etiology
High pitch, thin	Usually normal, occasionally impaired secondary to cognitive impairment	Usually normal	Unknown
Hoarseness secondary to hypohidrosis is common	Normal	Mild conductive hearing loss caused by chronic middle ear disease is possible secondary to cleft palate	Autosomal dominant
Normal	Normal	Normal	Autosomal dominant
Hoarseness secondary to anhidrosis	Normal	Late-onset progressive sensorineural hearing loss with high frequencies most severely affected	Autosomal dominant
Occasional hoarseness secondary to asymmetry of vocal cords	May be delayed and impaired by cognitive impairment	Normal	Unknown
Normal	Normal	Normal	Unknown
Normal onset, but late onset deterioration with possible periodic dysphonia	Normal	Late onset (after age 30) cochlear degeneration resulting in sensory hearing loss	Mitochondrial
Unknown	Normal	Conductive hearing loss caused by microtia of varying degree	Autosomal recessive
Normal	Severely impaired or absent in many cases	Conductive hearing loss secondary to chronic middle ear disease is possible	Etiologically nonspecific sequence with many possible genetic causes, including autosomal dominant inheritance

Major Features	Speech Production	Resonance
Holoprosencephaly (*continued*) form, microcephaly, anosmia, cognitive impairment, nasal anomalies, heart anomalies, single central incisor, cleft lip ± cleft palate, many other possible anomalies depending on etiology		
Homocystinuria Cognitive impairment, osteoporosis, dislocation of the eye's lens, tall and thin appearance in childhood, pectus excavatum or carinatum, frequent thrombosis and embolism, seizures, psychiatric disorders, maxillary arch collapse	Delayed and/or impaired secondary to cognitive impairment; in most severe cases, there may not be speech development	Normal
Hunter syndrome Mucopolysaccharidosis II with growth deficiency, cognitive deterioration when onset is early (type B), mild or no cognitive impairment when onset is late (type A), coarse facial features, contractures, macrencephaly, enlarged liver, chronic nasal discharge, chronic middle ear disease, delayed dental eruption, early death (childhood) when onset is early	Normal onset of speech, but gradual deterioration in early onset type (at about 2 years of age); sluggish articulation secondary to thickened tongue and lips	Often hyponasal secondary to chronic nasal congestion with thick mucus
Hurler syndrome Mucopolysaccharidosis I-H with growth deficiency, cognitive impairment, facial distortion with very coarse features, chronic mucus discharge from mouth and nose, macrencephaly, enlarged liver, chronic otitis and respiratory disease, early death usually by 10 years of age	Usually limited speech development	Hyponasality secondary to chronic nasal mucus
Hurler-Scheie syndrome Mucopolysaccharidosis I-H/S with growth deficiency, hernias, enlarged liver, clouding of the cornea, thickened skin, eventual cor pulmonale and congestive heart failure with death before 30 years	Normal early speech development with eventual articulatory difficulty secondary to chronic mucous secretion and thickening of the tongue and lips	Hyponasality eventually develops secondary to chronic nasal congestion
Hutchinson-Gilford syndrome (see Progeria)		
Hypochondroplasia Short stature, macrocephaly, short limbs, flaring of the metaphyses, spinal anomalies, abnormal pelvis, occasional cognitive impairment, cataract, strabismus	Usually normal but may be delayed if cognitive impairment is present	Hyponasality secondary to small nasal capsule caused by very short anterior cranial base
Hypohidrotic ectodermal dysplasia Thin fair skin, sparse fine hair, decreased sweating, absence of mucous glands in mucous membranes, hypo/anodontia, depressed nasal root, frontal bossing, small nose, large lips	Articulation may be impaired by missing or abnormal teeth	Normal
Incontinentia pigmenti syndrome (see Bloch-Sulzberger syndrome)		

Voice	Language	Hearing	Primary Etiology
			mapped to 7q36
Normal	Delayed and/or impaired, often severely, depending on the degree of cognitive impairment	Normal	Autosomal recessive
Wet hoarseness	Normal onset followed by deterioration in early onset form; mild delay in late onset form	Progressive conductive hearing loss with mixed loss in more severe cases	X-linked recessive mapped to Xp27.3
Wet hoarseness	Usually limited language development	Progressive conductive hearing loss	Autosomal recessive mapped to 4p16.3
Wet hoarseness	Normal	Progressive conductive hearing loss caused by mucous secretion in middle ear	Autosomal recessive mapped to 4p16.3
High pitch	Usually normal	Normal	Autosomal dominant mapped to mutation of fibroblast growth factor receptor 3 (FGFR3) gene at 4p16.3
Hoarseness secondary to dry vocal cords	Normal	Normal	X-linked recessive

Major Features	Speech Production	Resonance
Isoretinoin embryopathy (see Retinoic acid embryopathy)		
Iwashita syndrome Progressive motor deterioration with onset in childhood, decreased sensation, bilateral optic atrophy (onset in second decade), hearing loss	Normal onset with eventual articulatory deterioration in adolescence or early adult years	Normal
Jackson-Weiss syndrome Craniosynostosis of multiple sutures, medial deviation of big toes, possible soft tissue syndactyly, maxillary deficiency	Misarticulations secondary to maxillary deficiency and possible skeletal open-bite	Hyponasality possible
Johanson-Blizzard syndrome Growth deficiency, microcephaly, scalp defects, sparse hair which is upswept, pinched alar base with hypoplastic cartilages, hypo/anodontia, hypothyroidism, micropenis, pancreatic dysfunction, cognitive impairment in many cases, hearing loss	Possible delay if cognitive impairment is present; misarticulations secondary to missing teeth	Occasional cul-de-sac nasal resonance secondary to constricted nares
Johnson-McMillin syndrome Alopecia, micrognathia, facial asymmetry, small male genitalia, auricular anomalies, occasional cognitive impairment, occasional cleft palate, occasional dental anomalies	Possible speech delay if cognitive impairment is present; possible compensatory articulation if cleft palate is present; articulation distortion secondary to tooth anomalies	Possible hypernasality if cleft palate resulting in VPI is present
Kabuki make-up syndrome Cognitive impairment, wide palpebral fissures showing some conjunctiva at outer canthus, protuberant large ears, superiorly positioned eyebrows, short stature, cleft lip, cleft palate, scoliosis, short fifth fingers, heart anomalies, hip dislocation	Speech delay; compensatory articulation secondary to clefting is common	Hypernasality secondary to clefting and VPI
Kallmann syndrome Hypogonadism, anosmia, cleft lip, cleft palate, hearing loss	Compensatory articulation pattern secondary to clefting is an occasional finding	Hypernasality secondary to clefting
Kartagener syndrome Chronic sinusitis, situs inversus, male infertility, ciliary anomalies of the mucous membranes occasional eye anomalies	Normal onset and development	Hyponasality secondary to chronic nasal congestion and sinusitis
Kearns-Sayre syndrome Short stature, heart block, cardiomyopathy, ataxia, dementia, cognitive impairment, seizures, generalized myopathy, diabetes, renal dysfunction, retinitis pigmentosa, optic atrophy, ptosis, hearing loss, onset of neurologic, eye, and heart disorders before 20 years of age	Possible delay if cognitive impairment is present (under half of known cases); eventual decay of articulation skills with progressive neurologic degeneration	Normal
Keipert syndrome Hypertelorism, short large bulbous nose, downturned oral commissures,	Delayed speech secondary to cognitive impairment; possible articulatory impairment secondary	Normal

Voice	Language	Hearing	Primary Etiology
Normal	Normal onset	Progressive sensorineural hearing loss beginning in second decade of life	Autosomal recessive
Normal	Normal	Occasional conductive hearing loss secondary to compression of the middle ear space and chronic otitis	Autosomal dominant mutation in FGFR2 gene
Normal	May be delayed, impaired, or even absent depending on the presence and degree of cognitive impairment	Bilateral severe or profound sensorineural hearing loss common due to Mondini type anomaly; absent vestibular function	Autosomal recessive mapped to 17p13.3
Unknown	May be delayed or impaired if cognitive impairment is present	Conductive hearing loss secondary to middle ear fluid and/or external and middle ear anomalies	Autosomal dominant
Hoarseness	Language delay and impairment common secondary to cognitive impairment	Conductive hearing loss secondary chronic otitis media and/or malformed ossicles	Probably autosomal dominant
Normal	Mild impairment is possible	Approximately one third of cases have mild bilateral sensorineural hearing loss; conductive hearing loss may also occur in cases with clefts	Multiple causes including autosomal dominant, autosomal recessive, and X-linked recessive mapped to Xp22.3
Wet hoarseness secondary to chronic postnasal drip	Normal	Mild conductive hearing loss secondary to chronic serous otitis	Autosomal recessive
Normal	Possible delay and impairment if there is cognitive impairment; eventual deterioration with onset of dementia	Progressive high-frequency sensorineural hearing loss with onset just after ocular findings	Mitochondrial
Normal	Delayed and impaired secondary to cognitive	Sensorineural hearing loss of varying severity and laterality	Autosomal recessive

Major Features	Speech Production	Resonance
Keipert syndrome (*continued*) macrocephaly, broad distal phalanges of toes and fingers, cognitive impairment, hearing loss	to high frequency sensorineural hearing loss	
Keutel syndrome Chronic upper and lower respiratory infections, pulmonic stenosis, calcification of nasal, tracheal, and auricular cartilages, small nose with depressed nasal root, short distal phalanges of hands, occasional cognitive impairment, hearing loss, relatively small stature	Possible delay if cognitive impairment is present	Normal
KID syndrome (**K**eratits, **I**chthyosis, **D**eafness) Skin anomalies including keratitis on face, sparse hair, thick nails, photophobia, vascular keratitis of eyes, contracture of knees and heels, lesions of oral mucosa, hearing loss, small stature	Initially normal, but possible deterioration of articulation secondary to lesions of oral mucosa; possible "deaf" speech pattern if hearing loss is severe	Possible resonance disturbance secondary to hearing loss
Klinefelter syndrome (see 47 XXY under Chromosomal syndromes)		
Klippel-Trénauny-Weber syndrome Hypertrophy of one or more limbs, multiple hemangiomas, enlarged digits, facial asymmetry, eye anomalies, hemangiomas of the digestive tract, occasional cognitive impairment, growth disorder (both excessive and diminished)	Delayed when cognitive impairment is present (cognitive impairment usually accompanies facial asymmetry)	Normal
Kniest syndrome Short stature, barrel-shaped chest, joint enlargement and stiffness, kyphoscoliosis, inguinal and umbilical hernias, short clavicles, tracheomalacia, myopia, round face, hearing loss	Usually normal	Muffled oral resonance
Laband syndrome Gingival hypertrophy, coarse facies with large nose, absence or hypoplasia of distal phalanges of the hands and feet, absent nails, occasional cognitive impairment, synophrys, hirsutism	Articulation disorder related to placement problems because of gingival hypertrophy with dental spacing problems; possible speech delay secondary to cognitive impairment	Normal
LADD syndrome **L**acrimal (tearing) problems, **A**uricular anomalies, **D**ental anomalies, **D**igital anomalies	Normal	Normal
Langer-Giedion syndrome Bulbous nose, vertical maxillary excess, small stature, microcephaly, protuberant ears, sparse hair, loose skin in infancy, cone-shaped epiphyses in hands, multiple exostoses (bony projections) of long bones, hypotonia, cognitive impairment, hearing loss	Speech delay secondary to cognitive impairment	Normal
Larsen syndrome Multiple joint dislocations, frontal	Possible compensatory articulation secondary to cleft palate and VPI	Possible hypernasality secondary to cleft palate

Voice	Language	Hearing	Primary Etiology
	impairment		
Wet hoarseness	Possible delay if cognitive impairment is present	Sensorineural hearing loss, more severe in high frequecies; conductive component secondary to chronic respiratory infections may also occur	Autosomal recessive
Normal	Usually normal	Sensorineural hearing loss of variable severity which may be severe	Autosomal dominant
Hoarseness if hemangiomas involve the larynx	Delayed and impaired if cognitive disorders are present	Normal	Unknown
Hoarseness, thin voice	Normal	Both sensorineural and conductive loss have been found with conductive component secondary to otitis media	Autosomal dominant mutation in collagen 2 gene (COL2A1)
Normal	Possible language delay secondary to cognitive impairment	Normal	Autosomal dominant
Normal	Normal	Conductive hearing loss secondary to external and middle ear anomalies; occasional sensorineural hearing loss	Autosomal dominant
Normal	Language delay and impairment secondary to cognitive disorder	Progressive sensorineural hearing loss, moderate to severe	Autosomal dominant deletion at 8q24
Normal	Normal	Possible conductive hearing loss secondary to clefting and	Autosomal dominant

Major Features	Speech Production	Resonance
Larsen syndrome *(continued)* bossing, cleft palate, depressed nasal root, arachnodactyly, possible Robin sequence		and VPI
Lenz syndrome Microphthalmia, cognitive impairment, microcephaly, protuberant and mildly dysmorphic ears, kidney anomalies, digit anomalies (contractures and syndactyly), dental anomalies, cleft palate	Delayed speech with impaired articulation secondary to cognitive disorder and missing teeth; cleft palate may result in compensatory articulation	Possible hypernasality secondary to cleft palate and VPI
Lenz-Majewski syndrome Large fontanels and wide cranial sutures, hypertelorism, cognitive impairment, loose skin, hyperextensible joints, hypotonia, anomalous long bones, hypoplastic dental enamel, cryptorchidism, hearing loss	Lack or severe delay of speech development	Normal
LEOPARD syndrome Multiple *L*entigines, *E*lectrocardiographic conduct abnormalities, *O*cular hypertelorism, *P*ulmonic stenosis, *A*bnormal genitalia, *R*etarded growth, Sensorineural *D*eafness, occasional cognitive impairment	Possible articulation impairment secondary to hearing loss; possible delay secondary to cognitive impairment	Possible "deaf" speech type resonance if hearing loss is present at birth and severe
Lesch-Nyhan syndrome Self-mutilation, cognitive impairment, mild growth deficiency, gout, high uric acid levels	Normal onset followed by developing athetosis and dysarthria	Variable nasal and oral resonance abnormalities associated with dysarthria
Levy-Hollister syndrome (see LADD syndrome)		
Lop ears, micrognathia, conductive hearing loss Micrognathia, overfolded ears with large lobes, ossicular anomalies	Normal	Normal
Louis-Bar syndrome (see Ataxia telangiectasia syndrome)		
Lowe syndrome Cataracts, hypotonia, cognitive impairment, renal dysfunction, cryptorchidism	Usually severely delayed and impaired secondary to cognitive deficiency	Unknown
Maffucci syndrome Bone deformity, multiple severe hemangiomas, neoplasias	Articulation may be impaired by oral hemangiomas on tongue	Oral resonance may be impaired by oral hemangiomas
Mannosidosis Coarse facies, progressive cognitive deficiency, progressive ataxia, hypotonia, enlarged liver and spleen, macroglossia, hearing loss	Delayed speech onset; dysarthric articulation pattern based on both progressive CNS anomalies and enlarged tongue	Dysarthric pattern of oral and nasal resonance
Marden-Walker syndrome Cognitive impairment, microcephaly, flaccid facies, blepharophimosis,	Sigficantly delayed speech secondary to cognitive impairment; compensatory articulation	Hypernasal resonance possible secondary to clefting

Voice	Language	Hearing	Primary Etiology
		chronic middle ear disease	
Unknown	Delayed and impaired secondary to cognitive impairment	Normal	X-linked recessive
Unknown	Lack or severe delay and impairment secondary to cognitive impairment	Sensorineural hearing loss of varying severity is common	Suspected autosomal dominant
Normal	May be delayed or impaired if cognitive impairment is present	Sensorineural hearing loss of varying severity and varying age of onset (possibly present at birth)	Autosomal dominant
Tremulous voice with variable breath support	May be delayed in cases where cognitive deficiency is present	Normal	X-linked recessive caused by HPRT gene deletion at Xq26 → Xq27.3, the gene producing hypoxanthine-guanine phosphoribosyltransferase enzyme
Normal	Normal	Maximum conductive hearing loss in many cases, although a mild loss has also been found	Autosomal dominant
Unknown	Usually severely impaired	Normal	X-linked recessive, mutation in OCRL1 gene
Unknown	Normal	Normal	Unknown
Wet hoarseness	Delayed and impaired	High frequency sensorineural hearing loss, often severe	Autosomal recessive gene mapped to chromosome 19
Unknown	Delayed and usually severely impaired	Normal	Autosomal recessive

Major Features	Speech Production	Resonance
Marden-Walker syndrome (*continued*) anomalous auricles, arachnodactyly, joint contractures, cleft palate, failure to thrive, short stature	secondary to cleft palate and VPI possible	
Marfan syndrome Abnormal skeletal growth pattern with arachnodactyly, increased span, tall stature, hyperextensible joints, mitral valve prolapse, dilation of the aorta, aortic dissection, dislocated ocular lens, frontal bossing, prognathism, vertical maxillary excess, occasional cleft palate, temporomandibular joint disease	Occasional VPI secondary to cleft palate and VPI; occasional articulation disorder secondary to malocclusion, open-bite, limited oral opening	Occasional hypernasality secondary to cleft palate
Marinesco-Sjögren syndrome Small stature, microcephaly, cognitive impairment, ataxia, cataracts	Dysarthria	Assimilation hypernasality secondary to dysarthria
Maroteaux-Lamy syndrome Mucopolysaccharidosis VI with growth deficiency, coarse facies, corneal opacity, joint stiffness, hernias, macroglossia, macrocephaly, occasional hydrocephalus, chronic respiratory infections, early death from early childhood to teen years with two subtypes (A and B), A being more severe	Labored articulation related to thickened oral tissues and macroglossia	Hyponasality secondary to chronic nasal congestion
Marshall syndrome Short stature, short nose with severely depressed nasal root, myopia, cataracts, strabismus, skeletal anomalies, occasional cleft palate, maxillary and mandibular hypoplasia, hearing loss	Possible articulatory impairment secondary to malocclusion	Hyponasality related to small nasal capsule; hypernasality possible in cases with cleft palate, but this is an unusual speech finding
Marshall-Smith syndrome Large stature, accelerated skeletal maturation, cognitive impairment, tapered digits which are broad at the base, laryngomalacia, failure-to-thrive, upper and lower respiratory illness, early death	Most patients die before the development of speech	Nasal obstruction is common
Martin-Bell syndrome (see X-linked mental retardation)		
Maxillonasal dysplasia (see Binder syndrome)		
May-White syndrome Progressive ataxia beginning in the second or third decade of life, myoclonus, seizures, hearing loss	Normal onset and development with late deterioration	Normal
Melnick-Needles syndrome Prominent eyes, squared face, micrognathia, broad forehead, long neck, narrow thorax, scoliosis, relatively small stature	Normal	Normal
Miller syndrome Lower eyelid ectropion (notched lower lids), micrognathia, cleft palate ± cleft lip, anomalous auricles, limb anomalies, missing digits, hearing loss	Articulatory placement and production anomalies secondary to micrognathia; possible compensatory articulation pattern	Mixed hyper/hyponasality

Voice	Language	Hearing	Primary Etiology
Normal	Normal	Usually normal	Autosomal dominant fibrillin gene mutation mapped to 15q
Unknown	Delayed, with severe impairment and occasionally, no language development	Normal	Autosomal recessive
Wet hoarse	Delayed and impaired	Chronic middle ear fluid leads to conductive pathology	Autosomal recessive mapped to 5q11–q13
Occasional hoarseness	Usually normal	Sensorineural hearing loss of varying severity	Autsomal dominant
Hoarse cry	Most patients die before language development	Unknown	Unknown
Normal	Normal	Progressive sensorineural hearing loss preceding the onset of the neurological deterioration, usually in the moderate range	Probably autosomal dominant
Normal	Normal	Occasional conductive hearing loss secondary to chronic middle ear disease	X-linked dominant
Normal	Normal	Conductive hearing loss secondary to middle ear and/or external ear anomalies	Autosomal recessive

Major Features	Speech Production	Resonance
Moebius syndrome Inanimate face and oral structures, limb defects	Severe articulation impairment secondary to lack of animation of articulators	Muffled oral resonance
Mohr syndrome Relatively short stature, midline cleft of lip, broad nasal tip, hyperplastic frenulae, maxillary hypoplasia, cleft tongue, nodular tongue, occasional cleft palate, hearing loss	Articulatory impairment secondary to lingual anomalies; possible compensatory articulation secondary to cleft palate	Possible hypernasality secondary to cleft
Morquio syndrome Mucopolysaccharidosis IV is seen in two subtypes, A (severe) and B (mild) with growth deficiency, relatively normal facies with only mild coarsening, clouded corneas, severe joint and spine anomalies, dental spacing, liver enlargement, aortic regurgitation, inguinal hernia, hearing loss	Usually normal onset and early development	Occasionally hyponasal caused by chronic nasal obstruction
Muckle-Wells syndrome Nephritis, large rash over much of the body, limb pains, hearing loss	Normal	Normal
Muller-Zeman syndrome Severe cognitive impairment, severe psychomotor retardation, usually in infancy although, in some cases, onset is in childhood, progressive visual impairment, progressive contractures, hearing loss	Usually absent speech development	N.A.
Multiple endocrine neoplasia Neuromas beginning in the oral mucosa, multiple neoplasias, thin body build, thickened upper eyelids	Impairment of articulation related to multiple oral lesions which may be nodular and interfere with tongue placement	Oral resonance may be impaired; neuromas may also form on palate and interfere with velopharyngeal function
Multiple pterygium syndrome Webbing of the neck, at the elbows, behind the knees (popliteal), and fingers, cleft palate, short stature, downslanting palpebral fissures, micrognathia, Robin sequence, vertebral anomalies	Possible compensatory articulation secondary to cleft palate and VPI; articulatory placement abnormality secondary to micrognathia and malocclusion	Possible hypernasality secondary to cleft palate and VPI
Myotonic dystrophy (see Steinert syndrome)		
Nager syndrome Severe micrognathia, cleft or absent palate, absent or hypoplastic thumbs, radial anomalies, external and middle ear anomalies	Severe articulatory impairment including compensatory articulation secondary to clefting and severe tongue backing secondary to severe micrognathia	Mixed resonance abnormality with both hypernasal and hyponasal resonance disorders
Neurofibromatosis *NF I: Von Recklinghausen type* Café-au-lait spots on skin, eventual development of cutaneous neurofibromas, optic glioma, macrencephaly, heterotopias of the cerebral cortex, occasional heart anomalies, occasional cognitive impairment ranging from learning disabilities (common)	Occasional mild dysarthria or dyspraxia; speech delay if cognitive impairment is present	Hypernasality has been documented in a small percentage of cases

Voice	Language	Hearing	Primary Etiology
Normal	Delayed expressive language development	Normal	Autosomal dominant form mapped to 3q21→3q22, otherwise etiologically heterogenous
Normal	Normal	Conductive hearing loss caused by ossicular anomalies, especially of the incus	Autosomal recessive
Wet hoarseness	Normal onset and development	Mild or moderate mixed hearing loss with the larger component typically conductive	Autosomal recessive Type A mapped to 16q24 Type B mapped to 3p14
Normal	Normal	Progressive sensorineural hearing loss, first appearing in childhood, becomes severe in adult years	Autosomal dominant mapped to 1q44
N.A.	Usually absent language development	Progressive sensorineural hearing loss	Autosomal recessive
Hoarseness	Normal	Normal	Autosomal dominant microdeletion at 20p12.2
Thin voice probably secondary to short neck	Normal	Possible conductive hearing loss secondary to chronic middle ear disease related to clefting	Autosomal recessive
Normal	Normal	Conductive hearing loss caused by ossicular anomalies including fixation of the footplate of the stapes	Probable autosomal recessive
Occasional hoarseness	Occasional language delay and impairment if cognitive disorders are present	Normal	Autosomal dominant mapped to chromosome 17

Major Features	Speech Production	Resonance
Neurofibromatosis *(continued)* *NF I: Von Recklinghausen type* to mental retardation (uncommon), occasional facial asymmetry, skeletal anomalies		
NF II: Acoustic type Bilateral acoustic neuromas, hearing loss, café-au-lait spots on skin, eventual development of cutaneous neurofibromas, CNS tumors	Normal initially, may subsequently develop impairment if CNS tumors develop	Normal
NF III: Mixed type Shows elements of NFI and NFII, including café-au-lait spots on skin, CNS tumors, acoustic neuromas	Possible impairment if there is brain involvement, including dysarthria	Normal
NF IV: Variant type Variable findings not fitting into other categories, may include any of the elements of the other types of NF	Possible impairment if there is brain involvement	Possible hypernasality if there is CNS involvement
NF V: Segmental type Café-au-lait spots restricted to one segment of the body	Normal	Normal
NF VI: Café-au-lait type Only clinical feature is café-au-lait spots	Normal	Normal
NF VII: Late onset type Neurofibromas appear later in life, after 20 years of age, without café-au-lait spots	Normal	Normal
NF VIII: GI type Neurofibromas found only in the gastrointestinal tract	Normal	Normal
NF IX: Noonan type Combination of both NF and Noonan phenotype (see Noonan syndrome below)	Possible delay and impairment secondary to cognitive/CNS anomalies	Possible hypernasality
Noonan syndrome Small stature, cognitive impairment, low posterior hairline, webbed neck, pectus excavatum or carinatum, pulmonary stenosis, vertebral anomalies, hypoplastic male genitals, ptosis, downslanting eyes, vertical maxillary excess, occasional cleft palate (often submucous), hearing loss	Delayed or impaired if cognitive disorder is present; articulatory impairment secondary to malocclusion	Possible hypernasality if cleft is present
Oculo-auriculo-vertebral spectrum Facial asymmetry, spine anomalies, microtia, ocular anomalies, dermoid cysts, hearing loss, cleft palate ± cleft lip, facial paresis, occasional cognitive deficiency, occasional kidney anomalies, occasional heart anomalies, occasional limb anomalies	Misarticulation secondary to asymmetry of tongue motion, malocclusion, and possible compensatory articulation secondary to clefting	Hypernasality secondary to both clefting and pharyngeal asymmetry is common
Oculo-cerebro-cutaneous syndrome Asymmetric facies, multiple accessory skin tags, microphthalmia, eyelid defects, skin	In cases of severe cognitive impairment, there is no speech development, in milder cases speech	Hypernasality has been seen in several cases

Voice	Language	Hearing	Primary Etiology
Normal	Normal	Neural hearing loss secondary to acoustic neuromas	Autosomal dominant mapped to chromosome 22
Normal	May be impaired if there is CNS involvement	Neural hearing loss if acoustic neuromas are present	Sporadic, unknown
Normal	May be impaired if there is CNS impairment	Possible neural hearing loss	Unknown
Normal	Normal	Normal	Probably a somatic mutation
Normal	Normal	Normal	Autosomal dominant
Normal	Normal	Normal	Unknown
Normal	Normal	Normal	Autosomal dominant
Normal	Possible delay and impairment	Unknown	Unknown
Occasional hoarseness	Delayed or impaired if cognitive disorder is present	Occasional sensorineural hearing loss and/or conductive impairment	Autosomal dominant mapped to 12q22
Hoarseness caused by unilateral vocal cord paresis	Delayed and impaired in cases with cognitive impairment	Most cases have unilateral conductive hearing loss ranging from mild to severe, although bilateral conductive loss is also common secondary to middle ear anomalies; sensorineural loss of varying degree occurs infrequently	Heterogenous
Hoarseness has been seen in several cases	Expressive language may be absent or severely impaired in severe cases, delayed in	Conductive and sensorineural hearing loss may both be found	Unknown

Major Features	Speech Production	Resonance
Oculo-cerebro-cutaneous syndrome *(continued)* lesions, cognitive impairment	is delayed and articulation impaired secondary to facial skeletal anomalies	
Oculo-cerebro-renal syndrome (see Lowe syndrome)		
Oculo-dento-digital syndrome Microphthalmia, small corneas, small nose with pinched alar base, enamel hypoplasia, sparse hair with abnormal texture, broad lower jaw, minor skeletal anomalies, occasional cleft palate, occasional neuropathy	Dysarthria; articulation impairment secondary to dental anomalies	Hypernasality has been seen in several cases
Oculopharyngeal muscular dystrophy Late onset (after age 20 years) weakness of the facial and pharyngeal muscles including the eyelids and mandible	Gradual onset of dysarthria after onset of facial weakness	Hypernasal speech occurs after onset of mild dysarthria
Opitz syndrome Hypertelorism, hypospadias, cryptorchidism, cognitive impairment, hernias, cleft larynx, heart anomalies, cleft palate ± cleft lip, anal anomalies, renal anomalies	Delayed speech onset, possible compensatory articulation pattern secondary to clefting	Possible hypernasality secondary to clefting
Optico-cochleo-dentate degeneration (see Muller-Zeman syndrome)		
Oral-facial-digital syndrome *Type I* Hyperplastic frenula, median pseudo-cleft of the upper lip, lobulated tongue, cleft palate, palatal asymmetry, hypoplastic alar cartilages, digital anomalies, mild cognitive impairment, telecanthus, abnormal scalp hair, milia (small pimplelike lesions) of the ears, agenesis of the corpus callosum	Delayed onset secondary to cognitive impairment; compensatory articulation secondary to clefting and possible VPI; articulatory distortions secondary to anomalous tongue which may also interfere tongue placement	Hypernasality
Type II (see Mohr syndrome)		
Type III Lobulated tongue, polydactyly (postaxial), severe cognitive impairment, dental anomalies, small stature	Typically there is no speech development	N.A.
Type IV Cleft lip ± cleft palate, anomalous tongue, dysplastic tibia, anomalous digits, polydactyly, hyperplastic frenulae, cognitive impairment, club foot	Delayed speech onset in many cases secondary to developmental delay; articulatory impairment secondary to tongue anomalies; possible compensatory articulation	Hypernasality secondary to cleft palate
Type V Median notch or cleft of the vermillion of the upper lip, postaxial polydactyly, found only in Asian Indian individuals to date	Unknown, but presumed normal	Unknown
Type VI Cleft lip ± cleft palate, polydactyly, hyperplastic frenulae, cerebellar anomalies, severe cognitive impairment, hypertelorism, nystagmus	Usually no speech development	N.A.

Voice	Language	Hearing	Primary Etiology
	mildest cases		
Normal	Usually normal	Occasional mild conductive hearing loss secondary to chronic otitis media	Autosomal dominant
Normal	Normal	Progressive sensorineural hearing loss is possible in some cases	Autosomal dominant
Hoarseness	Delayed and impaired language development	Possible conductive hearing loss caused by chronic middle ear disease secondary to clefting	X-linked recessive and autosomal dominant cases have been reported with the dominant cases mapped to 22q
Normal	Delayed and mildly impaired	Possible conductive hearing loss caused by chronic otitis secondary to cleft palate	X-linked dominant
N.A.	Typically there is no expressive language	Unknown	Autosomal recessive
Normal	Language delay and impairment secondary to cognitive impairment	Conductive hearing loss in some cases	Autosomal recessive
Unknown	Unknown, but presumed normal	Unknown	Autosomal recessive
Unknown	Expressive language usually does not develop	Both sensorineural and conductive hearing loss have been found	Autosomal recessive

Major Features	Speech Production	Resonance
Type VII Hypertelorism, pseudocleft of the upper lip, lobulated tongue, renal dysfunction, cognitive impairment	Delayed	Unknown, presumed normal
Type VIII Lobulated tongue, median cleft upper lip, telecanthus, polydactyly, bifid or broad nasal tip, ankyloglossia, cognitive impairment	Delayed	Unknown
Oral teratoma Disruption of formation of the palate and oral cavity by interference with normal fusion by neoplastic mass (teratoma), cleft palate, jaw anomalies, skull base defects, possible cognitive impairment	Impaired articulation secondary to oral disruptions	Possible hypernasality secondary to cleft palate
Osler syndrome Small telangiectasias of the tongue, arteriovenous malformations and fistulae	Normal development, but possible dysarthria if arteriovenous anomalies cause strokes	Possible resonance abnormalities if arteriovenous anomalies cause strokes
Osteogenesis imperfecta *Type I* Bone fragility, blue sclerae, hearing loss, dental anomalies	Normal development	Normal
Type II Severe bone fragility with early death (prenatal or neonatal) occurring in essentially all cases	N.A.	N.A.
Type III Fragile bones, normal sclerae, found mostly in black South Africans	Unknown, presumably normal	Unknown, presumed normal
Type IV Fragile bones, easy bruising, opalescent teeth	Normal	Normal
Otodental syndrome Tooth anomalies, hearing loss	Normal	Normal
Oto-palato-digital syndrome *Type I* Prominent superior orbital ridge, hypertelorism, downslanting eyes, cognitive deficiency, small stature, abnormal digits with curvature spacing anomalies, cleft palate, Robin sequence, micrognathia	Delayed onset; possible compensatory articulation secondary to cleft palate and VPI	Hypernasality a possible finding secondary to cleft palate
Type II Short stature, hyertelorism, frontal bossing, micrognathia, broad thumbs, abnormal long bones, cleft palate, possible cognitive impairment, hearing loss, micrognathia	Possible compensatory articulation secondary to clefting and micrognathia	Possible hypernasality

Voice	Language	Hearing	Primary Etiology
Unknown	Language delay and impairment secondary to cognitive impairment	Normal	Unknown, possibly autosomal dominant
Unknown	Delayed and impaired	Unknown	X-linked recessive
Normal	Possible delay if cognition is impaired	Usually normal	Unknown
Normal at outset, possible disorder if stroke occurs	Normal development	Normal	Autosomal dominant
Thin voice, high pitch have been observed	Normal development	Conductive hearing loss has been related to fixation of the footplate of the stapes or fracture of the ossicles; sensori-neural and mixed hearing loss are also common, all of late onset	Autosomal dominant mutation in colagen 1 gene (COL1A1)
N.A.	N.A.	N.A.	Heterogenous with both autosomal dominant and recessive forms
Unknown	Unknown, presumably normal	Occasional conductive or mixed hearing loss	Heterogenous with both autosomal dominant and recessive forms
Normal	Normal	Late onset hearing loss, both conductive and sensorineural	Autosomal dominant
Normal	Normal	Sensorineural hearing loss with 1,000 Hz being the most severely affected frequency; onset variable from childhood to middle age	Autosomal dominant
Hoarseness has been noted	Delayed and impaired secondary to cognitive impairment	Conductive hearing loss secondary to ossicular malformations	X-linked recessive generally hypothesized, but autosomal dominant inheritance may be possible
Unknown	Usually normal although delay and impairment may be present if cognitive deficiency is a feature	Conductive hearing loss secondary to ossicular malformation in some cases	X-linked dominant

Major Features	Speech Production	Resonance
Pachyonchia congenita syndrome Thickened fingernails and toenails, dry skin, wet palms and soles, ichthyosis, boils, papular skin on knees and elbows, thickened laryngeal mucosa	Normal	Normal
Pena-Shokeir syndrome Growth deficiency, bulging eyes, telecanthus, microstomia, micrognathia, rocker bottom feet, arthrogryposis , pulmonary hypoplasia, cryptorchidism, gut anomalies, early death, severe cognitive deficiency	Speech rarely develops	N.A.
Pena-Shokeir Type II (see Cerebro-oculo-facial-skeletal syndrome)		
Pendred syndrome Goiter with sensorineural hearing loss	"Deaf speech" common	"Deaf speech" common
Perrault syndrome Ovarian dysgenesis in females, hearing loss	"Deaf speech" common	"Deaf speech" common
Pfeiffer syndrome Craniosynostosis, maxillary deficiency, hypertelorism, exophthalmus, broad thumbs, occasional choanal atresia or stenosis	Articulatory distortions secondary to maxillary deficiency, malocclusion and anterior skeletal open bite	Hyponasality
Pontobulbar palsy and sensorineural hearing loss Facial weakness, grooved tongue, vocal cord paresis, swallowing disorder, hearing loss, aspiration	Dysarthria	Hypernasality
Popliteal pterygium syndrome Cleft palate ± cleft lip, webbing of the space behind the knees (popliteal space), dysplastic toenails, external genital anomalies, lower lip pits	Compensatory articulation secondary to cleft palate and VPI	Hypernasality is common secondary to clefting
Prader-Willi syndrome Obesity, insatiable appetite, hypoplastic gonads, cryptorchidism, hypotonia, cognitive deficiency, small hands and feet	Delayed speech onset; articulatory impairment secondary to hypotonia	Hypernasality secondary to hypotonia which resolves with age
Progeria Premature aging, deficient subcutaneous fat, alopecia, brittle nails, progressive delayed dental eruption, early coronary artery disease and atherosclerosis, death before age 30 in most cases, high serum cholesterol	Normal	Normal
Proteus syndrome Multiple hamartomas, enlarged hands and feet, bony projections on skull, large head, cognitive deficiency in	Initially normal, then impaired by the presence of multiple cranial growths and distortion of the jaws and oral cavity	Hyponasality may occur secondary to nasal obstruction

Voice	Language	Hearing	Primary Etiology
Hoarseness	Normal	Normal	Autosomal dominant
N.A.	There is no language development	Unknown	Probably heterogenous with some autosomal recessive cases reported
Normal	Normal	Moderate to profound sensorineural hearing loss, more severe in the high frequencies with Mondini cochlear anomaly; decreased vestibular function	Autosomal recessive mapped to 7q31
Normal	Normal	Severe or profound sensorineural hearing loss	Autosomal recessive
Normal	Usually normal	Conductive hearing loss secondary to reduced size of middle ear and/or chronic middle ear disease	Autosomal dominant mutation in FGFR2 gene (fibroblast growth factor receptor 2) on 10q
Breathiness; hoarseness	Normal	Sensorineural hearing loss with usual age of onset in childhood	Autosomal recessive
Normal	Normal	Conductive hearing loss caused by chronic middle ear effusion secondary to clefting	Autosomal dominant
May be high pitched	Delayed and impaired	Normal	Deletion of 15q11–13 from paternal chromosome, or paternal 15q11 disomy
Thin, high pitch	Normal	Normal	Unknown; both autosomal dominant and autosomal recessive inheritance is possible
Normal	Normal in many cases, but in those with cognitive impairment language is disordered	Bony growths of cranium may block the external auditory canal resulting in conductive hearing loss	Unknown

Major Features	Speech Production	Resonance
Proteus syndrome *(continued)* about half of known cases, thought to be disease affecting Joseph Merrick (the *Elephant Man*)		
Pyknodysostosis Short stature, osteosclerosis, fragile bones, micrognathia with long term wearing of the mandibular condyles, hypoplastic clavicles, short stubby fingers, delayed eruption of the permanent teeth, abnormal teeth, occasional cognitive impairment	Normal	Normal
Rapp-Hodgkin syndrome Ectodermal dysplasia, cleft lip, cleft palate, hypohidrosis, sparse hair, hypoplastic or absent nails, missing and abnormal teeth, maxillary deficiency, hypospadias	Compensatory articulation pattern secondary to clefting and hypernasality; articulatory placement disorders secondary to clefting and maxillary deficiency	Hypernasality secondary to clefting is common
Refsum syndrome Retinitis pigmentosa, peripheral sensory and motor neuropathy, ichthyosis, hearing loss	Normal onset but probable late deterioration with onset of ataxia in adult years	Normal
Retinoic acid embryopathy Microtia, micrognathia, cleft palate, Robin sequence, hypertelorism, heart anomalies, brain anomalies, thymic hypoplasia/aplasia	Unknown (no long term follow-up is available), but severe cognitive impairment occurs in many cases and is probably incompatible with speech development	Unknown
Richards-Rundle syndrome Cognitive deficiency, ataxia, hypogonadism, nystagmus, deficiency of subcutaneous fat, joint contractures, hearing loss	Usually absent or severely delayed and impaired speech secondary to combined effects of cognitive disorder and hearing loss	Mixed resonance patterns consistent with hearing loss and poor motor control
Rieger syndrome Hypodontia, iris defects, maxillary deficiency, occasional hypospadias and hernias	Misarticulation secondary to Class III malocclusion	Normal
Riley-Day syndrome (see Dysautonomia)		
Robinow syndrome Frontal bossing, hypertelorism, wide palpebral fissures, short nose, macrocephaly, cleft palate ± cleft lip, progressive osteosclerosis of skull, shortening of the arms, brachydactyly, clinodactyly, vertebral anomalies, skeletal anomalies, small penis, cryptorchidism, minor female genital anomalies	Compensatory articulation possible in cases with clefts	Hypernasality common in cases with clefts; hyponasality may be seen in some cases related to mild nasal obstruction
Rothmund-Thompson syndrome Small stature, mottled and irregularly pigmented skin, cataracts, small hands with hypoplastic or missing thumbs, sparse hair, small teeth, occasional cognitive deficiency	Late onset in cases with cognitive deficiency; articulatory distortion secondary to dental anomalies	Normal

Voice	Language	Hearing	Primary Etiology
High pitch, thin	May be impaired in cases with cognitive impairment, otherwise normal	Normal	Autosomal recessive
Hoarseness secondary to hypohidrosis and dry vocal cords	Normal	Conductive hearing loss caused by chronic otitis media secondary to clefting	Autosomal dominant
Normal onset, but possible dysphonia in late adult years	Normal	Sensorineural hearing loss with onset in teen or early adult years, often beginning as asymmetric and progressing to severe, high frequency	Autosomal recessive
Unknown	Unknown (no long term follow-up is available), but severe impairment occurs in many cases and is probably incompatible with language development	Maximal conductive hearing loss in cases with grade III microtia or anotia. Sensorineural hearing loss is also likely in some cases	Fetal exposure to Vitamin A, and other medicines containing isoretinoin
Unknown	Severely impaired, often with no development of verbal language	When onset is early (in early childhood), sensorineural hearing loss progresses to severe; when late onset (teen years), progression is less severe	Autosomal recessive
Normal	Normal	Normal	Autosomal dominant mapped to 4q25, epidermal growth factor gene
Normal	Normal	Conductive hearing loss common in cases with clefts	Autosomal dominant
Occasional hoarseness	Delay and impairment in cases with cognitive deficiency	Normal	Autosomal recessive mapped to chromosome 8

Major Features	Speech Production	Resonance
Rubella embryopathy Cognitive impairment, growth deficiency, hearing loss, cataracts, glaucoma, small eyes, heart anomalies, enlarged liver, thrombocytopenia, skeletal anomalies, microcephaly	Speech development may be absent when cognitive deficiency is severe; speech may also be affected by sensorineural hearing loss	Normal when speech is present
Rubinstein-Taybi syndrome Beaked nose, downslanting eyes, hypertelorism, broad thumbs, cognitive impairment, very short stature, delayed bone maturation, strabismus, heart anomalies, cryptorchidism, nevus flammeus	Speech delay and dysarthriclike speech; some cases do not develop speech	Usually normal
Russel-Silver syndrome Very small stature, narrow face, delayed bone maturation, skeletal asymmetry, blue sclerae, café-au-lait spots, hyperhidrosis, hypoglycemia	Normal	Normal
Ruvalcaba syndrome Growth deficiency, late onset of secondary sexual characteristics, microcephaly, cognitive deficiency, brachydactyly, brachymelia, cryptorchidism, hypoplastic genitalia, small mouth, dental crowding	Delayed onset; misarticulations secondary to constricted maxilla and dental crowding	Normal
Saethre-Chotzen syndrome Craniosynostosis, soft tissue syndactyly, brachycephaly, occasional cleft palate	Normal, although cases with clefts may have compensatory articulation patterns	Usually normal, although cases with clefts may have hypernasality
Sanfilippo syndrome Mucopolysaccharidosis III with normal or slightly reduced height, cognitive deterioration, only mild coarsening of facial features, neurologic deterioration beginning in childhood before age 5	Early development may be relatively normal followed by rapid deterioration and vegetative state	N.A.
Scheie syndrome Mucopolysaccharidosis I-S, normal height, liver enlargement, mild facial coarsening	Normal	Normal or slightly denasal
Schwartz-Jampel syndrome Skeletal dysplasia, short stature, limited joint mobility, progressive tonic contractions of the facial muscles, progressive myotonia, kyphoscoliosis, occasional cognitive deficiency	Normal onset followed by some difficulty with articulation related to limited mouth movement and opening	Late onset oral and nasal resonance disorder secondary to progressive muscle contractures
Sclerosteiosis Progressive osteosclerosis with excessive bony overgrowth of craniofacial structures, clavicles, and pelvis, prognathism	Normal onset and development	Normal initially, followed by hyponasality with nasal obstruction
Seckel syndrome Very short stature, microcephaly, cognitive impairment, prominent beaked nose, micrognathia, posteriorly sloping forehead, hip dislocation, missing ribs, cryptorchidism	Very late or absent speech with occasional use of jargon	Normal

Voice	Language	Hearing	Primary Etiology
Normal	Delayed, impaired or absent expressive language secondary to cognitive impairment	Sensorineural hearing loss in nearly half of cases	Maternal infection with the rubella virus resulting in teratogenesis
Hoarseness is sometimes seen	Delayed, often severely with with some cases not developing expressive language	Normal	Deletion at 16p13.3
High pitch	Normal	Normal	Heterogenous, but linked to the long arm of chromosome 17 in some cases
Normal	Delayed and impaired secondary to cognitive impairment	Normal	Unknown
Normal	Normal	Conductive hearing loss in a small percentage of cases	Autosomal dominant mapped to 7p21.2
Hoarseness	Early development may be relatively normal followed by rapid deterioration and a persisitent vegetative state	Early hearing is presumed to be normal	Autosomal recesive
Hoarseness	Normal	Mild conductive hearing loss secondary to chronic otitis media	Autosomal recessive mapped to chromosome 4
High pitch	Normal	Normal except in cases with cognitive impairment (about 25% of cases)	Autosomal recessive
Normal	Normal	Sensory hearing loss secondary to bony overgrowth of cranial foramina and damage to auditory nerve	Autosomal recessive
High pitch	Very late onset or absent expressive language	Normal	Autosomal recessive

Major Features	Speech Production	Resonance
Sedlačková syndrome (see Velo-cardio-facial syndrome)		
Senter syndrome Growth deficiency, ichthyosis, dystrophic nails, anomalous teeth, corneal anomalies, cryptorchidism, hearing loss	Normal depending on degree of hearing loss	Normal
Seitelberger syndrome Neuroaxonal degeneration, dementia, spastic quadriplegia, optic atrophy, hearing loss	Early onset is normal followed by rapid deterioration in early child-hood so that all speech is lost	Normal early
Setleis syndrome Unusual facies with excessive soft tissue redundancy and multiple skin folds, small dysplastic areas of skin around the temples resembling forceps marks, thick lips	Early articulatory difficulties have resulted from redundancy of soft tissue around the lips causing distortions	Normal
SHORT syndrome Small stature, deficient subcutaneous fat, thin facies, Rieger anomaly, hyperextensible joints, delayed dental eruption	Delayed speech onset; articulatory distortions secondary to abnormal dental eruption	Normal
Shprintzen syndrome (see Velo-cardio-facial syndrome)		
Shprintzen-Goldberg syndrome Craniosynostosis, micrognathia, exorbitism,very short anterior cranial base, arachnodactyly, contractures, spinal anomalies, cognitive impairment, soft tissue hypertrophy, of palate, multiple abdominal hernias, soft pliable ears, pectus excavatum, airway obstruction	Severely delayed speech secondary to cognitive impairment; misarticulations secondary to malocclusion and hypertrophic soft tissue of the hard palate	Normal
Sialidosis An oligosaccharidosis (storage disease) with three forms differentiated by age of onset, the congenital form which is lethal, infant form which is characterized by severe cognitive deficiency, and childhood form which has normal early development followed by cognitive deterioration, mild facial coarseness, developing neuromuscular symptoms, tremors, myoclonus, and seizures	No speech development in congenital and infant forms; normal development in childhood form followed by neurologic degeneration and ataxia	Normal in childhood form at outset
Simpson-Golabi-Behmel syndrome Macrostomia, broad nose, cleft palate, polydactyly, cognitive deficiency, large stature, macrencephaly, vertebral anomalies, large cystic kidneys, gut anomalies	Delayed onset secondary to cognitive impairment; misarticulation secondary to poor oral motor coordination; possible compensatory articulation secondary to cleft palate	Possible hypernasality secondary to cleft palate
Sjögren-Larsson syndrome Ichthyosis, cognitive deficiency, short stature, spasticity	Delayed speech onset; dysarthria; absent speech development in severe cases	Dysarthric resonance pattern with mixed hyper- and hyponasality in severe cases

Voice	Language	Hearing	Primary Etiology
Normal	Normal	Sensorineural hearing loss of varying severity	Autosomal recessive
Normal	Early onset is normal followed by rapid deterioration in childhood	Late onset sensorineural hearing loss	Autosomal recessive
Normal	Language has been seen in one case	Normal	Autosomal recessive
Normal	Expressive language delay	Normal	Autosomal recessive
Hoarseness	Severe expressive language delay and impairment in many cases secondary to cognitive impairment	Normal	Unknown, although a mutation in a fibrillin gene is suspected
Normal in childhood form at outset with hoarseness developing late	No expressive language in congenital and infant forms; normal early development in childhood form followed by deterioration after onset of neurologic symptoms	Normal in childhood form	Autosomal recessive mapped to 16p21.3
Unknown	Delayed and impaired secondary to cognitive deficiency	Possible conductive hearing loss caused by chronic middle ear effusion secondary to cleft palate	X-linked recessive GPC3 gene mutation
Unknown	Delayed and impaired with no expressive language development in severe cases	Normal	Autosomal recessive mapped to 17p11.2, fatty aldehyde dehydrogenase gene

Major Features	Speech Production	Resonance
Sly syndrome Mucopolysaccharidosis VII with short stature, enlarged liver and spleen, facial coarseness, macrencephaly, skeletal and spine anomalies, inguinal hernia, mild cognitive deficiency with onset at approximately 2 years of age, all in childhood onset form. In congenital form, there is early death	Normal onset followed by later delay	Hyponasality is common
Smith-Lemli-Opitz syndrome Small stature, failure-to-thrive, cognitive deficiency, microcephaly, ptosis, low set ears, hypospadias, cryptorchidism, seizures, cleft palate, cataracts, occasional heart anomalies, feeding problems	Severely impaired or absent secondary to cognitive impairment	Possible hypernasality secondary to clefting if speech develops
Sotos syndrome Large stature, large size at birth, cognitive impairment, prominent broad forehead, hypotonia, early maturation, tall adult height, behavioral disturbances	Delayed onset of speech secondary to hypotonia and developmental delay; articulation distortion caused by dental spacing	Normal
Spondyloepiphyseal dysplasia Short stature, skeletal anomalies, cleft palate, Robin sequence	Possible compensatory articulation secondary to clefting	Possible hypernasality secondary to clefting
Steinert syndrome Muscle myotonia, vertical long face, poor facial animation, malocclusion with open bite, when late onset (inherited from father) there is male pattern baldness, personality and cognitive deterioration in adult years; when early onset, severe myotonia present from birth with possible cognitive impairment, developmental delay	In early onset form, delayed speech onset and severe articulatory impairment secondary to neuromuscular disease; in late onset form, articulatory impairment secondary to malocclusion and progressing myotonia	In early onset form, hypernasality is common from onset of speech secondary to primary muscle disease; in late onset form, hyperasality may be the first presenting symptom of the disease in early second decade of life
Stewart-Bergstrom syndrome Hand anomalies including curved digits with contractures, hearing loss	"Deaf speech" when hearing loss is severe	Normal
Stickler syndrome Round face, micrognathia, maxillary deficiency, cleft palate, Robin sequence, myopia, vitreoretinal degeneration, joint laxity, epiphyseal dysplasia, talipes equinovarus, anteverted nostrils	Articulatory distortion secondary to malocclusion; possible compensatory articulation secondary to clefting and VPI	Hyponasality secondary to small nasal capsule and small nasopharynx; possible hypernasality secondary to cleft palate and VPI
Sturge-Weber syndrome Large port-wine hemangioma usually on one side of the face, somatic hemangioma, limb enlargement, cognitive impairment, seizures, intracranial calcifications, malocclusion	Delayed onset secondary to cognitive impairment; articulation impairment secondary to malocclusion caused by unilateral maxillary hyperplasia	Hyponasality has been seen in some cases secondary to nasal obstruction

Voice	Language	Hearing	Primary Etiology
Wet hoarseness is common	Normal onset followed by delay and impairment	Conductive hearing loss secondary to chronic middle ear disease	Autosomal recessive mapped to chromosome 7
Hoarseness	Severely delayed and impaired or absent expressive language secondary to cognitive impairment	Normal	Autosomal recessive
Low pitch for age	Delayed and impaired secondary to cognitive impairment	Normal	Unknown
High pitch	Normal	Possible conductive hearing loss caused by middle ear disease secondary to clefting; occasional high-frequency sensorineural hearing loss	Autosomal dominant mapped to long arm of chromosome 12, collagen 2 gene mutation
Normal	Delay and impairment common in early onset form; normal in late onset form	Usually normal	Autosomal dominant with maternal inheritance resulting in early onset form and paternal inheritance resulting in late onset form; there is anticipation effect when multiple generations are affected
Normal	Normal	Sensorineural hearing loss, nonprogressive, ranging from mild to severe, unilateral or bilateral	Autosomal dominant
Normal	Normal	Occasional high frequency sensorineural hearing loss; conductive hearing loss caused by middle ear effusion secondary to clefting	Autosomal dominant mapped to long arm of chromosome 12, mutation in gene for collagen 2
Hoarseness	Delayed and impaired secondary to cognitive impairment	Normal	Unknown

Major Features	Speech Production	Resonance
Townes (or Townes-Brocks) syndrome Facial asymmetry, ear tags and pits, microtia, commissural cleft, digital anomalies, radial anomalies, anal anomalies, renal anomalies, hearing loss	Usually normal unless hearing loss is severe	Usually normal
Treacher Collins syndrome Micrognathia, absent or hypoplastic zygomas, defects of lower eyelids, absent lashes of inner two-thirds of lower eyelids, malar clefts, cleft palate, Robin sequence, cleft lip (uncommon), microtia, ossicular malformation, airway obstruction, choanal atresia, hearing loss	Misarticulations secondary to malocclusion and anterior skeletal open-bite; severe tongue backing secondary to severe micrognathia	Hyponasality secondary to nasal obstruction and small nasopharynx; occasional mixed resonance with VPI combined with nasal obstruction
Tricho-rhino-phalangeal syndrome Long pear-shaped nose, short mandibular ramus, large protuberant ears, sparse , hair thin fingernails, short stature, delayed bone maturation, cone-shaped epiphyses, Class II malocclusion	Articulation disorders related to placement from malocclusion; articulatory distortions	Normal
Tuberous sclerosis Seizures, cognitive impairment, angiofibromas (skin lesions, usually on face), dilated ventricles in brain, brain neoplasias, thickened calvarium, retinal lesions, renal neoplasias, cardiac rhabdomyomas, various other neoplasias in other parts of the body including the lungs and other organs, fibromas of the oral mucosa	Delayed onset secondary to cognitive impairment; slow, labored articulation with dysarthric quality in adult life	Usually normal although resonance may have a dysarthric quality of mixed hyper-/hyponasality

Turner syndrome (see Chromosomal Syndromes, 45XO)

Urbach-Wiethe syndrome Yellowish nodular lesions of the facial, neck, and hand skin, patches of balding, eye anomalies of fundus and vasculature, brain calcifications, laryngeal lesions, thickening of the tongue, other mucous membrane lesions of the mouth, occasional mental deterioration secondary to brain lesions	Usually normal onset with eventual articulatory impairment caused by mucosal lesions and thickening of the tongue	Usually normal although mild hyponasality may be seen if mucosal lesions obstruct the nasopharynx
Usher syndrome Hearing loss, retinitis pigmentosa with nightblindness followed by visual deterioration in adult life with blindness in approximately half of cases, occasional ataxia and mental illness; at least two subtypes have been delineated which are differentiated by the severity of the hearing loss and visual impairment	Speech often impaired by hearing loss which may be severe or profound	Resonance may be impaired by hearing loss
Van Buchem syndrome Osteosclerosis, compression of cranial nerves with sequelae	Normal	Initially normal, may become hyponasal secondary to nasal obstruction

Voice	Language	Hearing	Primary Etiology
Normal	Normal	Sensorineural hearing loss of variable severity	Autosomal dominant 16q12.1–16q13 deletion
Normal	Normal	Conductive hearing loss of varying degree ranging from mild to maximum depending on the degree of microtia; fixation of the footplate of the stapes is common; there is occasionally a sensorineural loss	Autosomal dominant mapped to long arm of chromosome 5 at 5q31.1, mutation in Treacle gene
Hoarseness is seen occasionally	Normal	Normal	Autosomal dominant deletion at 8q24.12
Hoarseness is common	Delayed and impaired secondary to cognitive deficiency	Normal	Autosomal dominant gene mapped to long arm of chromosome 9q34
Hoarseness is very common and is often present even in baby's cry, secondary to laryngeal lesions	Usually normal	Normal	Autosomal recessive
Normal	Language is affected only by hearing loss	Variable severity of sensorineural hearing loss depending on subtype of syndrome, ranging from moderate to profound, usually sloping to most severe in the high frequencies	Autosomal recessive with genes mapped to several different locations based on subtype with genes on 1q (type II), 3q21 (type III), chromosome 10 (type 1D), 11p15 (type 1C), 11q (type 1B), 14q (type 1A)
Normal	Normal	Late onset hearing loss, mixed or sensorineural due to osteosclerosis	Autosomal recessive

Major Features	Speech Production	Resonance
Van der Woude syndrome Cleft palate ± cleft lip, pits or mounds of the lower lip, absent premolars	Possible compensatory articulation secondary to VPI and clefting	Possible hypernasality secondary to clefting
VATER association *V*ertebral anomalies, imperforate *A*nus, *T*racheoesophageal fistula, *E*sophageal fistula, *R*enal anomalies, also heart anomalies, growth deficiency, limb anomalies, genital anomalies, occasional cognitive impairment	Usually normal, though may be delayed by presence and surgical repair of T-E fistula necessitating tracheotomy; occasional delay secondary to cognitive imapirment	Usually normal
Velo-cardio-facial syndrome Cleft palate, heart anomalies, facies characterized by a long nose with bulbous or dimpled tip and prominent root, puffy upper eyelids, allergic shiners, small ears with attached lobules and overfolded helices, learning disabilities, ADHD, eventual mental illness, scoliosis, hypo-calcemia, immune deficiency, vascular anomalies, kidney anomalies, feeding difficulties, hypotonia	Delayed onset; global glottal stop substitutions in cases with clefts or VPI	Severe hypernasality very common
Waardenburg syndrome Hearing loss, pigmentary anomalies of hair and skin (depigmentation), hetero-chromia iridium (two different colored eyes), occasional cleft lip ± palate, synophrys; has been subdivided into two types related to presence of wide spaced eyes as follows: 　Type I: telecanthus 　Type II: no telecanthus	Usually normal, though may be impaired by sensorineural hearing loss in most severe cases; occasional compensatory articulation in cases with clefts (less than 5%)	Usually normal, though may be hypernasal in cases with clefts
Weaver syndrome Overgrowth, advanced bone age, skeletal anomalies, hypotonia, delayed develop-ment, macrocephaly, broad forehead, large ears, deep set nails, broad thumbs	Delayed onset, sluggish articulation secondary to hypotonia	Usually normal although one case with hypernasality secondary to hypotonia has been seen
Werner syndrome Premature aging, hyperkeratosis and skin ulcerations with onset of premature aging in 20s or 30s, occasional cognitive and neurological impairment	Normal in most cases with delay in cases with cognitive impairment	Normal
Wildervanck syndrome Facial asymmetry, Klippel-Feil anomaly (cervical vertebrae fusion), Duane syndrome (eye motility disorder), hearing loss, occasional cognitive impairment, occasional cleft palate	May be normal, may be affected by sensorineural hearing loss and/or clefting	Possible hypernasality secondary to clefting; unusual oral resonance secondary to short pharynx caused by short neck and vertebral fusions
Williams syndrome Cognitive impairment, short stature, heart anomalies, hypercalcemia, microcephaly, large mouth, thick lips, microdontia, enamel hypoplasia, limited joint movement, scoliosis strabismus, hypertension, hyperopia	Echolalia, overtalkativeness	Normal

Voice	Language	Hearing	Primary Etiology
Normal	Normal	Possible conductive hearing loss caused by chronic middle ear disease secondary to clefting	Autosomal dominant mapped to 1q32
Aphonia or hoarseness secondary to T-E fistula, tracheotomy, and surgical repair	Usually normal	Normal	Etiologically nonspecific, probably a secondary developmental sequence, perhaps of vascular origin
High pitch	Delayed and impaired with specific deficits in auditory memory and processing	Conductive hearing loss caused by chronic middle ear disease secondary to both immune deficiency and clefting; sensorineural hearing loss found in approximately 15% and may be unilateral or bilateral, usually mild although moderate to severe cases have been seen	Autosomal dominant with deletion at 22q11.2 found in most cases
Normal	Normal	Variable degree of sensorineural hearing loss, ranging from mild to severe, usually flat or U-shaped audiograms; hearing loss more common in type II and may be progressive in type II	Autosomal dominant mapped to a PAX3 mutation, possibly at 2q37
Hoarseness seen in two cases	Delayed and impaired secondary to cognitive impairment	Normal	Unknown
Normal	Delayed and impaired in cases with cognitive impairment	Normal	Autosomal recessive
Hoarseness and breathiness have been observed	May be delayed and impaired secondary to cognitive impairment	Mixed or sensorineural hearing loss, occasionally purely conductive, occasionally unilateral, ranges from, mild to severe	Unknown
Usually normal though hoarseness has been observed	Language performance is not normal, but language structure is sophisticated; cliches are overused, perseverative nature to language use; friendly "cocktail party manner" conversation	Hyperacusis	Deletion at 7q11.23 encompassing elastin gene

Major Features	Speech Production	Resonance
Wolf-Hirschhorn syndrome (see Chromosomal Syndromes, 4p+)		
Xeroderma pigmentosa Skin hypersensitivity to sunlight, skin lesions and possible malignancy, occasional short stature, cognitive impairment, neuropathy, small genitals	Normal except in cases with cognitive impairment	Normal
X-linked mental retardation (Fragile X) Cognitive impairment, large testicles, mild short stature, small hands and feet, long narrow face, joint laxity	Delayed onset; dysfluency with classical stuttering and in some cases, "cluttering"; in more severe cases, nonsensical short bursts of perseverative or absent speech	Normal
Zinsser-Engman-Cole syndrome (see Dyskeratosis congenita)		
CHROMOSOMAL SYNDROMES		
45 XO (Turner syndrome) Short stature, webbed neck, short neck, low posterior hairline, lack of sexual development, shield-shaped chest, heart anomalies, renal anomalies, small nails, osteoporosis, pigmented nevi, occasional cleft palate, occasional cognitive impairment	Usually normal, but possible compensatory articulation in cases with clefting	Usually normal with occasional hypernasality in cases with clefts
Monosomy 21 Small stature, hypertonicity, failure-to-thrive, microcephaly, cleft palate ± cleft lip, large nose, micrognathia, micropenis, cryptorchidism, imperforate anus, thrombocytopenia	Usually absent speech development	N.A.
Triploidy Somatic asymmetry, iris coloboma, frontal bossing, growth deficiency, cognitive impairment, hypospadias, cryptorchidism, micrognathia, cleft lip ± cleft palate, early death in most cases	Often absent, may be present but delayed in mosaic cases	Hypernasality in cases with clefts who survive and develop speech
Tetraploidy Incompatible with life		
Trisomy 8 Cognitive impairment, agenesis of corpus callosum, high forehead, corneal opacities, strabismus, minor auricular anomalies, micrognathia, broad nose, digital contractures, heart anomalies, hydronephrosis, cryptorchidism, occasional cleft palate	Delayed and neurologically impaired	Hypernasality in cases with clefts
Trisomy 9 Severe cognitive impairment, failure-to-thrive, short palpebral fissures, skeletal anomalies, urogenital anomalies, incompatible with life	N.A.	N.A.

Voice	Language	Hearing	Primary Etiology
Normal	Normal except in cases with cognitive impairment	Progressive sensorineural hearing loss	Autosomal recessive mapped to 9q34.1
Normal	Delayed and impaired, with severe impairment or absent expressive language in severe cases	Normal	X-linked recessive several mutant genes have been found to cause mental retardation
Hoarseness has been seen in some cases	Usually normal, but may be delayed or impaired in cases with cognitive impairment	Conductive hearing loss possible secondary to chronic otitis, especially in cases with clefts	Deletion of entire X chromosome; there may also be mosaic cases with less severe phenotypes
Unknown	Usually absent language development	Unknown	Deletion of entire chromosome 21
Unknown	Usually absent, otherwise severely impaired in surviving cases or mosaics	Unknown	One entire extra set of chromosomes resulting in a 69XX or 69XY karyotype
Unknown	Delayed and impaired secondary to cognitive impairment	Usually normal	Extra chromosome 8, or mosaic
N.A.	N.A.	N.A.	Extra chromosome 9

Major Features	Speech Production	Resonance
Trisomy 13 Severe cognitive impairment and brain anomalies, cleft lip, cleft palate, micrognathia, heart anomalies, genital anomalies, polydactyly, microphthalmia, hypertonicity, renal anomalies, holoprosencephaly, incompatible with life	N.A.	N.A.
Trisomy 18 Severe cognitive deficiency and brain anomalies, hypertonicity, micrognathia, heart anomalies, renal anomalies, esophageal atresia, limb anomalies, loose neck skin, incompatible with life	N.A.	N.A.
Trisomy 21 (Down syndrome) Flat occiput, upslanting eyes, strabismus, small ears, large protruding tongue, short neck, micropenis, inguinal hernias, brachydactyly, short 5th finger, hyperextensible joints, obesity, cognitive impairment, small teeth, maxillary hypoplasia, heart anomalies, immune deficiency, blood disorders, T-E fistula, imperforate anus, occasional cleft palate ± cleft lip, airway obstruction, hypertrophic lymphoid tissue	Delayed onset; uncoordinated, labored articulation secondary to hypotonia and malocclusion combined with large tongue; dysfluency; rapid bursts of speech	Often hyponasal secondary to lymphoid tissue obstruction; occasionally hypernasal secondary to clefting
Trisomy 22 Heart anomalies, micropenis, cryptorchidism, ear tags, preauricular pits, large ears, facial asymmetry, cognitive impairment, rare with few reported cases	Unknown, presumed to be impaired secondary to cognitive impairment	Unknown
47XYY Tall stature, occasional cognitive impairment, large tooth size, excessive hostile or criminal behavior	Delayed speech with catch-up and eventual normal production	Normal
47 XXY (Klinefelter syndrome) (includes 48XXYY and 49XXXXY) Poor coordination, delayed social development, mental illness in adults, small testes, micropenis in 48XXYY and 49XXXXY, possible slight female characteristics, occasional cleft palate, occasional inguinal hernia, mild cognitive impairment possible, more common and severe in 48XXYY and 49XXXXY	Delayed speech development, eventual catch-up	Normal
47 XXX (Includes 48 XXXX and 49 XXXXX) Delayed or impaired social development, mild cognitive impairment, more severe in 48 XXXX and 49 XXXXX, growth deficiency in 48 XXXX and 49 XXXXX	Delayed onset	Normal

Voice	Language	Hearing	Primary Etiology
N.A.	N.A.	N.A.	Extra chromosome 13
N.A.	N.A.	N.A.	Extra chromosome 18
Hoarseness, low pitch	Delayed and often severely impaired	Usually normal although conductive loss secondary to chronic otitis with resulting intermittent conductive loss is common	Extra chromosome 21, may be mosaic cases who are less severely affected
Unknown	Unknown, presumed to be impaired secondary to cognitive impairment	Unknown	Extra chromosome 22
Normal	Delayed language early on with eventual normal development	Normal	Extra Y chromosome
Normal	Delayed language with eventual normal skills except in cases with cognitive impairment	Normal	Extra X chromosome(s) from nondisjunction
Normal	Delayed and impaired receptive and expressive language	Normal	Extra X chromosomes from nondisjunction

Major Features	Speech Production	Resonance
1q- Severe cognitive impairment and growth deficiency, microcephaly, strabismus, micrognathia, downturned oral commissures, heart anomalies, cleft lip ± cleft palate	Speech rarely develops	N.A.
1q+ Severe growth and developmental retardation, midface hypoplasia, broad forehead, heart anomalies, micrognathia, iris coloboma, low set ears, incompatible with life	N.A.	N.A.
2q- Severe growth and developmental retardation, macrocephaly, heart anomalies, cleft palate	Speech development has not been noted in reported cases	N.A.
2q+ Cognitive impairment, microcephaly, hypertelorism, prominent beaked nose, auricular anomalies, visual impairment, colobomas of iris, cleft palate	Unknown	Unknown
3p- Severe growth and developmental retardation, micrognathia, microcephaly, arched eyebrows, square face, polydactyly, heart anomalies, renal anomalies	No speech development has been reported	N.A.
3p+ Cognitive deficiency, usually very severe, brain anomalies including holoprosencephaly, cleft lip ± cleft palate, genital anomalies, heart anomalies, hypertelorism, large mouth, micrognathia	Unknown, although retardation is usually severe	Unknown
3q+ Severe cognitive deficiency, full eyebrows, heart anomalies, CNS malformations, upslanting eyes, microcephaly, irregular skull shape, cleft palate, short neck, minor hand anomalies, early death is common	There is usually no speech development	Usually absent speech development, but hypernasal resonance accompanies vocal production
4p- (Wolf-Hirschhorn syndrome) Low birthweight, hypotonia, severe cognitive deficiency and developmental delay, seizures, strabismus, high arched eyebrows, ptosis, iris coloboma, prominent nasal root, craniofacial asymmetry, ear tags, absent ear lobes, heart anomalies, cleft palate ± cleft lip, micrognathia, Robin sequence, kidney anomalies, early death common	Usually absent speech development	Usually absent speech development, but hypernasal resonance accompanies vocal production in cases with clefts
4p+ Cognitive deficiency of variable severity, small stature, microcephaly, short nose, large nasal tip, prominent and pointed chin, posteriorly rotated ears, micropenis in males, joint contractures, eye anomalies, hypertelorism	Delayed speech onset secondary to cognitive impairment; neurologic articulation impairment	Normal

Voice	Language	Hearing	Primary Etiology
High pitched cry	Expressive and receptive language are essentially absent	Unknown	Deletion of long arm, usually involving q24→q32
N.A.	N.A.	N.A.	Extra portion of long arm of chromosome 1
Unknown	Language development has not been noted in reported cases	Unknown	Deletion of 2q24→q32
Unknown	Unknown	Unknown	Extra chromosome 2q31→qter (terminal end)
Unknown	No language development has been reported	Unknown	Deletion of short arm of chromosome 3
Unknown	Unknown, although retardation is usually severe	Unknown	Duplication of 3p
Hoarse cry common	Severe impairment or absent expressive language; receptive language also severely impaired	Conductive hearing loss probable secondary to clefting and chronic infections	Duplication of 3q
Hoarse cry common	Severe impairment of both expressive and receptive language	Conductive loss probably common	Deletion of variable size at 4p16
High pitch	Delayed and/or impaired secondary to cognitive impairment	Normal	Partial trisomy of the short arm of chromosome 4

Major Features	Speech Production	Resonance
4q- Cognitive deficiency of variable severity, heart anomalies, short nose, low-set posteriorly rotated ears, cleft palate ± cleft lip, telecanthus, limited elbow extension, overlapping toes, minor auricular anomalies, early death common	Delayed speech onset secondary to cognitive impairment; lack of speech development in most severe cases; possible compensatory articulation in cases with clefts	Possible hypernasality in cases with clefts
4q+ Cognitive deficiency, heart anomalies, renal anomalies, microcephaly, posteriorly sloping forehead, downturned oral commissures, minor auricular anomalies, posteriorly rotated ears, umbilical hernia, inguinal hernia, minor hand and foot anomalies	Delayed speech onset; neurologic disorders of articulation development and production	Normal
5p- (cri-du-chat syndrome) High pitched cry in infancy, small stature, severe cognitive deficiency, severe hypotonia, microcephaly, orbital hypertelorism, downslanting eyes, posteriorly rotated ears, ear tags, prominent nasal root, micrognathia, heart anomalies, inguinal hernia, dislocated hips, failure to thrive with feeding difficulty, large bowel malrotation, small hands with joint contractures, occasional cleft palate ± cleft lip	Often absent speech development; if speech is present, severe delay in onset and gross articulatory impairment with neurologic basis for disorder; compensatory articulation secondary to cleft possible	Hypernasality possible if cleft is present
5p+ Severe cognitive deficiency, small stature, severe hypotonia, seizures, microcephaly, dolicocephaly (long skull), hypertelorism, upslanting eyes, low-set ears, occasional macroglossia	Often absent speech development; if speech is present, severe delay and severe unintelligibility with neurologic basis for impairment	Normal
5q- Severe cognitive deficiency, brachy-, cephaly coarse scalp hair, retrognathia, inguinal hernia, occasional cleft palate	Often absent speech development; if speech is present, severe delay and severe unintelligibility with neurologic basis for impairment; articulation may be disordered by cleft if speech is acquired	Hypernasality may be present in cases with clefts
5q+ Severe cognitive deficiency, low birthweight; microcephaly, hypertelorism, downslanting eyes, strabismus, large ears, micrognathia, preaxial polydactyly	Often absent speech development; if speech is present, severe delay and severe unintelligibility with neurologic basis for impairment	Normal
6p+ Cognitive deficiency, low birthweight, feeding problems, respiratory disorders, craniosynostosis, cataracts, microcornea, microphthalmia, short nose, microstomia, heart anomalies, renal anomalies, early death is common	Often absent speech development; if speech is present, there is severe delay	Normal

Voice	Language	Hearing	Primary Etiology
Normal	Delayed and impaired secondary to cognitive impairment; absent language development in most severe cases	Possible conductive hearing loss secondary to chronic otitis media in cases with clefts	Deletion of a portion of the long arm of chromosome 4
Normal	Delayed and impaired secondary to cognitive deficiency	Occasional conductive hearing loss	Partial trisomy of the long arm of chromosome 4
High pitched cry and voice common, but not universal	Severe impairment of both expressive and receptive language	Conductive hearing loss is common secondary to chronic otitis media in most cases	Deletion of a segment of the short arm of chromosome 5 at p14 →p15
High pitch	Severe impairment of both expressive and receptive language	Normal	Partial trisomy of a segment of the short arm of chromosome 5
Normal	Severe impairment of both expressive and receptive language	Normal	Deletion of a portion of the long arm of chromosome 5
Normal	Severe impairment of both expressive and receptive language	Normal	Partial trisomy of 5q31→qter (terminal end)
Hoarseness	Severe impairment of both expressive and receptive language	Normal	Partial trisomy of a portion of the short arm of chromosome 6

Major Features	Speech Production	Resonance
6q- Severe cognitive deficiency, microcephaly, upslanting eyes, cleft palate, micrognathia, possible Robin sequence, respiratory difficulties in infancy, hand anomalies, nail anomalies of fingers with nails growing out of both the palmar and dorsal surface of the digits, heart anomalies	Often absent speech development; if speech is present, there is severe delay; cleft palate may add to intelligibility problems if speech develops	Hypernasality secondary to cleft is possible if speech develops
6q+ Severe cognitive deficiency, microcephaly, short stature, cleft palate ± cleft lip, prominent forehead, downslanting eyes, down-turned oral commissures, low-set ears, joint contractures, scoliosis, talipes equinovarus, heart anomalies, genital anomalies	Often absent speech development; if speech is present, there is severe delay; cleft palate may add to intelligibility problems if speech develops	Hypernasality secondary to cleft is possible if speech develops
7p- Variable cognitive deficiency, microcephaly, craniosynostosis, cranial asymmetry, low-set ears, depressed nasal root, heart anomalies, genital anomalies, occasional cleft palate	Speech onset may be normal in cases with normal cognition; in cases with cognitive deficiency, delayed speech onset; possible compensatory articulation secondary to clefting	Hypernasality secondary to cleft palate is possible
7p+ Severe cognitive deficiency, hypertelorism, micrognathia, craniosynostosis, choanal atresia, talipes equinovarus, occasional cleft palate	Often absent speech development; if speech is present, there is severe delay	Hyponasality secondary to coanal atresia or stenosis; possible hypernasality secondary to cleft palate
7q- Severe cognitive deficiency, small stature, prominent forehead, cleft palate ± cleft lip, severe hypotonia, heart anomalies, micro-penis, hypospadias, occasional holoprosencephaly	Often absent speech development; if speech is present, there is severe delay; possible further impairment of articulation secondary to clefting	Hypernasality secondary to cleft palate is possible
7q+ Cognitive deficiency, small stature, prominent forehead, short nose, cleft palate, early death is common	Delayed speech onset secondary to cognitive deficiency; possible compensatory articulation secondary to cleft palate and VPI; in some cases, there is no speech development	Possible hypernasality secondary to clefting and VPI
8p- Cognitive deficiency, small stature, microcephaly, heart anomalies, genital anomalies, minor auricular anomalies, epicanthi, depressed nasal root	Delayed speech onset secondary to cognitive deficiency	Normal
8p+ Severe cognitive deficiency, absent corpus callosum, heart anomalies, genital anomalies, cleft palate, frontal bossing, depressed temporal region, round face, downturned oral commissures, short neck	Often absent speech development; if speech is present, there is severe delay; possible further impairment of articulation secondary to clefting	Hypernasality secondary to cleft palate is possible

Voice	Language	Hearing	Primary Etiology
Hoarseness	Severe impairment of both expressive and receptive language	Possible conductive hearing loss secondary to chronic otitis media	Deletion of a portion of the long arm of chromosome 6
High pitch	Severe impairment of both expressive and receptive language	Possible conductive hearing loss secondary to chronic otitis media	Trisomy of a portion of the long arm of chromosome 6
Unknown	Language may be normal in cases with normal cognition; language delay and/or impairment is likely in cases with cognitive impairment	Possible conductive hearing loss secondary to chronic otitis media in cases with clefts	Deletion of a portion of the short arm of chromosome 7
Unknown	Absent language development in most cases, severely impaired in those who develop language	Possible conductive hearing loss caused by chronic otitis media secondary to clefting	Trisomy of a portion of the short arm of chromosome 7
High pitch	Language may be normal in cases with normal cognition; language delay and/or impairment is likely in cases with cognitive impairment	Possible conductive hearing loss secondary to chronic otitis media in cases with clefts	Deletion of a portion of the short arm of chromosome 7
Unknown	Language delay and impairment secondary to cognitive deficiency	Possible conductive hearing loss secondary to chronic middle ear disease	Partial trisomy of long arm of chromosome 7
High pitch	Delayed and impaired secondary to cognitive deficiency	Normal	Deletion of a portion of the short arm of chromosome 8
Thin voice secondary to short neck	Absent language development in most cases; severe language delay and impairment in rest of cases	Possible conductive hearing loss secondary to chronic otitis media in cases with clefts	Trisomy of a portion of the short arm of chromosome 8

Major Features	Speech Production	Resonance
8q+ Cognitive deficiency of variable severity, short nose, mild hypertelorism, abnormal skull shape, low-set ears, pectus excavatum or carinatum, scoliosis, occasional cleft palate	Delayed speech onset in milder cases, absent speech development in most severe cases; possible compensatory articulation secondary to cleft palate and VPI	Possible hypernasality secondary to cleft palate and VPI
9p- Cognitive deficiency, trigonocephaly, hypertelorism, upslanting eyes, microstomia, ear lobe anomalies, heart anomalies, webbed neck, micrognathia, omphalocele or umbilical hernia, inguinal hernia, arachnodactyly, occasional cleft palate	Delayed speech onset in mildest cases; articulatory impairment secondary to both malocclusion and neurodevelopmental abnormalities; possible compensatory articulation secondary to cleft palate and VPI	Possible hypernasality secondary to clefting and VPI
9p+ Broad forehead, hypertelorism, large nasal tip, macrostomia, large ears, short neck, cognitive deficiency, finger joint contractures, minor skeletal anomalies, delayed bone age, delayed closure of anterior fontanel, strabismus, heart anomalies, occasional cleft palate ± cleft lip	Delayed speech onset in most cases; possible compensatory articulation secondary to clefting	Possible hypernasality secondary to clefting
10p+ Severe cognitive deficiency, dolicocephaly, prominent forehead, downslanting eyes, prominent nasal root, hyperextensible joints, cystic kidneys, cleft lip ± cleft palate	Speech does not develop	N.A.
10q+ Severe cognitive deficiency, heart anomalies, renal anomalies, small stature, cleft palate, micrognathia, possible Robin sequence, prominent forehead, arched eyebrows, epicanthi, finger contractures, cryptorchidism	Often absent speech development; if speech is present, there is severe delay; possible further impairment of articulation secondary to clefting and micrognathia	Hypernasality secondary to cleft palate is possible
11p- (see Aniridia-Wilms tumor syndrome)		
11q- Cognitive deficiency, small stature, heart anomalies, minor ear anomalies, joint contractures, thrombocytopenia (low platelets)	Variable delay and impairment secondary to cognitive deficiency; neurogenically based articulation impairment	Normal
11q+ Cognitive deficiency of variable severity, hypertonia, small stature, craniofacial asymmetry, anal anomalies, heart anomalies, hip dislocation, cryptorchidism, ear tags and pits	Variable delay and impairment secondary to cognitive deficiency; neurogenically based articulation impairment	Normal
12p+ (12p tetrasomy) Severe cognitive deficiency, respiratory disorders, small stature, hypotonia, sparse hair, coarse facial features, high forehead, fleshy auricles, short neck, supernumerary nipples	Speech does not develop	N.A.

Voice	Language	Hearing	Primary Etiology
Unknown	Delayed and impaired secondary to cognitive deficiency	Normal	Trisomy of a portion of the long arm of chromosome 8
Normal	Delayed and impaired secondary to cognitive deficiency	Occasional conductive hearing loss which may be exacerbated by chronic otitis media	Deletion of a portion of the short arm of chromosome 10
Thin voice secondary to short neck	Delayed and impaired in all cases although impairment is highly variable and related to the degree of cognitive impairment	Possible mild conductive hearing loss secondary to clefting and narrow external ear canals	Trisomy of a portion of the short arm of chromosome 9
N.A.	There is no language development	Unknown	Trisomy of a portion of the short arm of chromosome 10
High pitch	Absent language development in most cases; severe language delay and impairment in rest of cases	Possible conductive hearing loss secondary to chronic otitis media in cases with clefts	Trisomy of a portion of the long arm of chromosome 10
Normal	Delayed and impaired secondary to cognitive deficiency	Normal	Deletion of a portion of the long arm of chromosome 11
High pitch	Delayed and impaired secondary to cognitive deficiency	Normal	Trisomy of a portion of the long arm of chromosome 11
Weak cry high-pitched cry	Language does not develop	Sensorineural hearing loss	Tetrasomy of a portion of the short arm of chromosome 12

Major Features	Speech Production	Resonance
13q- Frontal bossing, microcephaly, triangular skull shape, short neck, broad nasal root, microphthalmia, iris and retinal coloboma, severe cognitive deficiency, large ears, retinoblastoma, microcephaly, occasional holoprosencephaly	Usually absent speech development	N.A.
14q- Severe cognitive deficiency, severe hypotonia, seizures, dilated lateral ventricles, large low-set ears, long narrow face, micrognathia	Usually absent speech development	N.A.
14q+ Cognitive deficiency, small stature, cleft palate, micrognathia, possible Robin sequence, downturned oral commissures, hypogonadism, heart anomalies, pulmonary anomalies	Delayed and impaired speech development which may be severe with further impairment of articulation secondary to clefting and micrognathia	Hypernasality secondary to cleft palate is possible
15q- Cognitive deficiency of variable severity, but usually severe, small stature, heart anomalies, telecanthus, delayed bone age, thumb position anomalies	Speech does not develop in many cases; in milder cases speech onset is delayed and speech impaired neurogenically	Normal
15q+ Severe cognitive deficiency, hypotonia, short stature, joint laxity, seizures, heart anomalies, scoliosis, pectus excavatum, micrognathia, short neck	Often absent speech development; if speech is present, there is severe delay; possible further impairment of speech production may be caused by micrognathia and malocclusion	Abnormal oral resonance secondary to short neck
16q- Cognitive deficiency, small stature, hypotonia, microcephaly, high forehead with metopic ridging, occasional cleft palate, micrognathia, possible Robin sequence, small appearing eyes, short neck, polydactyly, occasional heart anomalies	Delayed and impaired speech development which may be severe with further impairment of articulation secondary to clefting and micrognathia	Possible hypernasality secondary to clefting and VPI
17p+ Severe cognitive deficiency, small stature, microcephaly, small eyes, broad nasal root, low-set ears, short webbed neck, finger flexion abnormalities, small male genitalia	Speech does not develop in many cases; in milder cases speech onset is severely delayed and speech is neurogenically impaired	Unusual oral resonance secondary to short neck
18p- Cognitive deficiency, small stature, microcephaly, maxillary deficiency, telecanthus, strabismus, downturned oral commissures, retrognathia, short neck, micropenis, cryptorchidism, occasional cleft palate ± cleft lip, occasional holoprosencephaly, occasional heart anomalies	Delayed speech onset; in most severe cases, no speech development; possible compensatory articulation pattern secondary to clefting	Possible hypernasality secondary to clefting

Voice	Language	Hearing	Primary Etiology
Hoarse, shrill cry	Severe receptive and expressive language impairment	Normal	Deletion of a portion of the long arm of chromosome 13 at q31→q32
Weak cry	Severe impairment or absent language development	Normal	Deletion of a portion of the long arm of chromosome 14
High pitch	Impaired language development with severe language delay in many cases	Possible conductive hearing loss secondary to chronic otitis media in cases with clefts	Trisomy of a portion of the long arm of chromosome 14
High pitch	Language does not develop in many cases; in milder cases, language is delayed and impaired	Normal	Deletion of a portion of the long arm of chromosome 15
High pitch	Language does not develop in many cases; in milder cases, language is severely impaired	Normal	Trisomy of a portion of the long arm of chromosome 15
High pitch	Language is frequently severely impaired	Possible conductive hearing loss secondary to clefting and chronic otitis media	Deletion of a portion of the long arm of chromosome 16
High pitch	Language does not develop in many cases; in milder cases, there is severe language delay and impairment	Normal	Trisomy of a portion of the short arm of chromosome 17
Normal	Delayed and impaired secondary to cognitive impairment; in most severe cases, there is no language development	Normal except for cases with chronic otitis media secondary to clefting	Deletion of a portion of the short arm of chromosome 18

Major Features	Speech Production	Resonance
18q- Cognitive deficiency (often severe), hypotonia, small stature, seizures, microcephaly, maxillary deficiency, strabismus, nystagmus, iris and/or retinal coloboma, downturned oral commissures, hearing loss, widely spaced nipples, genital anomalies, inguinal hernias, heart anomalies, cleft palate ± cleft lip, rib anomalies, talipes equinovarus, spina bifida occulta	Delayed speech onset; in most severe cases, no speech development; possible compensatory articulation pattern secondary to clefting; articulation placement disorder secondary to maxillary deficiency	Possible hypernasality secondary to clefting
22q- (22q11—see Velo-cardio-facial syndrome)		

Voice	Language	Hearing	Primary Etiology
Low pitch	Delayed and impaired secondary to cognitive impairment; in most severe cases, there is no language development	Sensorineural, mixed, and conductive loss of varying severity have all been found	Deletion of a portion of the long arm of chromosome 18

APPENDIX

⊓

NORMATIVE DATA

A: Length and Weight Norms for Female Children from Birth to 36 Months (3 Years) of Age.

B: Head Circumference and Weight to Length Proportion Norms for Female Children from Birth to 36 Months (3 Years) of Age.

C: Length and Weight Norms for Male Children from Birth to 36 Months (3 Years) of Age.

D: Head Circumference and Weight to Length Proportion Norms for Male Children from Birth to 36 Months (3 Years) of Age.

E: Height and Weight Norms for Female Children from 2 Years to 18 Years of Age.

F: Weight to Height Proportion Norms for Female Children from 2 Years to 18 Years of Age.

G: Height and Weight Norms for Male Children from 2 Years to 18 Years of Age.

H: Weight to Height Proportion Norms for Male Children from 2 Years to 18 Years of Age.

Appendixes A through H were adapted from data published by P.V.V. Hamill, T. A. Drizd, C. L. Johnson, A. F. Reed, and W. M. Moore. Physical growth: National Center for Health Statistics percentiles. *American Journal of Clinical Nutrition, 32,* 607–629, 1979. Reprinted courtesy of Ross Laboratories.

I: Head Circumference Norms for Males and Females.

J: Ocular Norms for Proportion of Inner Canthal Distance (measure B) to Outer Canthal Distance (measure A).

K: Inner Canthal and Outer Canthal Distance Norms.

L: Outer Canthal Distance Norms.

M: Middle Finger Length Norms.

N: Palmar Length Norms.

O: Total Hand Length Norms.

P: Proportion of Middle Finger to Palmar Length Norms.

Q: Ear Length Norms.

Appendix II-A

LENGTH AND WEIGHT NORMS FOR FEMALE CHILDREN FROM BIRTH TO 36 MONTHS (3 YEARS) OF AGE

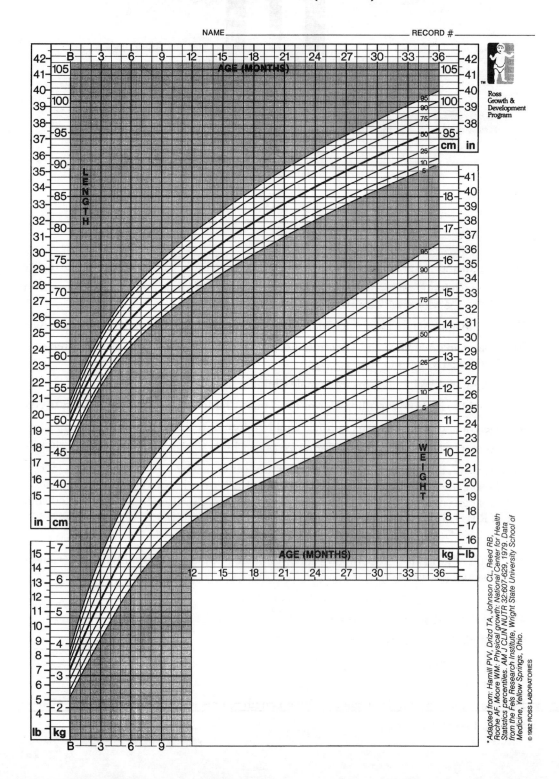

Adapted from: Hamill PVV, Drizd TA, Johnson CL, Reed RB, Roche AF, Moore WM: Physical growth: National Center for Health Statistics percentiles. AM J CLIN NUTR 32:607-629, 1979. Data from the Fels Research Institute, Wright State University School of Medicine, Yellow Springs, Ohio.
© 1982 ROSS LABORATORIES

Appendix II-B

HEAD CIRCUMFERENCE AND WEIGHT TO LENGTH PROPORTION NORMS FOR FEMALE CHILDREN FROM BIRTH TO 36 MONTHS (3 YEARS) OF AGE

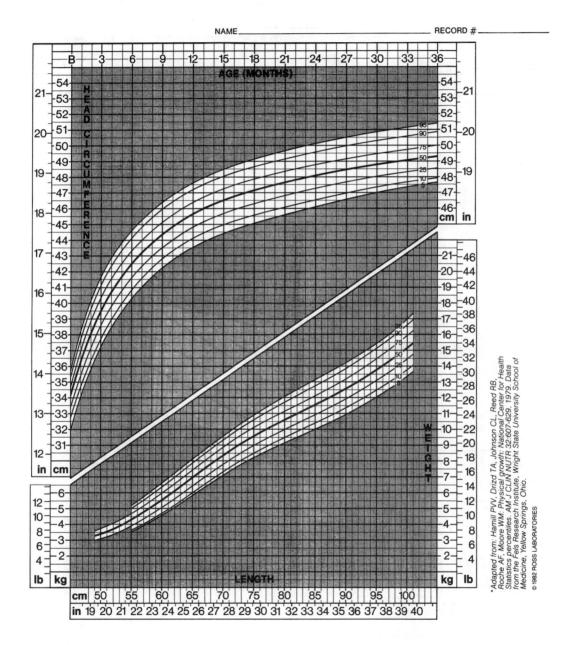

NAME_____ RECORD #_____

*Adapted from: Hamill PVV, Drizd TA, Johnson CL, Reed RB, Roche AF, Moore WM: Physical growth: National Center for Health Statistics percentiles. AM J CLIN NUTR 32:607-629, 1979. Data from the Fels Research Institute, Wright State University School of Medicine, Yellow Springs, Ohio.

© 1982 ROSS LABORATORIES

Appendix II-C

LENGTH AND WEIGHT NORMS FOR MALE CHILDREN FROM BIRTH TO 36 MONTHS OF AGE

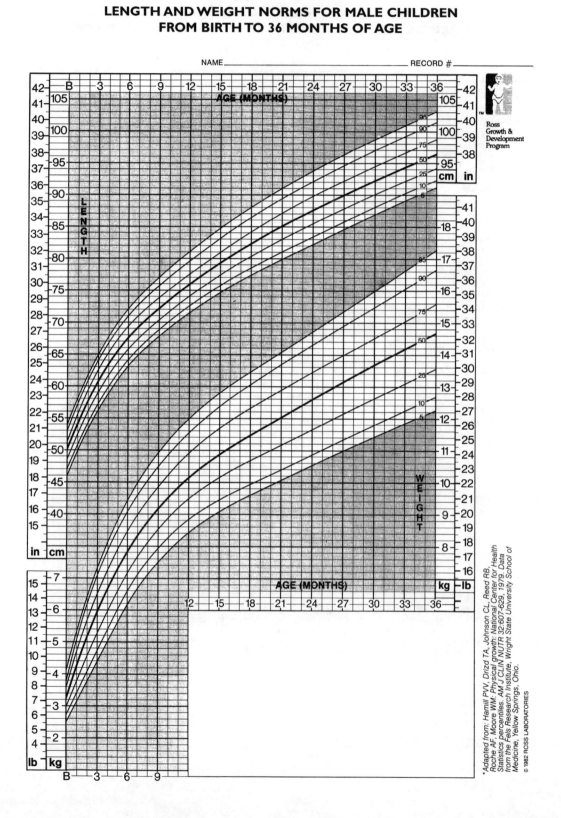

Adapted from: Hamill PVV, Drizd TA, Johnson CL, Reed RB, Roche AF, Moore WM: Physical growth: National Center for Health Statistics percentiles. AM J CLIN NUTR 32:607-629, 1979. Data from the Fels Research Institute, Wright State University School of Medicine, Yellow Springs, Ohio.

© 1982 ROSS LABORATORIES

Ross
Growth &
Development
Program

Appendix II-D

HEAD CIRCUMFERENCE AND WEIGHT TO LENGTH PROPORTION NORMS FOR MALE CHILDREN FROM BIRTH TO 36 MONTHS (3 YEARS) OF AGE

NAME_____   RECORD #_____

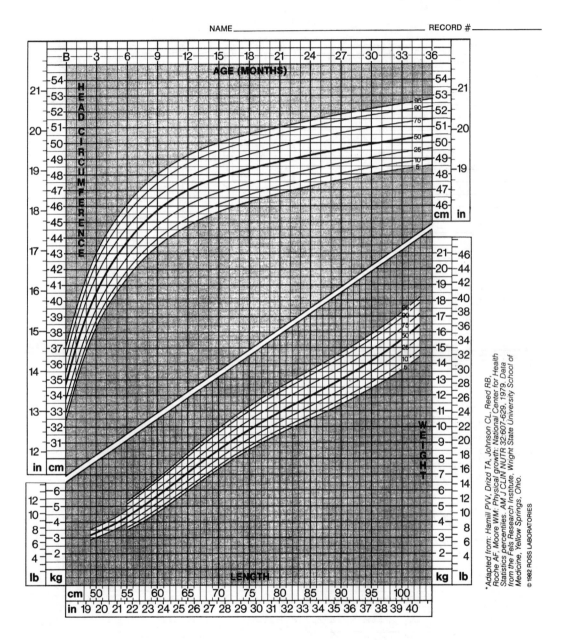

*Adapted from: Hamill PVV, Drizd TA, Johnson CL, Reed RB, Roche AF, Moore WM. Physical growth: National Center for Health Statistics percentiles. AM J CLIN NUTR 32:607-629, 1979. Data from the Fels Research Institute, Wright State University School of Medicine, Yellow Springs, Ohio.

© 1982 ROSS LABORATORIES

Appendix II-E
HEIGHT AND WEIGHT NORMS FOR FEMALE CHILDREN
FROM 2 YEARS TO 18 YEARS OF AGE

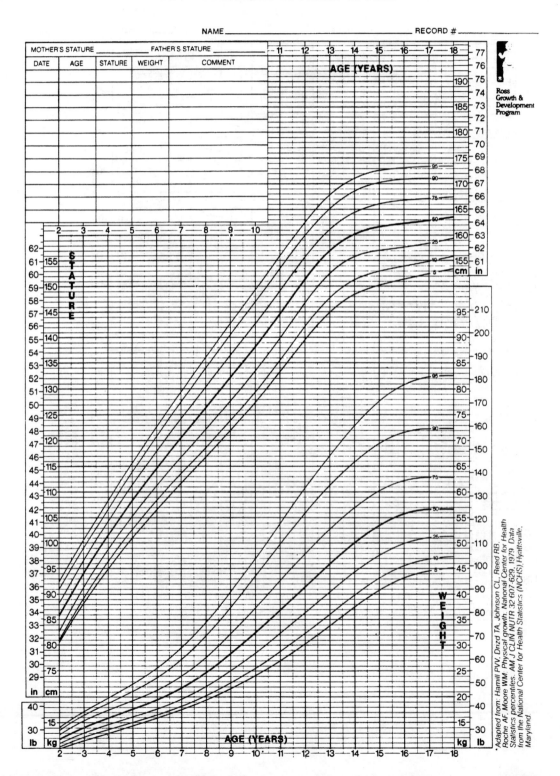

Adapted from: Hamill PVV, Drizd TA, Johnson CL, Reed RB, Roche AF, Moore WM. Physical growth: National Center for Health Statistics percentiles. AM J CLIN NUTR 32:607-629, 1979. Data from the National Center for Health Statistics (NCHS), Hyattsville, Maryland.

Appendix II-F

WEIGHT TO HEIGHT PROPORTION NORMS FOR FEMALE CHILDREN
FROM 2 YEARS TO 18 YEARS OF AGE

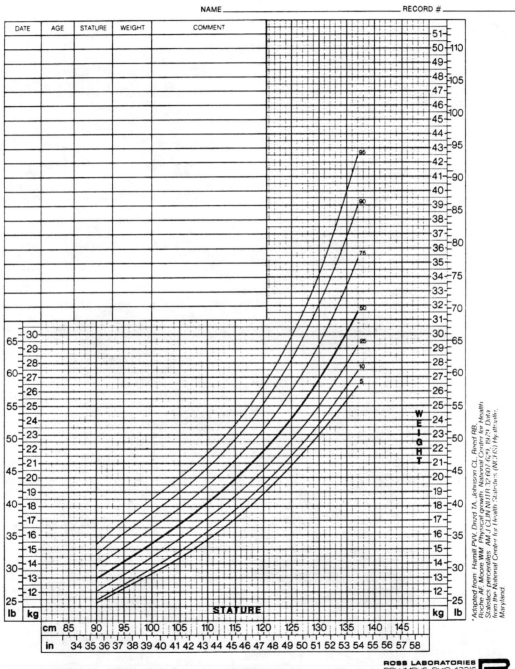

NAME _____   RECORD # _____

Adapted from: Hamill PVV, Drizd TA, Johnson CL, Reed RB, Roche AF, Moore WM. Physical growth: National Center for Health Statistics percentiles. AM J CLIN NUTR 32:607-629, 1979. Data from the National Center for Health Statistics (NCHS) Hyattsville, Maryland.

SIMILAC Infant Formulas
in vivo performance
closest to mother's milk

ISOMIL Soy Protein Formulas
When the baby can't take milk

ADVANCE Nutritional Beverage With Iron
Instead of 2% lowfat milk

ROSS LABORATORIES
COLUMBUS, OHIO 43216
DIVISION OF ABBOTT LABORATORIES USA

G108(0.05) JANUARY 1986   LITHO IN USA

Appendix II-G

HEIGHT AND WEIGHT NORMS FOR MALE CHILDREN FROM 2 YEARS TO 18 YEARS OF AGE

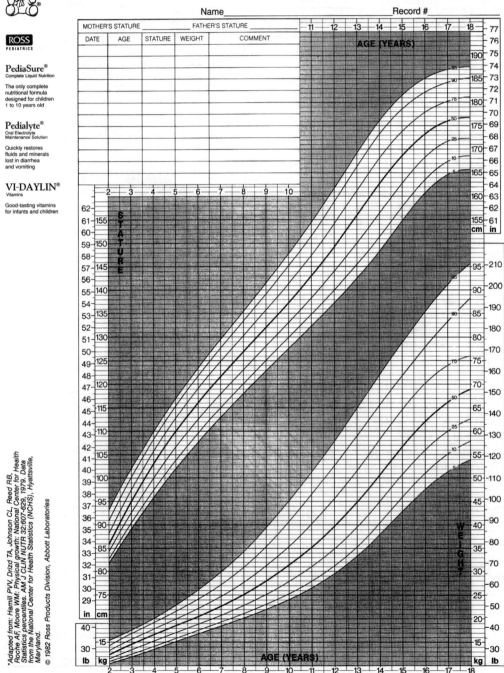

Appendix II-H

WEIGHT TO HEIGHT PROPORTION NORMS FOR MALE CHILDREN FROM 2 YEARS TO 18 YEARS OF AGE

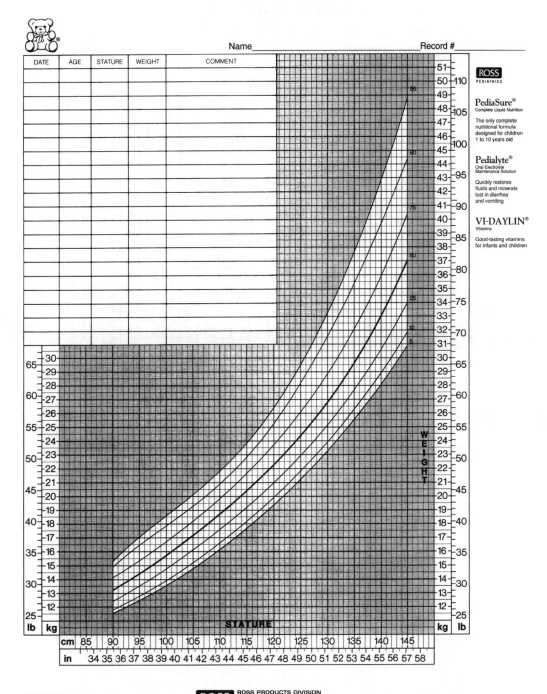

51212 09892WB
(0.05)/JUNE 1994

ROSS PRODUCTS DIVISION
ABBOTT LABORATORIES
COLUMBUS, OHIO 43215-1724

LITHO IN USA

Appendix II-I

HEAD CIRCUMFERENCES
FOR MALES AND FEMALES

HEAD CIRCUMFERENCES

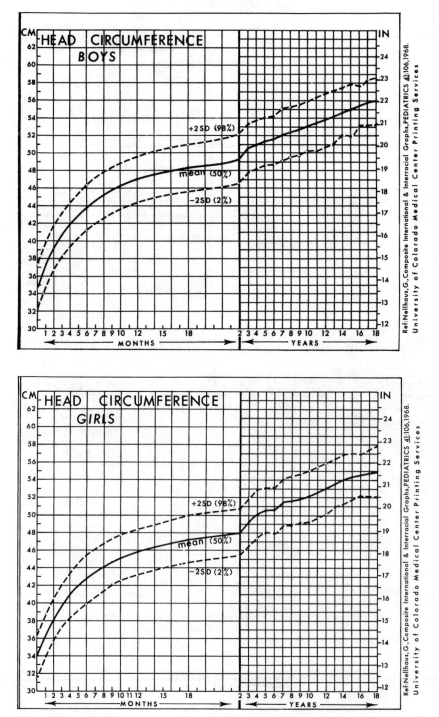

Appendix II-J

OCULAR NORMS FOR PROPORTION OF INNER CANTHAL DISTANCE (MEASURE B) TO OUTER CANTHAL DISTANCE (MEASURE A)

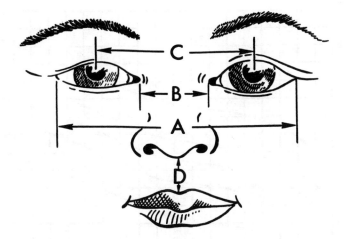

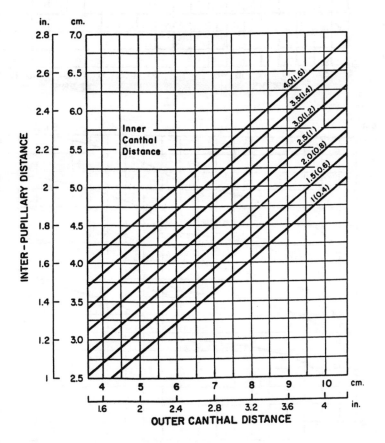

Appendix II-K
INNER AND OUTER CANTHAL DISTANCE NORMS

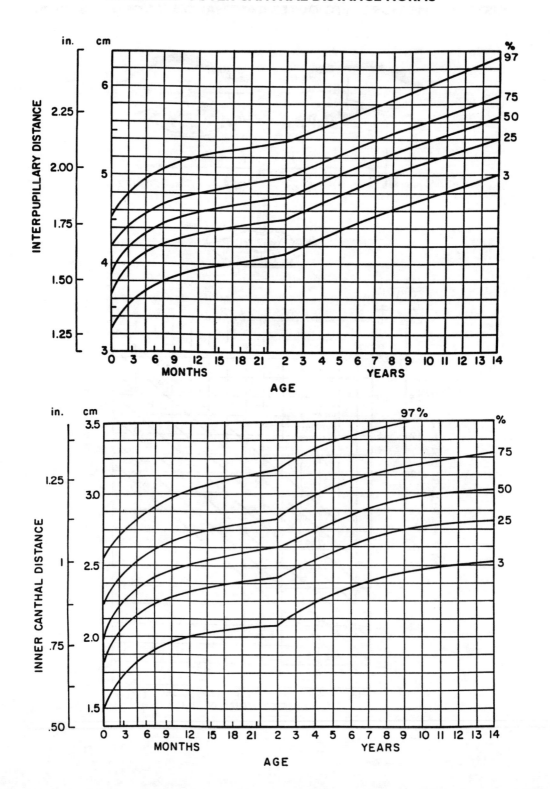

Appendix II-L
OUTER CANTHAL DISTANCE NORMS

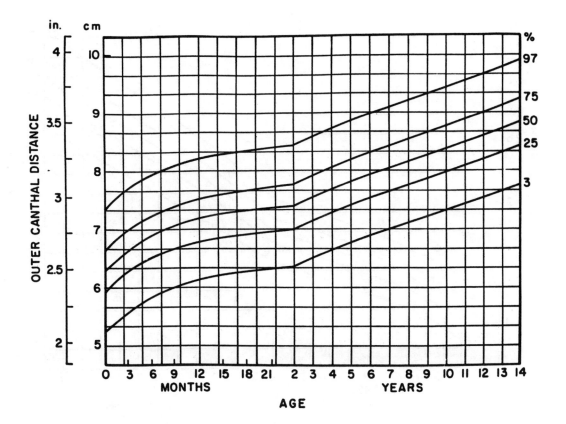

AGE

Appendix II-M
MIDDLE FINGER LENGTH NORMS

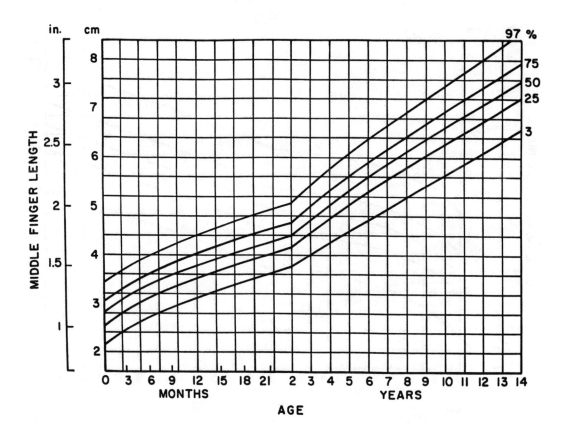

Appendix II-N
PALMAR LENGTH NORMS

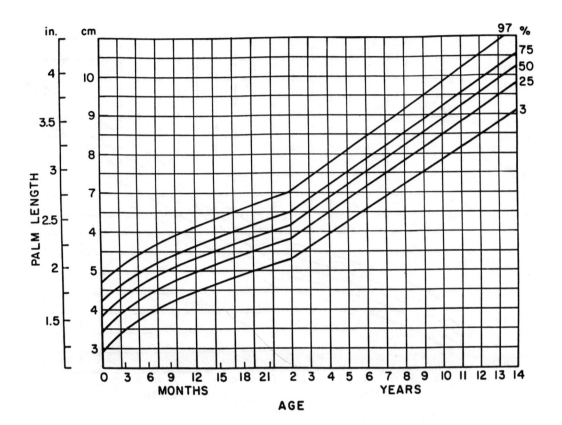

Appendix II-O
TOTAL HAND LENGTH NORMS

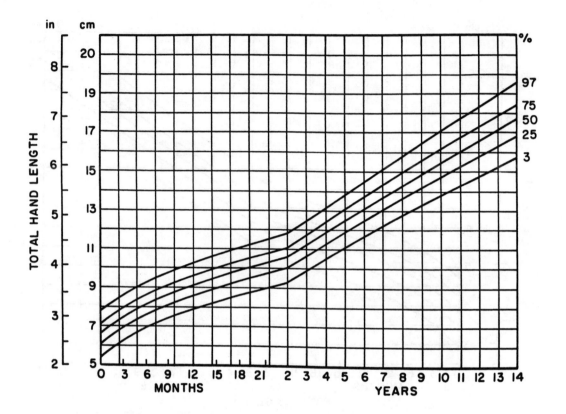

Appendix II-P
PROPORTION OF MIDDLE FINGER TO PALMAR LENGTH NORMS

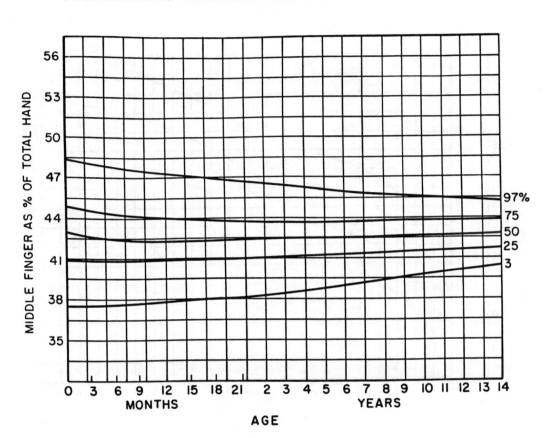

Appendix II-Q
EAR LENGTH NORMS

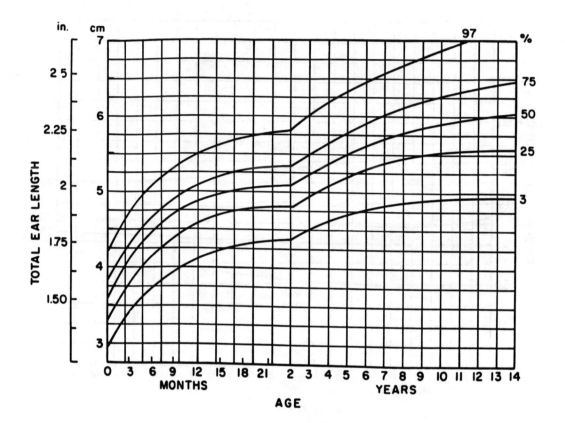

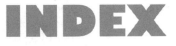

INDEX

Numbers in *italic type* refer to figures.

NOTES

NOTES

NOTES

NOTES